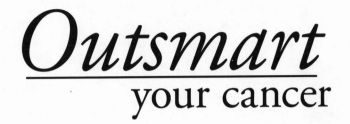

Outsmart
your cancer

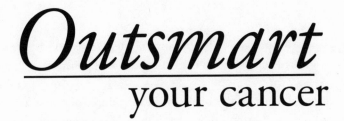

Outsmart
your cancer

Alternative Non-Toxic Treatments That Work

SECOND EDITION

Tanya Harter Pierce, m.a., mfcc

THOUGHTWORKS PUBLISHING
2009

First Edition: September 2004 (448 pp.)
Second Edition: August 2009 (528 pp. plus Audio CD)

Typesetting by www.FionaRaven.com

ISBN-13: 978-0-9728867-8-9
ISBN 0-9728867-8-8
LCCN 2003104206

ATTENTION CORPORATIONS, UNIVERSITIES, COLLEGES, AND PROFESSIONAL ORGANIZATIONS: Quantity discounts are available on bulk purchases of this book for educational, gift purposes, or as premiums for increasing magazine subscriptions or renewals. Special books or book excerpts can also be created to fit specific needs. For information, please contact Thoughtworks Publishing at info@outsmartyourcancer.com or (888) 679-2669.

Disclaimer

Tanya Harter Pierce is *not* a physician and none of the information in this book should be construed as "medical advice." The author is merely presenting her findings, as would an investigative journalist. Thus, the material in this book should be used for educational and informational purposes only. Each person must make his or her own decisions about treatment. Prior to making those decisions, anyone who has cancer or suspects he or she may have cancer, should consult with a qualified physician.

A conscientious effort has been made to only present information that is accurate and truthful in this book. However, the author cannot be held responsible for inaccuracies that may be found in her source material. She is also not responsible for any changes in ingredients or reduction in quality of any of the products mentioned in this book, should that occur. Moreover, this is not a comprehensive survey of *all* non-toxic cancer treatments available.

Note: The alternative non-toxic approaches presented in this book are not approved by the FDA as treatments for cancer.

Acknowledgments

My most abundant and never-ending gratitude goes to my husband, David Pierce. Without his total support and belief in me, I would not have been able to write this book. He not only supported me in a myriad of ways, but also gave me excellent editorial input on every chapter. Next, I send my love to Yahtzee, my devoted dog who gave me joyful companionship through all aspects of this work until she passed just before the 2nd Edition went to print. Her sweetness and special personality kept me going and grounded me in the important things of life.

I also want to thank my brother, Craig, who introduced me to some important sources of alternative cancer treatment information, and to express warm gratitude to my sisters, Margo and Kathy, and my mother, Bonnie, for their enthusiasm and encouragement about my project. And I sincerely thank the many medical professionals and other experts who graciously reviewed or provided important input to specific sections of this book.

Finally, I deeply appreciate and applaud the efforts of all the pioneering physicians, scientists, medical researchers and authors who went before me and wrote books, articles, and Internet postings to share their knowledge of alternative cancer therapies. To *all* of them I say, "Your commitment and courage will never be forgotten!"

Table of Contents

For additional information
and to read and listen to MORE
cancer recovery testimonials,
please visit :

www.OutsmartYourCancer.com

Introduction

The writing of the First Edition of this book came about quickly and unexpectedly. I was suddenly jolted into cancer treatment research when a family member of mine was diagnosed with cancer in 2001. Since conventional medicine could not offer the likelihood of a long-term cure, I decided to try to help out by looking into alternative options. As a recently retired Marriage, Family, Child Counselor, I had the time to collect information. And, though I am not a doctor or other type of medical practitioner, my Master's degree in clinical psychology gave me some formal background for evaluating scientific studies and methodology.

What I discovered in my search amazed me. The alternative treatments I read about were *fascinating* and I was surprised that I had not heard anything about these powerful non-toxic methods. This was particularly surprising to me since I had spent years looking into alternative medicine which I then used to treat my own chronic health challenges. When I found out about the incredible recoveries alternative non-toxic cancer treatments were achieving, I was stunned!

Why hadn't I read about or heard of these effective approaches through the media? Why was it that no one else close to me knew about them either? At first, I did not have the answers to these questions. But the one thing I knew was that people with cancer should *not* have to spend months and months, like I did, to discover this information for themselves.

I also uncovered widespread misconceptions about alternative cancer treatments. For instance, I learned that alternative approaches to cancer do *not* just involve juicing lots of carrots and taking supplements from a local health food store to strengthen one's immune system. I found out that the successful approaches involve *much* more powerful methods than that, and often directly *kill* cancer cells without the help of the immune

⸛. Some, in fact, target cancer cells in such specific ways that they ⸛ more like drugs and can't be done along with other alternative approaches because the different methods would counteract each other. I also discovered that for many of these approaches, the way they work has been proven by rigorous scientific research performed by highly respected physicians, brilliant biochemists, and Nobel Prize-winning scientists. Effective alternative approaches to cancer *are* obtainable today, and they are *not* bogus methods developed by quacks and kooks as the public has been led to believe.

I never intended at first to write a book. I merely wanted to evaluate as much information I could and report on it to family and friends. However, it soon became clear that the collection of information had a life of its own and quickly multiplied into more than I had bargained for. When I finally decided to produce a book, my goal became to present the material in a way that readers could easily understand and to answer such questions as, "What are the most common alternative cancer treatments?" . . . "How effective are they?" . . . "How do they work?" . . . "Where can I obtain these treatments?" . . . and . . . "Why doesn't my doctor tell me about these options?" These questions and more are answered in the following pages. The various approaches are presented in a somewhat chronological order, starting with the alternative treatments that were developed first, and include key historical aspects of each one.

During my search, I spoke to over a hundred people who had recovered from their cancer using the alternative treatments presented in this book, and between the First and Second Edition communicated with many more. In the treatment chapters, you will read amazing recovery stories for yourself. Some of these stories were borrowed from other publications with permission. Most, however, are case histories I collected personally from cancer survivors.

All of the alternative approaches to cancer discussed in this book are methods that *should* have been evaluated by and accepted into mainstream medicine years ago. Unfortunately, that did not happen. In the following chapters, you will learn many of the reasons why.

Four years have elapsed since the printing of the First Edition, and a great deal of *new* information has been added to the Second Edition. Two completely new chapters have been added (Chapter 17 and Chapter 20), significant sections of various chapters have been re-written and improved with new information, and all chapters have been updated. Plus, in keeping with the fact that this book is the *definitive* source of information on the Protocel® formula, a great many new tips and explanations have been added to Chapter 12 which discusses how to use Protocel® for *best* results. On top of all of that, a new audio CD has been inserted into the back of the book that contains helpful information about alternative versus conventional methods and presents testimonials from people who courageously used non-toxic approaches to cure their own cancer. I hope readers will be inspired listening to these testimonials. There is nothing so convincing as hearing these types of stories from everyday people in their own words!

Though I cannot counsel you on the decision you should make for your own particular medical situation, my hope is that this book will save you valuable time in your own search for answers. And if you have been told that conventional medicine cannot offer you a long-term cure, then this book may provide you with much-needed hope.

I sincerely wish you the very best on your path to recovery!

Tanya Harter Pierce, M.A., MFCC

"... That Wisdom may finish what Knowledge did start ..."

—Astarius

From the invocation "Let There Be" on the CD "Spirit Rap"
©2000 by Astarius Reiki-Om, www.astarius.com

Section One

Understanding Cancer

1

The Cancer Reality Today

If you are facing a cancer diagnosis, the first thing you should know is that there *is* hope in the world of alternative, non-toxic treatments. And I am referring to very *real* hope—not the "false hope" that is so often offered in the guise of chemotherapy and radiation. Tens of thousands of people have declined conventional medicine, either as soon as they were diagnosed or after conventional methods failed, and used alternative methods instead to overcome their cancer. These people have then gone on to live normal, healthy lives!

The second thing you should know is that you are far from alone. Right now, one in every two to three Americans will develop life-threatening cancer at some point in their lives. This estimate comes primarily from the official American Cancer Society figures of 1996, which predicted that 40 percent of all Americans will develop life-threatening cancer. This statistical estimate has been confirmed by other researchers as well, many of whom believe the 40 percent figure to be *conservative*. Overall, cancer rates have been rising at an alarming rate for the past 100 years. In recent years, the rate of lung cancer incidence has been going down due to fewer people smoking, but the rates of virtually all other types of cancer are still increasing.

Whenever a person finds themselves facing a cancer diagnosis, time is of the essence. There are urgent decisions to make, and you need treatment information fast. You may have various doctors, relatives, or friends

3

pushing you to quickly get your surgery, chemotherapy, and/or radiation. They may even say things like, "If you don't do this now, you will die!" If this is happening to you, try to remember that these people are pushing you because they care about you and are, themselves, scared. And they are right when they say that you need to take action *very soon*.

But you deserve to know that everyone in America is strongly influenced—even brought up all their lives—to think that conventional treatments are the only answers to cancer. Surgery, chemotherapy, and radiation are commonly called "The Big Three" of mainstream cancer treatment, and most doctors think these are the only answers.

Unfortunately, there are serious problems with these conventional treatment approaches. Of the three, surgery is definitely the most effective. Surgery can sometimes bring about long-term recovery when cancer is caught early and is in an area where the entire cancerous area can be cut out. This is particularly true for early cancers where an *entire* organ or body part can be removed, such as a kidney, thyroid gland, testicle, or uterus. But for the *majority* of cases, the cancer has already metastasized (spread to other areas of the body) by the time a person is diagnosed. And, for those cases, surgery cannot get all of the cancer cells. Many researchers believe that surgery can even *promote* metastasis in some cases.

Chemotherapy and radiation have even *worse* long-term recovery rates than surgery. This is largely because they resort to toxic methods of "bludgeoning" a person's cancer to death. These toxic treatments harm healthy parts of a person's body along with the cancer, thereby making long-term recovery difficult.

The good news is that, even if you have been diagnosed with cancer that has already metastasized, there *are* alternative options to conventional treatments. And they often have better track records, in general, than what mainstream medicine is offering. I know many people who were told by their doctor that their late-stage or metastasized cancer was incurable, only to completely recover later by using a non-toxic, alternative approach! In fact, you may find after reading this book that your biggest difficulty is not in finding a good alternative treatment approach to cancer, but in deciding which one to use because there are so many to choose from.

There are very important reasons why alternative treatments for cancer often have better track records than conventional ones. Most importantly, alternative, non-toxic approaches work in ways that do not harm normal, healthy cells of the body. They do this by focusing on those aspects of cancer cells that are significantly different from healthy cells. These approaches treat cancer as a "whole-body" disease and work *with* a person's immune system to attack the cancer cells everywhere, even the free-floating individual cells. This is different from mainstream practices, which focus primarily on just treating tumors (which may represent most of the cancer cells in a person's body, but not all), and use toxic treatments that can seriously damage the body's immune system and vital organs.

In other words, conventional medicine tries to *bludgeon* your cancer to death with toxic treatments that can be extremely harmful to your body, while alternative methods use non-toxic approaches to *Outsmart Your Cancer*!

Benefits of Non-Toxic Approaches

The most obvious benefit of using a non-toxic approach to cancer is that, by doing so, a person does not damage healthy parts of his or her body while trying to recover from their illness. Chemotherapy and radiation can damage virtually any cells they come in contact with and may have extremely serious long-term side effects such as liver, kidney, nerve, and heart damage. These side effects can often be life-threatening in and of themselves. Other side effects, such as chronic weakness, may result from damaged adrenals and/or thyroid glands, and this can reduce a person's quality of life.

Besides general bodily damage that can be caused, many cancer patients are not even told by their doctors that some common conventional treatments for cancer are themselves *carcinogenic*. The fact is that some chemotherapy agents are known carcinogens, and the chemotherapy treatment given to many patients to put their cancer into remission may directly cause a *secondary* cancer to develop in that person a few years later. Radiation can also cause cancer, which has been well-known since radiation techniques were first developed. Though surgery is not considered carcinogenic, it may cause the spread of cancer to other parts of the body.

Moreover, at some point, the use of a toxic treatment for cancer may enable the cancer to spread *even faster* in a person's body. This is because that person's immune system and other natural defense mechanisms have been so weakened by the treatment itself, the body can no longer fight off the cancer. So it only makes sense that using a toxic treatment for cancer can work against long-term recovery by giving the body more damage to recover from.

But there is another benefit of non-toxic approaches that is critical to long-term recovery from cancer, yet is little understood. This is the benefit that comes from *continual use* of a treatment. The importance of this particular benefit cannot be overstated. Conventional toxic approaches, such as chemotherapy and radiation, do not allow for continual use because they are so toxic, continual use would kill the patient before the cancer could! For this reason, toxic treatments are always administered with doses spaced out. This necessity to space out the administration of a toxic treatment is not optimally effective since one of cancer's best abilities is to grow new cells *fast*. Thus, in-between toxic treatment administrations, while the patient's body is recovering from the treatment, the cancer cells are recovering too. And those cancer cells that grow back the fastest are those cells that have some amount of "resistance" to the treatment. In other words, the treatment itself selects for the proliferation of resistant cancer cells in a person's body. This type of resistance has become more and more evident with the use of antibiotics causing antibiotic-resistant bacteria. In the case of chemotherapy use, this type of dynamic may result in what are called "multi-drug-resistant" cancer cells, or MDR cells.

With non-toxic treatments, however, these vicious dynamics are avoided. Non-toxic approaches do not harm the body and therefore allow for continual use. When a cancer treatment is non-toxic and can be administered continually every day, resistant cells are not promoted. In fact, a non-toxic approach can be done every single day for months or years. This allows the treatment approach to work in the body "24/7" and *never* gives the cancer cells a chance to grow back in ever more virulent forms.

Also, non-toxic approaches can often be continued for years *after* one has achieved remission, if a person chooses to. This gives people a way to help ensure that their cancer does not come back!

The Bigger Picture

To sum up the bigger picture of conventional versus alternative cancer treatments today, I have come up with what I call the "three basic truths." They are:

1. Conventional treatments have failed
2. Successful alternative treatments abound
3. The "disbelief factor" is alive and well

First Basic Truth—Conventional Treatments Have Failed

It is commonly accepted by many reputable cancer researchers that the conventional "war on cancer" has failed. In fact, it has failed so miserably that the conventional cancer industry has had to resort to "fudging" their cure-rate statistics so the public will continue to think they are doing a good job! (By "cancer industry," I mean the part of organized medicine devoted to cancer research, treatment, and education, which is led primarily by the National Cancer Institute [NCI], the American Cancer Society [ACS], the Food and Drug Administration [FDA], the American Medical Association [AMA], a few large centers throughout the country such as Memorial Sloan-Kettering Cancer Center in New York, and various pharmaceutical companies that produce cancer drugs.)

Once we clear away the fudged statistics and get down to the true reality, however, we find that current conventional medical treatments for cancer can only bring about real cures (long-term survival) for a very small percentage of cancer patients. People with primary cancer (cancer that has not yet metastasized) have the best chance of survival with conventional treatments, where they may have about a 10 to 15 percent chance of long-term recovery if the cancer is caught early and is in an area of the body that allows for total surgical removal. But most cancer patients are not lucky enough to be diagnosed with primary cancer. In the United States, between two-thirds and three-fourths of all cancer patients have cancer that had *already metastasized* by the time they were first diagnosed. And when it comes to conventional medical treatments for metastasized cancer, many researchers agree that the long-term survival rate for these patients is less than 1 percent. (In some cases, it is as low as one-tenth of a percent.) When it comes to the long-term effectiveness of chemotherapy in general, some highly respected cancer researchers believe it is effective in only 2 to 3 percent of all cancers.

You might say, "Wait a minute; I heard that 40 to 50 percent of all cancer cases today are being cured by mainstream medicine. I also heard that *most* cancers, when caught early enough, are curable." Well, I believe that you heard that because these are the typical types of figures the cancer industry likes to advertise. But the truth is that when you hear a statistic like "40 to 50 percent cure rate" or "most cancers are curable if caught early," you are being presented statistics that have been incredibly *fudged and manipulated*. I learned about the official fudging tactics from a variety of sources, but primarily from the in-depth work done by two prominent cancer researchers: Ralph W. Moss, Ph.D., and Lorraine Day, M.D.

Ralph Moss is a highly renowned cancer researcher who has written numerous books including *The Cancer Industry, Questioning Chemotherapy*, and *Cancer Therapy: The Independent Consumer's Guide to Non-Toxic Treatment and Prevention*. Moss began his cancer research when he was hired as a science writer at New York's Memorial Sloan-Kettering Cancer Center in 1974. There, he was able to observe the workings of the cancer industry from the inside. But according to Moss, his employment at Memorial Sloan-Kettering ended when he would not go along with the advertising of misleading information to the public. Over the years since then, he has diligently researched the *real* truth for the public, which he has carefully quoted and documented in his books. In an ever-growing circle of people researching the truth about cancer treatments, Ralph Moss is considered to be a leading authority.

Dr. Lorraine Day is an orthopedic trauma surgeon who rose to the position of chief of orthopedic surgery at San Francisco General Hospital. In 1992, Dr. Day's life changed dramatically when she was diagnosed with breast cancer that had already metastasized. Though she was pressured by specialists to undergo a mastectomy followed by chemotherapy and radiation, she chose *not* to receive those treatments because she knew so much about the severe damage to her body they could cause. Instead, she immediately started looking into other ways to treat herself, and eventually was able to completely heal and overcome her advanced cancer by drastically changing her diet and through other natural steps.

Dr. Day details her amazing story and reveals the results of her own in-depth research into cancer treatments in her numerous videos which can all be purchased from her website (www.DrDay.com). One of Dr. Day's videos reveals the stark truth about conventional cancer treatments and their side effects and real cure rates. It is called *Cancer Doesn't Scare Me Anymore*, and I highly recommend it. (See ordering instructions at the end of this chapter.)

Taken primarily from research done by both Dr. Moss and Dr. Day, the six *big ways* official cancer cure rates and statistics have been "fudged" are the following:

1. **By the way "cure" is defined.** The current cancer authorities, such as the ACS, NCI, and FDA, have all chosen to define "cure" as alive five years after diagnosis.[1] This official definition does not mean "cancer free," nor does it mean "healed of your disease," which is what most people think the word "cure" means.

To give you a better idea of what I am talking about, we can look at the true story of one female cancer patient. In this woman's battle against breast cancer, she did all the conventional approaches—surgery, radiation, and chemotherapy. Unfortunately, the woman did *not* survive. She died, full of cancer, five years and two weeks after her diagnosis. To add insult to injury, her husband found out later that his beloved wife was listed as a "cure" on the official ledgers, because she had died two weeks *after* the five-year mark. Thus, because of the American Cancer Society's definition of "cure," many patients who live five years after their cancer diagnoses are listed as "cured"—*even though they still show evidence of having cancer, or even though they die from their cancer.*[2] Thus, the definition of "cure" is the first big fallacy of official cancer cure-rate statistics, and may be the biggest official fudging tactic used.

2. **By simply not including certain groups of people, or certain types of cancer.** This is one of the hardest fudging tactics to believe. It means that, at times, the official cancer authorities have been able to make their statistics look better than they really are by simply not including certain groups of people in their statistics who tend to show lower recovery rates than other groups. These groups might be less likely to recover for socio-economic or other reasons.

   I was shocked when I discovered this could include *all non-white Americans*. According to Ralph Moss, two prominent medical researchers who published their findings in the *New England Journal of Medicine* stated that the NCI "generally reports whites-only figures. Nonwhites . . . are kept in a separate category, untallied with the main group."[3] Moss states that "NCI's solution is to list them in separate (but equal) charts, and then to present the white charts as the norm."[4] Moreover, the NCI has also been known to greatly improve its advertised cancer cure rates by simply omitting *all lung cancer patients* from their statistics![5] (It seems that the NCI sees lung cancer as different from other cancers because of its connection to cigarette smoking.) Yet, according to the American Cancer Society, lung cancer is the leading cause of cancer death for both men and women. Thus, in some statistics, the National Cancer Institute simply does not include the type of cancer that causes more deaths than any other type. Both of the above tactics of omission can only be called "biased selection," and yet these statistics are presented as representative of all patients and *all* life-threatening cancers.

3. **By including types of cancer that are not life-threatening.** The cancer authorities were able to improve their publicized cure rates even more when they took this brilliant step years ago. This tactic involves including cancers in their statistics that are easily treatable and not life-threatening, such as simple skin cancers. According to Dr. Douglas Brodie, "Five-year survivals of non-melanoma skin cancers, localized cancers of the cervix, and some other non-spreading (metastasizing) cancers detected early in specific sites, have been 'curable' (that is, amenable to five-year absences of symptoms) since the days of Ptolemy."[6]

   As will be covered in Chapter 19, ductal carcinoma in situ (DCIS) is now included in breast cancer statistics. DCIS is really more of a "pre-cancerous" state that many experts believe should not even be classified as cancer, and is 99 percent curable. Yet, DCIS now comprises about 30 percent of all breast cancer diagnoses in the United States and is included in the cure-rate statistics for life-threatening breast cancer as well. Thus, easily treatable skin cancers and DCIS are types of *non*-life-threatening cancers that are included in statistics used to imply what a patient's chances of recovering from *life-threatening* cancers are. This tactic is like adding the risk of being killed by a bicycle or someone on a skateboard when compiling the statistical likelihood of being killed in a car crash!

4. **By allowing earlier detection to imply longer survival.** This tactic is subtle but important. Over the decades, one of the aspects of cancer medicine that *has* improved because of improved technology is that of earlier detection. Advances in technology have allowed doctors and researchers to detect cancer on average about six months earlier than they used to be able to detect it. With the definition of cure being "alive five years after diagnosis," earlier detection has, by itself, added many new patients to the conventional "cure" list.

   What is *not* accurate, however, is to claim that these improved statistics reflect *improved life expectancy* because of better treatment methods. In other words, because tumors are getting diagnosed at earlier stages than before, and because of the way "cure" is officially defined as a time deadline following diagnosis, long-term survival rates may *look* better now than they did years ago. But the reality is that no improvement in long-term survival has occurred at all.

5. **By deleting patients from studies who die too soon.** This is a particularly treacherous way the cancer industry manipulates statistics.

What this means is that it has become an acceptable practice in official cancer studies with human patients to simply drop a patient from the records if he or she dies from cancer before the treatment protocol is considered to have been completed. According to Dr. Lorraine Day, this means that "if a cancer patient dies on day 89 of a prescribed 90-day course of chemotherapy, he or she would just disappear from the list of treated patients and would not be listed as a failure."[7] Yet, if a patient in the control group (those *not* getting the specified treatment) dies at *any* time, that patient is listed in the study as a death from cancer. This is a double standard that shows an institutional lack of integrity and is definitely *not* consistent with true scientific method.

6. **By using an adjustment called "relative survival rate."** This was a variant on the five-year survival statistic that the official cancer industry created and adopted in the 1980s to help them claim that the war on cancer was being won. According to Ralph Moss, "Relative survival rates take into account the 'expected mortality figures.' Put simply, this means that if a person hadn't died of cancer he might have been run over by a truck, and that must be factored into the equation."[8]

These *adjusted* rates are used in a very misleading way because they are presented to the public as representative of mainstream medicine's ability to help a cancer patient recover from their life-threatening cancer. But, in truth, the relative survival rate adjustment is just one more way that cancer cure-rate statistics are manipulated to make conventional treatments look better than they really are.

The above six major fudging tactics are the real back story behind the "official" cancer cure-rate claims currently being advertised to the public. It is only by using these types of extreme statistical manipulations and a totally misleading definition of "cure" that the cancer industry can make bogus statements like *40 to 50 percent of all cancers are curable.* It takes very little research to see that these statistics are not real, and that conventional medicine has failed in the arena of cancer treatment.

Because these tactics are now institutionally ingrained in mainstream cancer treatment and research, the conventional data available start out distorted from the get-go. Therefore, the real data needed to figure out the "true" conventional cure-rate statistics for cancer just aren't available. However, we don't need those data to know that we are in the midst of a very serious problem. All we need to know is that in just one year (1996), more people in the United States died of cancer than the number of U.S. soldiers who died in all of World War II, the Korean War, and the entire Vietnam War combined![9] This is quite a sobering thought. Another is that Americans are dying of cancer at a rate approximately equivalent to ten September 11th terrorist attacks every month!

So, in the bigger picture, the first basic truth is "conventional cancer treatments have failed."

Second Basic Truth—Successful Alternative Treatments Abound

How many times have we heard television commercials that imply the pharmaceutical companies are working very hard to find a cure for cancer? Yet, you will discover in the following pages that many successful treatments for cancer have already been developed. They just don't get publicity since they are labeled "alternative." To put it briefly, the cancer treatments that have been relegated to the alternative world have generally involved natural forms of treatment that could not be patented or otherwise controlled by the big multi-billion-dollar cancer industry. This huge industry is run by powerful pharmaceutical companies and even bigger corporate cartels. Its profits are threatened by any natural or individually owned treatment that can't be patented or controlled by big business for profit.

The truth is that there have been many highly successful cancer treatments developed over the past century that *should have been incorporated into mainstream medicine.* Most of them were developed and pioneered by highly respectable physicians or scientists—not quacks or con artists. The best of the alternative, non-toxic treatments for cancer have had blatantly higher success rates than conventional treatments, and these success rates reflect real cures, not phony redefined cures! But these successful cancer treatments have been suppressed to one degree or another, and many misconceptions about alternative cancer treatments have flourished as a result.

One misconception is that, in order for treatments to be suppressed, there must be some kind of centrally located, "conspiracy" going on with little evil men in dark clothes wringing their hands and tittering "hee-hee" while eagerly anticipating peoples' deaths. This is not at all how it works. The suppression has been carried out in many different ways by many different organizations and is simply the result of business economics and common unethical tactics that tend to occur when large money interests are involved in any field.

Surgery, chemotherapy, and radiation involve billions of dollars of profit for the industries that supply them. Moreover, the current system for new drug development and approval by the FDA is set up such that the cost of developing and bringing a new cancer drug to market is close to a billion dollars. (Common costs are 700 to 800 million dollars in the United States.) Without a patent, this type of cost investment is not economically feasible for a pharmaceutical company. This means that, since any treatment made up of natural ingredients is not patentable, a natural form of treating cancer will never be pursued by a drug company. Unfortunately for the public, the most successful treatments for cancer either involve natural substances or are privately owned and patented by creative individuals who were willing to think out of the box to develop something totally new. What they have to offer is always going to be an economic threat to the multi-billion-dollar cancer establishment.

Thus, to say that there is a conspiracy to suppress alternative cancer treatments is like referring to industries that pollute the environment as joining in a conspiracy to sacrifice the well-being of our natural ecology. That would be ludicrous and would show a total lack of understanding that the way big businesses get where they are is by being profit-motivated. When it comes to the environment, it is true that some of the tactics used by industries to circumvent environmental protection laws or public safety may seem conspiratorial, especially if they involve falsifying paperwork, paying off Congress, or illegally dumping waste under the cover of darkness. But that does *not* mean there is a broad conspiracy by big business to pollute the environment. In the same way, there is no broad conspiracy by big business to suppress alternative cancer treatments. In both cases, big businesses are just doing what they do best—*protecting their profits.*

Another misconception about alternative treatments for cancer in general is that they simply involve going to the nearest health food store and buying everyday types of supplements. If you find it hard to believe that doing this would be a successful way to overcome such a powerful health challenge as cancer, your instincts are right. This is *rarely* how it is done. Most of the successful alternative approaches involve much more powerful treatments than that, and often revolve around very innovative methods that require the help of an experienced alternative practitioner or a knowledgeable support group to be done properly.

There is actually an amazing human story going on in the world of alternative cancer treatment these days. With conventional medicine failing most cancer patients, more and more people are turning to alternative medicine every year to save themselves. And large numbers of them are winning! They are beating their cancer even though conventional medical experts are claiming that what they are doing cannot be done. They are beating their cancer even though the big insurance companies are not recognizing or paying for the treatments they are using. They are beating their cancer because they are "outsmarting" their cancer with alternative, non-toxic treatments that work. Thus, the second basic truth of the cancer reality today is that "successful alternative treatments abound."

Third Basic Truth—The "Disbelief Factor" Is Alive and Well

Another widely held misconception about alternative cancer approaches is that, if they really worked better than the current conventional approaches, doctors and clinics everywhere would be using them. This misconception is at the heart of what I call the "disbelief factor." The disbelief factor is a dynamic that occurs in people's minds when they say, "If there really are natural, non-toxic treatments for cancer that can bring about real, long-term cures, even in cases of late-stage metastasized cancers, then why aren't all doctors using these treatments?"

Finding it hard to understand why all doctors are not using the most effective and least toxic treatments for cancer is not the problem. The real problem arises when a person finds this so hard to believe that he or she simply can't accept the possibility that there could be alternative approaches out there that really work. And when they are told there *are*, they often don't listen at all because it is just too preposterous to believe. This is the disbelief factor at work.

For those people with cancer who let the disbelief factor win, it is a tragic situation. Their disbelief keeps them from doing any further research on their own. They trust their doctors, not knowing that their doctors have only been taught the mainstream treatments and usually know nothing of the alternative ones. What these people don't realize is that most doctors are just people who *also* have a hard time believing in alternative treatments, and who ask, "If these treatments really work, why wasn't I taught them in medical school?"

And patients usually do not realize that, even if their doctor did think an alternative treatment for cancer would help them, in most U.S. states that doctor is *not* legally allowed to prescribe or even recommend anything other than the big three of surgery, chemotherapy, and radiation. That is why cancer patients who are doing alternative treatments will so often hear from their conventional doctor monitoring them, "Just keep doing whatever it is you are doing!" These oncologists often don't even want to know what the patient is doing that is working because they know they can't prescribe it anyway. Unfortunately, the legal straightjacket that conventional oncologists are in only contributes to the prevalence of the disbelief factor. The fact that the disbelief factor is alive and well is the third basic truth of the cancer reality today.

As you can see, the "bigger picture" of cancer treatment in modern countries such as the United States puts cancer patients at a disadvantage. The almost total separation between conventional and alternative therapies requires patients to do their own homework if they are to make a fully informed decision about their treatment. The good news, however, is that there *are* excellent alternative approaches available. But before we delve into those approaches, there are two basic questions to answer first: "Why so much cancer?" and "What causes it?"

Resources:

Book

Ralph W. Moss, Ph.D. *The Cancer Industry*. New York: Equinox Press, 1999.

Video

Lorraine Day, M.D. *Cancer Doesn't Scare Me Anymore*. To order, call (800) 574-2437, or visit Dr. Day's website: www.drday.com.

2

Why So Much Cancer
and What Causes It?

More and more people who have never smoked, who do not drink heavily, and who have exercised and been health conscious all their lives are being diagnosed with cancer. And they are wondering how this could have happened to them. It is common for a person's first question after diagnosis to be, "Why me?" When they find out that they are far from alone, then the questions become, "Why so much cancer?" and "What causes it?"

It seems that if we listen to doctors, pharmaceutical companies, or advertisements on television about cancer clinics and treatments, we come away with the idea that cancer is some sort of *mysterious affliction* that no one completely understands. Other than knowing that too much sun exposure can cause skin cancer, smoking too much can cause lung cancer, and drinking too much can cause liver or kidney cancer, we somehow get the idea that, for just about any other case, the medical profession is "stumped" as to what causes cancer. What the public does not know, however, is that it is only the conventional medical world that is stumped. Researchers and practitioners who have been relegated to the alternative no man's land have been putting important pieces of the cancer puzzle together for decades and have already proven a number of key causes. Understanding these causes is important for the cancer patient because it moves cancer out of the realm of "something I can't fight" into the realm of "something I have control over."

Is Cancer Genetically Caused?

What about cancer being genetically caused? We hear so much about modern cancer research focusing on genes and how certain people are "predisposed" to cancer because of their family history. In fact, looking at cancer as a genetically inherited disease has become so common that some women who have never been diagnosed with cancer are actually considering having both of their breasts surgically removed because they have a family history of breast cancer. This incredibly extreme preventive measure exhibits a powerful belief that cancer is genetic!

Although it is certainly possible that a predisposition to a few cancers may be genetically inherited, I will go out on a limb here and say that most cancers are not a result of genetic inheritance. In her video, *Cancer Doesn't Scare Me Anymore* (mentioned in Chapter 1), Dr. Lorraine Day presents two compelling reasons why we must assume that most cancers are *not* genetically inherited. Her first reason is based on the incredible rate at which cancer incidence has risen over the past century. As an example, she refers to how the incidence of breast cancer has risen dramatically since the early 1900s. Yet, those were the days of our grandmothers. Since the women of today are so closely linked genetically with their grandmothers, if breast cancer were a genetically inherited disease, then the grandmothers would have about the same basic rate of incidence as their granddaughters. But the grandmothers of today's women had a much *lower* incidence of breast cancer than today's women. As recently as the 1960s, about 1 in every 20 American women developed breast cancer. Now, just 45 years later, about 1 in every 8 American women are developing breast cancer. If breast cancer were a genetically inherited disease, there would be no way of explaining this dramatic increase in incidence over just 45 years, between one generation of mothers to their daughters.

There are many other examples of dramatic rises in cancer rates as well. For instance, Dr. Stoff and Dr. Clouatre wrote in their book, *The Prostate Miracle*, that between 1985 and 1996, prostate cancer diagnoses in this country rose from about 85,000 cases per year to over 317,000 cases per year.[1] This huge increase was over a mere 11-year period! And the incidence rate of non-Hodgkin's lymphoma has nearly *doubled* since the early

1970s. Both breast cancer and prostate cancer have been strongly linked to pesticide exposure, and non-Hodgkin's lymphoma has been strongly linked to herbicide exposure. Thus, it would seem much more likely that pesticides and herbicides are bigger contributors to these types of cancers than genetic inheritance. Moreover, *all* cancer incidence rates have risen over just a few generations. This sort of rise in all types of cancer would not be happening if cancer were primarily genetically caused.

Dr. Day's second reason to not assume that cancer is primarily an inherited disease is based on the reality that different groups of people around the world show different incidences of various types of cancers depending on what lifestyle or diet they are engaged in. In countries where certain types of cancer are particularly rare, the incidence of these cancers increases when people from those countries adopt a Western diet. But attributing cancer to dietary factors alone is misleading. As you will see, there are many environmental and common lifestyle factors that can contribute to the development of cancer. For example, cigarette smoking may be the single *biggest* causal factor to cancer in our modern world today. It has been estimated that a whopping 30 percent of all cancer deaths in the United States are attributable to tobacco smoke. This means that if everyone were to suddenly stop smoking, deaths from cancer would reduce by about one-third!

The confusing issue is that cancer does, to a certain extent, involve the genes in cells. But that does not mean it is an *inherited* condition. For instance, genes in cells can mutate as a result of being hit by radiation or because of damage caused by some sort of toxin. Nutritional deficiencies can also contribute to gene damage. Robert Barefoot and Carl Reich, M.D., make the point in their book *The Calcium Factor* that chronic calcium deficiency in a person's diet can precipitate a condition around cells whereby carcinogens are more able to penetrate the cell walls and thereby gain access to and cause mutations of genes.

Moreover, researchers have proven that there are certain genes that can promote the growth of cancer (oncogenes) and certain genes that can inhibit the growth of cancer (tumor suppressor genes), and that *the activity of these oncogenes and tumor suppressor genes can be turned on or off by various physiological factors.* This is critical for people to understand. There are many things in our *inner* physiological environment that can either promote or suppress the actions of certain genes within cells. So, yes, cancer does involve genes, but that does not mean that cancer is genetically inherited. When it comes to cancer, gene activity simply reflects the dynamic state of genes in their interrelationship with the body's inner environment.

This is not to say that a predisposition to cancer is never inherited. There may be a very small percentage of cases involving some inherited factor. But very little has been proven about this to date, and what the evidence proves much more powerfully is that genetic inheritance is not a significant cause of cancer. When cancer appears to run in families, it is more likely that there are other factors, such as diet, lifestyle, ways of dealing with emotional stress, and so forth, that family members have in common which are contributing to the development of cancer.

In general, the approach in modern medical science today is to look for just "one thing" that causes a particular illness. This may be partly why the search for an inherited genetic cause of cancer is so popular. However, a great deal of evidence points to cancer as a "multi-factorial" disease. This means that many factors usually go into the development of cancer for any particular person. I have come to look at these multiple factors as falling into two general categories: (1) "triggers," and (2) "deficient control mechanisms."

Triggers and Deficient Control Mechanisms

To understand how triggers and deficient control mechanisms contribute to the development of cancer, I'd like to use the analogy of a forest fire. What if someone were to ask the question: "What causes forest fires?" Looking for just one answer would be silly. We all know there are *many* things that can "trigger" a forest fire—a commuter throwing a lit cigarette out the car window into roadside brush; a camper allowing embers from a camp fire to blow up into the limbs of an overhanging tree; a bolt of lightning during a storm that hits a tree and causes it to ignite; or sunlight shining through a discarded piece of glass just the right way, causing some pine needles to ignite. These are all examples of factors that can trigger a forest fire.

But does a forest fire occur *every* time one of these triggers happens? No. This is because there are *also* many factors that will determine whether or not the initial spark will turn into a raging forest fire or not. I refer to these factors as "control mechanisms."

Some of the control mechanisms in the forest fire analogy may involve humans actively putting the fire out before it becomes big enough to be classified as a forest fire. But many of the control factors can happen without human involvement at all, and these would be factors in the environment around where the initial trigger, or spark of fire, occurred. For instance, environmental control mechanisms for the above examples might be: not enough brush and wind occurs along the roadside to fan a fire, so the commuter's cigarette spark is short-lived and burns itself out; the embers from the camper's fire have blown into the tree leaves of a very healthy, moist tree, so the fire never gets started in the first place; the bolt of lightning during the storm starts a tree blazing, but the accompanying rain drenches the tree and puts the fire out; or the sunlight shining through the glass starts a wisp of smoke in some pine needles, but the area is damp and surrounded by large rocks so the small fire has no where to spread and dies out quickly.

In this way, we can see that there are many "triggers" that can cause a spark that could result in a forest fire, but there are also many environmental "control mechanisms" that could stop that spark from turning into something that rages out of control and causes great destruction. *So too with cancer.* There are many common triggers, such as random errors in cell replication, or too much exposure to ultraviolet radiation, radioactive fallout, pesticides, and other environmental toxins. But there are also many natural control mechanisms within our bodies to keep these sparks from turning into raging forest fires of cancer.

Most medical practitioners and researchers agree that, in fact, we all probably have cancer cells developing in each of us all the time, but our bodies are able to dispose of them before they rage out of control. In other words, a healthy body can normally defend itself quite well against the development of cancer because it knows how to deal with these natural occurrences.

But life in the modern world has *skewed the balance between triggers and control mechanisms for cancer.* On the one hand, modern industrialized societies have introduced countless potent carcinogens and other toxins into our air, food and water, so that our bodies now have to deal with many more triggers to cancer than ever before. And on the other hand, modern industrialized societies have created highly processed, less than optimum foods and, through advertising, have promoted eating habits that result in poor nutritional support to our bodies. This lack of vital nutritional support can cause our own natural control mechanisms to become compromised and deficient.

The sad reality is that there are many *more* triggers to the development of cancer in humans than ever before in history, and peoples' control mechanisms are generally more deficient than ever before as well. There is just no getting around it. When we ask the question—"Why so much cancer and what causes it?"—the simplest answer is *modern living*.

A Disease of Modern Living

"Modern living" is obviously a broad reference, but it can be easily broken down into the categories of diet, environment, and lifestyle. For each of these categories, there are numerous factors that can contribute to cancer. Some are cancer-causing triggers, others are deficient control mechanisms. Briefly listed, some of the most important cancer-contributing factors of modern living are the following:

Modern Diet

- Not enough fresh fruits and vegetables
- Too many cooked and processed foods
- Foods grown in depleted soils
- Not enough essential fatty acids
- Too much refined sugar and refined flour
- Artificial sweeteners
- Excessive soda, coffee, or tea consumption
- Chronic dehydration (not enough water)

Modern Environment

- Pesticides
- Herbicides
- Chlorine byproducts (from chlorinated water and other sources)
- Fluoride
- Asbestos
- Fiberglass
- Nuclear radiation (from nuclear tests done decades ago)

Modern Lifestyle Choices and Treatments

- Cigarette smoking
- Birth control pills
- Hormone replacement therapy for menopause
- Common medical and dental X-rays

- Toxic teeth (from dangerous dental practices)
- Childhood vaccines
- Chronic stress
- Prescription drug use

This is *not* a comprehensive list by any means, but it is enough to give you an idea of the types of factors today that can contribute to cancer. Now, let's look in a little more detail at these factors. (Each item above is listed in **bold** where it first appears in the following text.)

Diet

One of the biggest problems with the modern American diet today is that it typically involves a huge **deficiency of fresh fruits and vegetables.** Our modern diet has unfortunately developed around speed, ease, and the profitability of the foods being sold. People living fast and on-the-go lifestyles don't generally have a chance to carry fresh fruits and vegetables around wherever they go, so they must rely on **cooked and processed foods**, which are easier to carry around or prepare quickly. Cooking destroys important natural enzymes that aid the body in assimilating nutrients, and highly processed foods are practically devoid of much-needed vitamins, minerals, fiber, and phytochemicals. Fresh fruits and vegetables, on the other hand, provide us with many different nutrients that help our bodies defend against the development of cancer.

When we, in modern industrialized countries, *do* eat fresh fruits and vegetables, we are often eating produce that was grown in **depleted soils.** The more and more commonly occurring soil depletion results from over-cropping and the use of chemical fertilizers that do not maintain a proper balance of minerals in the soil. This means that even our fresh fruits and vegetables may be deficient and imbalanced in their mineral content.

Essential fatty acids are another nutritional category critical to the healthy functioning of the body yet very deficient in the common modern diet. Two of the most important are the omega-3 and omega-6 fatty acids. These are called "essential" because the human body cannot biosynthesize them; therefore, they must be obtained through diet. The omega-6 fatty acids are primarily found in nuts and seeds, and the omega-3 fatty acids are primarily found in fish. When you think about it, seeds, nuts, and fish have been common dietary staples for humans for eons. Yet they are not abundant in the modern Western diet.

When we don't get enough vital nutrients, the cancer control mechanisms in our bodies cannot function optimally. But problems with the modern diet are not only defined by deficiencies. For instance, there is an overabundance of certain foods such as refined sugar. **Refined sugars and refined flours** (which are metabolized like sugar in the body) are hundreds of times more prevalent in the common modern diet than in the natural diets humans thrived on for millennia. This overabundance of refined sugars and flours contributes to all kinds of physical problems. One problem is that, if cancer does get started, lots of sugar in the diet may help the cancer to thrive because *cancer loves sugar.*

If a person tries to reduce his or her sugar intake, however, he or she often does this by replacing white sugar with **artificial sweeteners** such as aspartame (the sweetener used in NutraSweet, Equal, and Spoonful). Aspartame is one of the most common artificial sweeteners used today, and yet it was found to cause various types of primary brain tumors in rats when studies were done in the 1970s. Even though these studies showed a very clear connection between aspartame and brain cancer, the FDA approved its use as a tabletop sweetener in July 1981. Two years later, in July 1983, aspartame was approved for widespread use in diet beverages as well. One year after that, the number of human brain tumors in the United States suddenly increased by 10 percent! There are currently more than 5,000 aspartame-containing products on the market today, and it is estimated that over 200 million people in the United States consume it.

Aspartame is comprised of 10 percent methanol, 40 percent aspartic acid, and 50 percent phenylalanine. Methanol has been proven to cause damage to the optic nerve which can cause blindness, and aspartic acid has been proven to create holes in the brains of mice. Phenylalanine breaks down into diketopiperazine (DKP), a tumor-causing agent.

The creation of DKP in the body is one way aspartame can trigger cancer. Another way is partly related to what happens to aspartame when it exceeds 86 degrees Fahrenheit, as it often does when, for instance, diet drinks are being shipped in hot trucks or stored in hot warehouses. At higher than 86 degrees, the methanol (wood alcohol) in aspartame converts to formaldehyde and then to formic acid. Both formaldehyde and formic acid are potent carcinogens. In fact, formaldehyde is categorized in the same class of deadly poisons as cyanide and arsenic. On the other hand, when methanol occurs naturally, as it does in fruits, it is always in the presence of ethanol. Ethanol keeps methanol stable and prevents it from breaking down into formaldehyde and formic acid. But the methanol in aspartame is "free" methanol, and thus unstable.

Therefore, not only does the methanol break down into carcinogenic agents, but the ingredient found in largest quantity, phenylalanine, also breaks down into a direct tumor-initiating substance. The brain seems to be particularly susceptible to these types of damaging substances and *some neurosurgeons have found high levels of aspartame in brain tumors after the tumors were surgically removed and examined.*

But brain cancer is not the only type of cancer aspartame has been linked to. Animal tests performed between 1971 and 1974 proved that aspartame caused mammary tumors (breast cancer) in rats. Nutritionist Janet Starr Hull, Ph.D., wrote a revealing book on the dangers of aspartame called *Sweet Poison*. In it, she lists the names of researchers and their universities who have published studies on aspartame. According to Dr. Hull, testicular cancer and endometrial (uterine) cancer have also been associated with aspartame. And in 2005 and 2007 the Ramazzini Foundation in Bologna, Italy completed animal studies that indicated a link between aspartame and the development of leukemia and lymphoma in both male and female rats and mammary gland tumors (breast cancer) in female rats. (The link to breast cancer, of course, had already been found in the earlier 1970s studies.)

Thus, it appears that staying away from aspartame is one way to help oneself avoid cancer. And parents may want to be extra diligent about checking the ingredients list of anything sweet they give their children. For instance, aspartame is commonly used now to sweeten children's syrups, antibiotics, and vitamins. Given the high rate of brain cancers and leukemias in children these days, aspartame could certainly be a contributing factor that needs to be avoided.

Besides cancer, aspartame causes over 90 different documented adverse side effects. These side effects include debilitating MS type symptoms, seizures, coma, blindness, birth defects, and death. Some experts believe that aspartame was the primary cause of the "Gulf War Syndrome" suffered by so many American troops. This is because thousands of pallets of diet drinks were shipped to Desert Storm troops where they were left to sit for weeks at a time in 120-degree Fahrenheit heat. Dr. Hull states that out of 90 independently-funded studies, 83 of them found one or more problems caused by aspartame. But out of the 74 studies funded by the aspartame industry (e.g., Monsanto, G.D. Searle, and ILSI), every single one of them claimed that no problems were found.

Sodas are now one of the most common beverage alternatives to water. But they are either high in sugar or high in aspartame or some other artificial sweetener. They are also high in phosphorus, which can disrupt the mineral balance of the body. And many sodas contain caffeine, which is a diuretic. All caffeinated drinks, whether they are sodas or **coffee or tea**, can actually contribute to **chronic dehydration**. Good, clean water is much more important to drink than many people realize. None of the cells of the body can work at optimum functioning levels if they are chronically dehydrated, and many experts believe chronic dehydration can contribute to cancer by causing cell damage.

So, the common modern way of eating and drinking in the Western world is full of nutritional deficiencies and, at the same time, complicated with an overabundance of harmful substances. This type of diet contributes to "deficient control mechanisms." And when an overload of toxins barrages the body on a daily basis for year after year, there are going to be problems. Unfortunately, most of these toxins come from our environment, which includes our air, water, and foods we eat. And more of these toxins are directly carcinogenic than most people realize.

Environment

This category of cancer-causing factors is probably the worst offender. In our modern world, we are surrounded by toxins in our air, water, and soil. We eat, drink, and breathe them on a regular basis. For instance, we breathe in countless petrochemical molecules every day from smog if we live in a normal industrialized city. But some of the worst chemicals, and *most* carcinogenic, are often the ones we don't ever see, feel, or taste.

One primary source of these invisible chemicals is **pesticides**. Pesticides are amply sprayed onto our food crops and are also used for household or garden insect control. I, like many others, used to have the misconception that pesticides can be removed from our produce once we get the produce home from the grocery store and thoroughly wash it. This is not true. The pesticides sprayed onto crops get *into* our foods. These dangerous substances cannot be completely removed by washing the fruit or vegetable before eating it because they are *absorbed into* the fruit or vegetable as it grows. This happens in large part as a result of the pesticides being washed into the soil around the crops and then being absorbed by the plants as they take up water and nutrients from the soil.

Thus, no matter how much we wash our fruits and vegetables, we will be eating pesticides unless we buy only "organic" produce from reputable sources. But even those people who are conscientious about buying only organic foods will probably also be ingesting at least some pesticides. This is because, through rain and irrigation runoff, pesticides have contaminated virtually all of our surface and ground water.

Pesticides are similar to artificial sweeteners in that small exposures to them may be considered harmless, but daily exposure over many years is a very different story. Many of the carcinogenic compounds in pesticides do not easily break down over time, and tend to build up in the body, where they are stored in the fat cells. This can cause a *cumulative* buildup over the years. Many pesticides produce a potent estrogenic effect, which means they mimic estrogen in our bodies. (More details on their relationship to cancer are covered in Chapter 19.) Because so many of the pesticide chemicals have estrogenic properties, they can be a *big* factor in numerous cancers of the body where sex hormones play a role—such as cancers of the breast, uterus, ovaries, and prostate.

In 1978, Israel enacted a strict ban of certain pesticides that had been linked to breast cancer. Previous to this, the occurrence of breast cancer in Israel had been steadily rising. Over the next 10 years, after banning these pesticides, breast cancer incidence in Israeli women dropped sharply. (There was an 8 percent overall decline, and a 30 percent drop in breast cancer deaths for women under age 44.)[2] And this decline in breast cancer incidence and mortality occurred while these same rates in the rest of the world were climbing, and while other negative factors in Israel, such as alcohol consumption, fat intake, and insufficient dietary amounts of fruits and vegetables, were increasing.

The 1976 Israeli study that had identified these pesticides found them to occur at much higher concentrations in the malignant tissues of women with breast cancer when compared to normal breast tissues. Over the years following the ban, there was a corresponding noticeable drop of these same pesticides in Israeli cow's milk and *Israeli women's breast milk*. Thus, these carcinogenic pesticide chemicals were clearly associated with breast cancer. The fact that these chemicals have been found in mother's milk also indicates they can be passed on to infants through breast feeding. This scary possibility may be one explanation of why so many young children these days are developing cancer.

One of the pesticide chemicals that Israel banned in 1978 was DDT, which has been linked to breast cancer by many different studies since the 1970s. Most people don't know, however, that DDT is still showing up in our environment here in the United States. For instance, in 1996, 80,000 tons of dirt containing DDT were dredged from Richmond Harbor in the San Francisco Bay at a site that had previously been a pesticide packaging plant.[3] The plant had conveniently dumped much of its residue into the bay. After dredging up this massive amount of dirt, the U.S. government decided to get rid of it by having it moved and buried in a landfill in Arizona. At some point in the future, the DDT in this landfill is probably going to leach into the surrounding Arizona groundwater and become a toxic contaminant to humans and animals once again.

But the use of pesticides on crops is not the only way we are exposed to pesticide carcinogens. A recent *Science News* article highlighted a study that showed a link between "household" pesticide use and childhood leukemia. According to the article, written by J. Pickrell, a team of researchers from the University of California at Berkeley interviewed families in Northern California over a four-year period (1995–1999). Among these families were 324 children age 14 years or younger. Half of these children were already diagnosed with leukemia (mostly acute lymphoblastic leukemia), and the other half were free of cancer. What these researchers found was that:[4]

- Families of the children who had developed leukemia were about *three times as likely* to have employed the use of a professional exterminator in their home than the families who did not have a child with cancer.

- The highest risk to children appeared to occur when a professional exterminator was employed while the child was two years old.

- Whenever a mother was exposed during pregnancy to any kind of household pesticide, the risk of her unborn child later developing leukemia was *twice* as high as for mothers who were *not* exposed to household pesticide use during pregnancy.

Thus, regularly spraying our homes for cockroaches, ants, fleas, or other pests may put us in danger of developing cancer in a similar way that large-scale spraying of food crops can.

Herbicides that are sprayed on lawns and crops to kill weeds also can contribute to cancer. For example, one of the most widely used herbicides in the world, a chemical called "2,4-D" has undergone scrutiny as a contributor to cancer in humans. Used in lawn products since 1944, 2,4-D is particularly good at killing dandelion weeds, which plague parks, residential lawns, and golf courses, but it has also been heavily used on commercial crops.

A revealing *Los Angeles Times* newspaper article from June 1, 2002, written by Emily Green, stated that Kansas crop workers who had been working with 2,4-D had a higher than normal rate of non-Hodgkin's lymphoma. This article also reported that the overall incidence of non-Hodgkin's lymphoma had increased in farm workers by 75 percent over the previous 20 years and that some statisticians have now linked heavy wheat growing regions of the United States (which are notable for their use of 2,4-D) to higher incidences of cancers of the esophagus, stomach, rectum, throat, pancreas, larynx, prostate, kidney, and brain.

According to the *Times* article, one reason the carcinogenic effect of this herbicide may have gone unnoticed for about 50 years is that the effect only surfaces as a result of combining different ingredients together. In other words, by itself, 2,4-D is virtually biologically inert, but when it is *mixed* with other common ingredients in weed killer products it can combine with other chemicals to become deadly. Yet, this weed killer is still commonly sold for residential lawns and gardens and used by many people who have no idea how cancer-causing it may be.

Smog, pesticides, and herbicides are all sources of environmental toxins that most of us are aware of to at least some degree. But many of the most carcinogenic environmental pollutants we are exposed to on a daily basis are ones that most of us *are not at all aware of.* The biggest invisible culprits may be chlorine byproducts, fluoride, asbestos, fiberglass, and nuclear radiation. In the following paragraphs, these carcinogens will be introduced briefly. But since they are such important issues, they will be discussed in more detail in the Appendix of this book as well.

Chlorine byproducts, also called "organochlorines," are unnatural compounds that are created as a result of the chemical interaction between chlorine and organic material. They occur largely as a result of chlorinating public water supplies, but they also occur in our daily lives from other chlorine sources. According to a joint study conducted by Harvard University and the Medical College of Wisconsin, the simple act of drinking chlorinated water accounts for about 15 percent of all rectal cancers and about 9 percent of all bladder cancers. These add up to about 10,700 cases of cancer every year in the United States that are suspected to be due to drinking chlorinated water alone.[5]

More details about chlorination are discussed in the Appendix, but it is worth noting here that one category of chlorine byproduct, called "dioxins," has been referred to by scientific experts as *the single most carcinogenic type of manmade chemical known to science*. Read the Appendix to see how you may be ingesting dioxins every time you eat beef or dairy products, or even every time you drink a cup of coffee.

Fluoride is currently a controversial issue. But it appears to be controversial only on the *political* level, not the scientific level. To researchers who have studied it, there is no doubt that fluoride is an extremely hazardous substance to everyone's health in many ways.

Besides many other serious health problems, fluoride has now been linked to human cancers of the bone, bladder, liver, mouth, and lung, and it may contribute to other cancers as well. Dean Burk, Ph.D., former chief chemist of the National Cancer Institute, has been quoted as saying, "In point of fact, fluoride causes more human cancer deaths, and causes them faster, than any other chemical." Even Proctor and Gamble (the makers of Crest toothpaste) presented studies to the U.S. Public Health Service that showed fluoride to be a cancer-causing agent *at the lowest concentrations used*.

The public was fooled into accepting water fluoridation because the original tooth-decay prevention tests were done using calcium fluoride, or CaF_2. Calcium fluoride is the type of fluoride found naturally in water and plants. Yet, the type of fluoride that got added to public water supplies and toothpaste was *sodium fluoride*, or NaF. As opposed to calcium fluoride, sodium fluoride is highly toxic, but it is still the type of fluoride added to many public water sources and common dental products.

Unfortunately, even if you *don't* drink fluoridated water or use fluoridated toothpaste, that does not mean you are not being exposed to toxic sodium fluoride. Through water sources, it has now contaminated many of our foods and numerous commercial beverages such as sodas, juices, teas, beer, and wine. Exposure to fluoride contamination in modern countries is virtually inescapable. (See the Appendix for more information on the history of fluoridation and studies that link it to cancer.)

Another environmental cancer-triggering substance most people rarely think about is **asbestos**. We have heard bad things about it and have also heard that it has been largely banned and regulated. However, what we don't know is that a great deal of asbestos is *still* in our environment. Countless buildings all over the United States still contain asbestos insulation that releases microscopic fibers into the air. This includes countless modern skyscrapers and tens of thousands of children's schools. The microscopically small fibers from asbestos get into the air we breathe and take an incredibly long time to settle out of the air. They are also virtually indestructible. Once breathed into the body or ingested into the intestinal tract, these fibers can irritate cells and eventually cause cancer.

Virtually every man, woman, and child in industrialized countries has now been exposed to asbestos-contaminated air, no matter where they live or work. It has been estimated that in the 20th century asbestos killed something like 300,000 asbestos workers, and countless other people whose cancers and other illnesses are suspected to have been asbestos related. According to cancer researcher Ralph W. Moss, Ph.D., some officials in our government have estimated that possibly 10 to 15 percent of all cancer deaths in this country are due to asbestos! (For more details on asbestos and cancer, please refer to the Appendix.)

It took many years before the use of asbestos was regulated in the United States, but as it was phased out, many manufacturers turned to the use of **fiberglass** instead. Fiberglass has not been studied as much as asbestos, but many researchers believe it may be *just as cancer-causing*. This is a controversial subject as well, but if fiberglass is as carcinogenic as asbestos, then we are in big trouble because approximately 90 percent of all the homes in America use fiberglass insulation. Air circulating through air condition and heating vents can pick up and circulate microscopic pieces of this material from the insulation packing. It is as yet unknown as to how much fiberglass pollution is in the air we breathe. (For more details on fiberglass and cancer, please refer to the Appendix.)

Last but not least, in our look at major environmental cancer-causing factors we rarely think about, we come to **nuclear radiation**. Back in 1954, a Hollywood movie called *The Conqueror* was filmed on sand dunes outside of St. George, Utah. This location was about 150 miles downwind from atomic bomb testing sites. For three months, crew members and stars including John Wayne, Susan Hayward, Agnes Moorehead, and producer Dick Powell breathed in dust that was laced with radioactive fallout. Of the total 220 people involved with that film's production, 91 had contracted cancer by 1980 and half of them died of the disease. Those who died of cancer included John Wayne, Susan Hayward, Agnes Moorehead, and Dick Powell.[6]

We cannot be sure that radiation from nuclear fallout was the only cause of these actors' deaths, but the rates of cancer incidence in some areas of Utah have been so high that, in 1990, Congress officially apologized to the citizens of Utah and other areas downwind from nuclear testing. (See the Appendix for more details.)

Of course, you may be thinking, "Why would nuclear radiation be a factor in cancer today? After all, we're not testing nuclear bombs anymore, and we're not in a war involving nuclear weapons." The answer is that, during the 1950s and 1960s about a thousand nuclear devices were test-detonated in the Nevada desert as well as in a few other places around the United States, and the nuclear fallout from those tests is still affecting us today. Many of the detonations were carried out underground, but 184 were atmospheric, above-ground tests.[7] Radioactive nuclear fallout was then wind-blown over just about every part of the United States. Moreover, the tests in the United States were not the only sources of nuclear fallout exposure. It is probable that Americans were also exposed to fallout blown over the Pacific from the World War II detonations at Hiroshima and Nagasaki, test detonations carried out in the Pacific, test detonations carried out in the Soviet Union, and from nuclear power plant disasters such as Chernobyl and Three-Mile Island.

This wind-blown fallout from domestic tests, as well as from sources abroad, resulted in a great deal of "direct" radiation exposure to many people who later developed cancer. But it also settled onto our crops and into our soil and water. Since many of the damaging radioactive substances that settled into our water and soil have a very long half-life, they are still affecting us today. We still breathe them into our bodies when dust blows through the air, and we still ingest them through our crops and drink them in through our water.

The important thing to remember about nuclear fallout is that some of the radioactive substances take only about 30 years to deteriorate, but other radioactive substances take *thousands* of years to deteriorate. This means that they keep on emitting radioactivity for a very long time. In other words, the fact that test detonations have stopped does *not* mean radiation exposure has stopped.

Once ingested, these radioactive compounds can get stored in various places in our bodies and keep on radiating. That is why nuclear fallout is capable of causing so many different types of cancers over a very long period of time. Even the National Cancer Institute finally admitted in a government report in 1997 that fallout from bomb tests carried out in the 1950s could have caused up to 75,000 cases of cancer. And since the NCI was only looking at the effects of *one* of the many radioactive isotopes generated, nuclear fallout has probably caused more like hundreds of thousands of cancers in humans. (For more details on nuclear radiation and cancer, please refer to the Appendix.)

Modern Lifestyle Choices and Treatments

This is a very important category of modern living because it involves cancer-causing factors we have control over. It is also a very disturbing category, since it highlights some big cancer-causing triggers that we may unwittingly *choose* to subject ourselves to without realizing that we are greatly increasing our chances of developing cancer by doing so.

Without a doubt, the first of these factors to look at is **cigarette smoking**. The director of the Harvard Center for Cancer Prevention has estimated that *tobacco smoke alone accounts for about 30 percent of all cancer deaths in the United States.*[8] Only about one-third of these cancer deaths involve tobacco-related lung cancer. This is because cigarette smoking has also been linked to cancers of the head, neck, mouth, throat, vocal cords, bladder, kidney, stomach, cervix, pancreas, and even to leukemia. Of the lung cancer cases that *are* tobacco-related, an estimated 20 percent of them are due to "passive" exposure. In other words, about 3,000 lung cancer deaths occur each year in the United States among *non-smokers* who have been passively exposed to tobacco smoke.[9]

According to W. John Diamond, M.D., and his co-authors of the book *An Alternative Medicine Definitive Guide to Cancer*, the cancer-causing ability of cigarette smoking was known to the tobacco industry back around 1950. Among a number of studies linking cigarette smoke to cancer incidence, in December 1953, researchers at the Sloan-Kettering Institute in New York published the alarming results of one scientific study involving laboratory animals. This study showed that when cigarette smoke condensate was simply "painted" onto the skin of mice, 44 percent of the mice developed cancer.[10]

It is a sobering thought that the number of cancer deaths in the United States could be cut by one-third if people just stopped smoking cigarettes.

One of the *next* biggest cancer-triggering modern lifestyle choices has to do with the use of synthetic hormones by women. Many modern women have chosen to use **birth control pills** or to take synthetic hormones for relief from menopause symptoms. Whether or not long-term use of birth control pills can cause cancer is still a controversial subject, but there is a great deal of research indicating it *can* be a contributor—at least for young women who start their use of the pill before age 20. On the other hand, the cancer-causing ability of synthetic **hormone replacement therapy** (HRT) for women dealing with menopause has been well established.

The following is a quote from Dr. Walter Willett, M.D., chairman of the Department of Public Health at Harvard Medical School. He refers to the current common HRT prescriptions of Premarin and Provera in the following statements:

> The downplaying of the risk of using animal-derived and synthetic HRT is even more despicable. The spin doctors calmly stated that for every 10,000 women on HRT during one year, only eight more will have invasive breast cancer, only seven more will have a heart attack, only eight more will have a stroke, and only 18 more will have blood clots. Sounds benign, doesn't it? It does, until you do the math.
>
> There are 8 to10 million women currently using HRT. Using conservative numbers, that adds up to 6,400 cases of invasive breast cancer, 5,600 heart attacks, 6,400 strokes, and 14,400 cases of blood clots to organs such as the lungs. That adds up to 32,800 cases of drug-induced morbidity *each year*![11]

And the above quote only refers to conservative estimates for HRT-induced breast cancers, though HRT-induced uterine cancer has *also* been well-established. (This will be discussed in more detail in Chapter 19.)

Another choice common to modern living is the use of X-rays. It has been estimated that approximately 78,000 people every year develop cancer as a direct result of having been given **medical and dental X-rays**. Some researchers believe that a majority of breast cancer occurrences may be caused by medical X-rays given for diagnosing chest and lung problems, or spinal-related back and neck problems.

One of the most insidious sources of contributing factors to cancer, unfortunately, may be the field of modern dental practices. The subject of **toxic teeth** is still controversial, but evidence linking cancer with dangerous dental practices exists. The most common dental practices that have been linked to cancer are: (1) silver/mercury fillings, (2) nickel-alloyed stainless steel used in certain types of crowns, and (3) root canal procedures. Many alternative practitioners who specialize in treating cancer agree that it can be important to deal with one's toxic teeth for a better chance of recovery from cancer. Not everyone has toxic teeth, but those who do may not know it. This is because toxic teeth don't always display clear warning signs, such as pain in the mouth or abnormal shading on X-rays. (Chapter 21 presents more details on toxic teeth and what you can do about them.)

Possibly one of the saddest realities today is that the common practice of administering **childhood vaccines** may be introducing carcinogenic substances into millions of children and contributing to pediatric cancers. This subject is also very controversial, but some researchers have come up with information that is quite alarming.

One couple whose two-year-old son was diagnosed with the most common type of pediatric brain cancer—medulloblastoma—did their own informal research, which they posted on the Internet at www.our alexander.org/burton.htm. These parents went through agony when their small son was diagnosed and suffered through two brain operations and then chemotherapy. After their little boy Alexander died, these parents tried to figure out why he might have gotten cancer. He had been a strong child, and no one in his family, going back three generations on both his parents' sides, had ever developed cancer.

Alexander's parents researched how long medulloblastoma tumors generally take to grow, then looked into what had happened in the months just before that time. From their son's medical files, Alexander's parents discovered that just before this tumor had most likely started growing, Alexander had gotten numerous pediatric vaccines. Then his parents researched the available material on these vaccines, particularly on the DPT, IPV, OPV, and Hepatitis B vaccines. What they found out was horrifying.

Taken from www.ouralexander.org/burton.htm, here are some of the facts Alexander's parents discovered:

- There are six ways that vaccinations may cause cancer, directly or indirectly.

- Standard medicine really doesn't know if vaccines are carcinogenic or not, because no official studies have ever been done on this. In fact, according to Alexander's parents, "*None* of the vaccines injected into children have ever been tested for their carcinogenic (cancer causing), mutagenic (mutation causing), or teratogenic (developmental malformation causing) potential."

- Most vaccines contain carcinogenic chemicals in them, usually in the form of mercury derivatives, aluminum, and/or formaldehyde. If a parent were found injecting any of these substances into a child, they would be charged with child abuse. Yet these potent carcinogens are in most childhood vaccines.

- Vaccines sometimes contain viruses, or bacteria that contain viruses, and some viruses have been associated with certain cancers. Also, vaccinations for one type of virus can carry *unexpected* viruses in them that may come from the animals used to create the vaccine. For example, the polio vaccine of the 1950s and 1960s that was injected into millions of children was found to carry an unexpected virus from the monkey kidney cells that were used to culture the polio vaccine. This monkey virus, called SV40, was found to *definitively* cause cancer. In fact, in studies with young hamsters that were injected with SV40, 80 percent of them developed brain cancer! When this was discovered, polio vaccine manufacturers switched to a different type of monkey to avoid the SV40 virus, but in the meantime, millions of young people had already been injected with it. In 1995, the authors of one study on human brain tumors who published their results in the *Journal of the National Cancer Institute*, stated, ". . . we found SV40 DNA sequences in five of six choroid plexus papillomas, eight of eleven ependymomas, three of seven astrocytomas . . . None of the 13 normal brain tissues were positive for SV40 DNA."[12]

The possibility that many children may be developing cancer as a result of vaccines given to them to avoid illnesses that are less critical than cancer is simply horrifying and is an issue that desperately needs to be more prevalent in the public's awareness.

Another common aspect of modern life that is connected to lifestyle choices is stress. **Chronic stress** is probably the most common type of modern stress, as opposed to the type of stress generated by a single, temporary crisis. Chronic stress can result from a lifestyle that creates daily situations where a person is *constantly* feeling as though he or she is racing against the clock or on the edge of a crisis. Mothers and fathers who try to juggle full-time jobs while raising children and dealing with extracurricular school activities, busy freeway driving, and so forth, are prime targets of chronic stress.

But even *without* fast-paced lifestyles, certain personality traits alone can sometimes generate chronic stress. These tend to be the personality traits, or learned behavioral patterns, involving how we communicate with other people and deal with our emotions. People who chronically "stuff" their anger, frustration, or fear and don't know how to get their emotional needs met are often suffering on a physiological level from chronic stress.

High levels of chronic stress can negatively affect the body's defenses in many ways. It can cause higher than optimum stress hormones to be produced by the body on a daily basis, which can create an imbalance in other hormones. The adrenals are the glands that respond to stress the most and they release stress-related hormones. If they are chronically stressed over time, they can eventually become fatigued or even burn out to a point where they are no longer able to produce their hormones in optimum levels. This can then lead to pH imbalance, poor digestion, and reduced effectiveness of the thyroid gland, among other problems. Chronic stress can even deplete the body's stores of vitamin C, because this vitamin is used up to create some of the stress hormones that the body generates. Along with other weakening effects of environmental triggers and deficient control mechanisms in the body, many cancer researchers believe that chronic stress can actually be a powerful factor in contributing to the development of cancer.

Finally, one fast-growing area of lifestyle choices that can trigger cancer is that of common **prescription drug use**. Some types of commonly prescribed drugs such as cholesterol-lowering medications are now being linked to an increased risk of cancer. It is not always easy to prove whether a prescription drug can cause cancer or not, but all you have to do is listen carefully to the many pharmaceutical ads on television in order to get an idea of the magnitude of this issue. A large number of drugs that are advertised for non-life threatening conditions actually have "lymphoma" stated as one of the possible side effects in these commercials. What much of the public *doesn't* know is that lymphoma is a *life-threatening* form of cancer! For anyone diagnosed with lymphoma, a 50% chance of being alive 5 years after diagnosis is a common prognosis, and there is little assurance of being cured anytime after those 5 years. It is obvious that Big Pharma is counting on people not understanding what lymphoma is, and of course lymphoma is not the only type of cancer that many of these drugs can cause.

Is It All Doom and Gloom?

It is clear that, although cancer has been around for thousands of years, and has occurred in humans, animals, and even plants for millennia, the *frequency* of cancer today has put cancer into the category of a disease of modern living. After reading about so many possible cancer-promoting factors in the modern world, it is no wonder that many people who have eaten well, exercised, and otherwise lived conscientiously healthy lives are developing cancer. But the purpose of this chapter is *not* to promote a "doom and gloom" attitude. In fact, a doom and gloom feeling is *already* alive and well with so many of us seeing our friends and loved ones succumbing to cancer at such a high rate.

On the contrary, the purpose of this chapter is just the opposite. Understanding something is the first step toward releasing fear about that thing and also toward conquering it. Too many people are being diagnosed with cancer today and feeling totally confused as to why it happened. They also may feel guilty or bad about themselves. Since there appears to be no reason why they should have gotten cancer, they may even feel they are being divinely punished in some way. Under these circumstances, they may give up all hope of surviving the disease.

But, as we have seen, there are very clear reasons why so many people are developing cancer today and there are very clear things each one of us can do to help ourselves avoid a cancer diagnosis or cancer recurrence (besides using a treatment approach.) We can stay away from toxic dental practices, stop ingesting aspartame, avoid toxic household pesticide spraying, and say no to non-bioidentical hormones, vaccines and prescription drugs, to name a few. There are also things we can do collectively as a public to help ensure better health for our children. We can stand up for our rights *not* to have pesticides, dioxins, nuclear radiation, fluoride, asbestos, or fiber glass in our environment, food, and water.

It is up to us to *not* fall prey to the two big conventional medicine lies: 1) that cancer is some sort of mysterious affliction that nobody really understands, and 2) if you have a family history of cancer, that proves it's genetic and runs in your family. These two lies simply make people feel they are powerless to do anything about cancer.

In actuality, cancer is really quite well understood, but you won't find this understanding in conventional medicine—you'll find it by looking into alternative non-toxic treatments. And there is a very good reason for this. Because alternative approaches are non-toxic, they cannot rely on a toxic shotgun type of method. They have to "outsmart" cancer by targeting common characteristics of all cancer cells. This brings up the question, "How different are different types of cancer?"

How Different Are Different Cancers?

Is lung cancer a whole different disease from liver cancer or uterine cancer or prostate cancer? Are leukemias, bone cancers, lymphomas, kidney cancer and bladder cancer all different diseases? The simple answer is that *conventional* medicine tends to look at cancers in different parts of the body as different diseases. But in the *alternative* cancer treatment field, cancer is cancer no matter where it is.

What you will discover in the following pages is that, once cancer develops in the body, it basically involves the same mechanics and cell functioning *wherever* it occurs. Although there are some minor differences among differently diagnosed cancers, these differences are minimal compared to the similarities that all cancers share. And the differences that *do* show up appear to result more from the fact that different types of body cells and body locations are involved in different diagnoses of cancer. Thus, rather than say there are different "types" of cancer, it would be more accurate to say there are different "manifestations" of cancer.

One minor difference the location of cancer can cause is the *speed* at which the cancer cells grow. This difference is linked to the type of cell involved in that particular system of the body. For instance, cancers of the blood, such as leukemia, replicate faster than many other cancers simply because blood cells normally have the characteristic of replicating more quickly than other cells. Another minor difference is that cancers in sexual organs are generally much more affected by the sex hormones of the body than other cancers are. This is for the obvious reason that normal cells of sexual organs tend to have more receptor sites for those types of hormones, so when those cells become cancerous, they still have receptor sites.

And yet another minor difference that may be caused by the location of cancer in the body is the circulatory system that is involved. For instance, cancers of the lymph system and brain are in areas of the body that have unique circulatory characteristics and this may affect how well, or how quickly, medicines or nutrients from the blood can get to these types of cancer.

However, if we look at the most important characteristics of cancer on the basic level of cellular structure and functioning, different types of cancer are not significantly different. In other words, *all malignant cancer cells share important common characteristics* no matter where they occur in the body. Understanding these common characteristics can help take the mystery out of cancer—but more importantly, understanding the common characteristics and mechanics of *all* cancer cells provides the keys to understanding how to *outsmart* your cancer. The final key is provided by the fact that non-toxic treatments can safely be administered over long periods of time, 24 hours a day and 7 days a week. In this way, cancer cells are never given the chance to grow back in between treatments as they are with toxic chemotherapy or radiation.

Different non-toxic approaches may target different characteristics of cancer, but the outcome is always the same. In other words, they *outsmart* and defeat the cancer by either naturally blocking some aspect of the cancer cells' ability to function, by naturally strengthening the body's own ability to overcome the cancer, or both. In the next section, you will read about 21 different strategies that others have used to *outsmart* their cancer over the past 100 years. These are not *all* of the alternative strategies that have ever been used, but they are approaches that have exhibited some of the longest and most successful track records and are largely still available to people within the United States.

To give the reader a historical sense of these remarkable approaches, they are presented in a somewhat chronological order. The first two non-toxic methods for cancer that were widely used in the U.S. were herbal therapies in the early 1900s. These herbal approaches were observed to work and are still working for many people today, but they have *not* been well understood as to their mechanism of action. Even without full scientific understanding, however, the herbal therapies of the early 1900s were working better than conventional treatments for cancer today. Later approaches tended to be more completely understood and scientific explanations are presented in those chapters along with studies and case stories.

If you are currently dealing with a cancer diagnosis, there *is* hope in the world of alternative, non-toxic treatments.

Section Two

Alternative

Non-Toxic Treatments

3

The Hoxsey Therapy

We begin our in-depth look at alternative, non-toxic cancer treatments with an herbal approach called "the Hoxsey therapy." Herbal treatments are documented as the oldest type of approach to cancer and have been used with success for thousands of years by indigenous people all around the world.

In recent years, modern science has proven that many herbs do, in fact, have cancer-fighting properties. They have been shown to support the body's immune system, improve blood circulation, strengthen the functioning of major organs, and enhance the efficient elimination of toxins, among other things. They can act very much like a potent drug as well. For instance, some herbs have direct cytotoxic effects on the cancer cells themselves, while not harming other cells of the body. Other herbs have been shown to inhibit a tumor's ability to produce new blood vessels to feed itself, thereby strangling the tumor's system of nourishment. And still other herbs have anti-microbial properties. Thus, herbs are often referred to as "nature's medicine" and the Hoxsey therapy for cancer is a wonderful example of this.

The Hoxsey therapy was the first widely used alternative non-toxic treatment for cancer in the modern United States. Still obtainable today, it is a treatment that consists of an herbal topical salve, an herbal topical powder, and an herbal internal tonic. Though many people have never heard of it, this treatment approach was very successful and was actually used by tens of thousands of Americans in the early to mid-1900s. Around 1953, at the height of the Hoxsey therapy, the main Hoxsey clinic in Dallas, Texas had 12,000 patients and was the largest private cancer center in the world. There were also subsidiary clinics in 17 other states.

History

The history of the Hoxsey therapy is a colorful one. Harry Hoxsey, an American man born in 1901, was the person responsible for the widespread use of the Hoxsey therapy for cancer. But the herbal remedy had started farther back in time, and had been passed down to Harry by his great-grandfather, John Hoxsey. It was John Hoxsey, a horse breeder in Illinois, who developed the herbal remedy in the mid-1800s. According to the story as Harry told it, in 1840 his great-grandfather John had a stallion that was expected to die as a result of having developed a cancerous lesion on its leg. This horse had been one of John's favorites, so when the horse had to be put out to pasture, he kept an eye on it. He noticed that the horse exhibited atypical behavior by grazing primarily on one clump of shrubs and flowering plants. He also noticed that the horse's cancer completely healed after a number of months and the stallion made a full recovery.

Curious about his horse's amazing return to health, John picked samples from the plants on which the stallion had been grazing. Through experimentation, he developed an herbal tonic, salve, and powder from them. Some think John Hoxsey may have also gotten input from some of the local Native Americans about the use of these plants, but no one knows for sure. He then started using these remedies to treat other horses suffering from external cancers or other types of lesions. John's herbal mixture proved to be quite successful, and word spread quickly until horse breeders were bringing their horses to him from as far away as Indiana and Kentucky.

John Hoxsey's herbal mixtures were eventually passed down to Harry's father, a veterinarian. Harry's father used the herbal remedies to treat animals with cancer and other conditions. But he started to quietly use the herbal treatments to help humans with cancer as well.

When Harry was eight years old, he began assisting his father in administering these treatments to some of the local people. These were generally people who had no other hope for recovery, and the Hoxsey remedies were having success. Just before his father's death, Harry, the youngest in a family of 12 children, was entrusted with the secrets of how to prepare the remedies and was given the responsibility to carry on the family's healing tradition.

Harry wanted to do this and enjoyed helping people. He decided to become trained as a doctor so he could legally administer the remedies to cancer patients. But coming from a poor coal-mining family, he had to work very hard to start saving money for medical school. Kenny Ausubel wrote the most in-depth and well-documented book about the history of the Hoxsey therapy, titled *When Healing Becomes a Crime: The Amazing Story of the Hoxsey Cancer Clinics and the Return of Alternative Therapies*. According to Ausubel, Harry did *not* want to treat any person with cancer until he had obtained his medical license. But while Harry was saving up for his medical training, people with life-threatening cancer who had heard about the success of his father's remedies kept coming to him and *begging* him to treat them. He tried to avoid doing this, but eventually treated some of them out of the goodness of his heart.

Unfortunately, Harry later discovered that his efforts to get a medical license would never be successful because, as a result of treating some of these desperate cancer patients without a license, Harry was blackballed from entry into medical schools.

Finally, one physician convinced Harry that he could legally administer his remedies to cancer patients as long as he was working as a medical technician under the supervision of a licensed physician. Since he couldn't get a medical license, Harry agreed to do this and began helping people with cancer under the official supervision of various different doctors. He was just in his early twenties, but he was a bright and energetic young man. The Hoxsey remedies were very successful, which brought more and more cancer sufferers to his door. Then, in 1924, when Harry was only 23 years old, he opened the first official Hoxsey Cancer Clinic in Dallas. It was operational into the 1950s and eventually became the biggest private cancer center in the world.

The Hoxsey therapy was mostly known for its success with external tumors on the surface of the body. People with external cancers were treated with an herbal paste applied directly onto the tumor and given a liquid herbal tonic to drink as well. People with internal cancer that showed no external signs were just given the tonic. Certain dietary changes were also recommended to patients in general, along with a few nutritional supplements. The ingredients of Hoxsey's internal tonic are well known, with most sources saying it was made up of potassium iodide, licorice, red clover, burdock root, stillingia root, berberis root, pokeroot, cascara, prickly ash bark, and buckthorn bark. Though it was not proven at the time, botanists have since found all of the herbs in the Hoxsey tonic to have various anti-cancer properties. And the external salve contains bloodroot, which has been used by Native Americans to treat cancer for centuries.

But Harry Hoxsey was a renegade self-taught healer, and because he was not a doctor of medicine, he was constantly being arrested for practicing medicine without a license. Technically, he ran his treatment facilities legally because he always maintained a supervising physician with a valid license. But despite this fact, and maybe because established doctors felt threatened by him, Harry Hoxsey is said to have been arrested more times than any other person in medical history!

According to Ausubel and others, the *biggest* reason that Harry Hoxsey kept getting arrested was because the powerful head of the American Medical Association, Morris Fishbein, was out to get him. They claim that Fishbein wanted to buy Hoxsey's remedies from him, but Hoxsey refused. Thereafter, it is well documented that the ruthless Fishbein conducted a personal vendetta against Hoxsey.

Unfortunately for Hoxsey, the American Medical Association was just coming into its own as a powerful organization, and Morris Fishbein was not only the head of this organization, but also editor of the *Journal of the American Medical Association (JAMA)*. This journal was becoming a powerful force, and Fishbein used it as his primary vehicle for discrediting the Hoxsey therapy. In numerous articles over many years, Fishbein pronounced Hoxsey's cancer treatment as nothing but quackery. Journal articles also ridiculed and discredited any physician who chose to endorse Hoxsey's therapy. In this way, it soon became political suicide for a doctor or other medical expert to even consider using the Hoxsey treatment. The AMA's adamant disapproval of Hoxsey also seemed to be what prompted many of his arrests for practicing medicine without a license even though Harry always worked legally under the supervision of a licensed physician.

What kept saving Hoxsey was the success of his treatment as well as his own tenacious character. Virtually every time Harry was arrested, groups of his cancer patients would gather outside the jail as a show of support. The crowds got bigger and bigger, and people brought Hoxsey homemade food and sang hymns outside the jailhouse all day long. Eventually, the wardens would release him.

The success of Hoxsey's cancer treatment was also what kept getting him acquitted in the many court trials he had to go through. According to Ausubel, in one case, a local deputy sheriff refused to serve Hoxsey with a subpoena, even though he was ordered to do so, because the deputy sheriff himself was undergoing treatment for cancer with Hoxsey. In another case, Hoxsey was acquitted in a trial because 12 of the jury members were either former patients of Hoxsey's or had relatives or friends who had been helped by him. In yet another court battle, the trial ended favorably for Hoxsey because the presiding judge had been raised by a relative Hoxsey's father had cured of cancer.[1] Even several senators endorsed Hoxsey's cancer therapy. And over the many years he was charged with practicing medicine without a license, not a single cancer patient ever testified against him.

One of Harry Hoxsey's vehement opponents in Texas was Al Templeton, assistant district attorney. Over a two-year period, Templeton had Harry arrested more than 100 times. But in an ironic twist of fate, the district attorney's younger brother, Mike Templeton, came down with cancer of the intestine. He went through conventional treatment and a colostomy. But when his cancer was still there and began growing again after the surgery, Mike's conventional doctors told him there was nothing more they could do for him. At this point, Mike secretly went to the Hoxsey clinic for treatment and ended up completely recovering from his cancer. Upon hearing of his younger brother's unexpected cure, Al Templeton reversed his attitude toward Harry. After years of continually arresting him, Templeton became Harry Hoxsey's lawyer and began legally defending him in court instead!

A Texas nurse named Mildred Nelson also believed Harry Hoxsey to be a quack at first. Mildred was trained in conventional medicine and tried to talk her own mother out of receiving the Hoxsey therapy for cancer in 1946. Mildred's mother, Della Mae, was in a desperate situation. According to Ausubel,

> Ranch wife Della Mae Nelson had uterine cancer that had been extensively treated with twenty units of X-ray and thirty-six hours of radium. She was so badly burned from the radiation that she couldn't even pull a sheet over her body for a year after. Wasted to eighty-six pounds, she was bleeding internally, so severely impaired that she had to learn to walk all over again. Then the cancer recurred.[2]

When Della Mae's cancer recurred, her conventional doctors told the family there was nothing more they could do for her. Against her daughter's wishes, Della Mae then sought treatment at the Hoxsey clinic in Dallas. She, too, completely recovered from her cancer as a result of the Hoxsey therapy. (Della Mae Nelson died about 50 years later, in 1997, at the age of ninety-nine. She had outlived most of the conventional doctors and nurses that had treated her). Needless to say, Mildred was finally convinced that Hoxsey's herbal treatment was effective and went to work for Hoxsey's Dallas clinic as a nurse. Mildred's father was subsequently also treated for cancer by Hoxsey, and he completely recovered as well.

Mildred found Harry Hoxsey to be a compassionate, admirable man with many talents. She recalled that he had a photographic memory and never forgot a patient's name or face. She also said, "He had a sixth sense if somebody was sick. He seemed to have almost a psychic thing of what would work for this particular person."[3] Hoxsey claimed to achieve about an 85 percent success rate for cancers that were external and about an 80 percent cure rate for patients with internal cancer that had *not* been already treated with prior surgery or radiation.[4] Many of the bus and taxi drivers in the local area were so used to transporting and talking to people who were getting well at the Hoxsey clinic, they claimed it was where they would go if they got cancer.

During the time that Hoxsey's treatment was showing great success, however, conventional treatments for cancer were beginning to become a very big business. By the 1950s, conventional cancer treatment had already become focused on surgery, radiation, and the fast-growing field of chemotherapy. Some people believe that Morris Fishbein was not the only obstacle to Hoxsey's Therapy, but that the inexpensive and unpatentable Hoxsey therapy threatened the emerging cancer industry's big profits and stimulated opposition from many sources. The favorite approach from the conventional medical establishment was to label Hoxsey a "quack" or a "hoaxer." These statements went completely against the facts, which unequivocally showed that Hoxsey's treatment not only worked for a wide variety of cancer cases, but worked *better* than conventional methods of the day.

Since most quacks are in it for the money, if Hoxsey *was* a quack, he wasn't a very good one. All of the Hoxsey clinics admitted and treated any cancer patient who came to them, even *those that could not pay*. Ausubel's book documents numerous times when Hoxsey exhibited generosity to his patients above and beyond the call of duty, including fully treating people who had used up their last dime on bus fare to get to the clinic. Many times Hoxsey then drove them to a local place where they could stay. In reality, Hoxsey was following the advice his father had given him when he handed the responsibility of the family remedies over. His father said:

> Now you have the power to heal the sick and save lives. What I've managed to do in a tiny part of this state, you can do all over the country, all over the world. I've cured hundreds of people. You can cure thousands, tens of thousands.
>
> But it's not only a gift, son; it's a trust and a great responsibility. Abe Lincoln once said God must have loved the common people because he made so many of them. We're common, ordinary people. You must never refuse to treat anybody because he can't pay. Promise me that![5]

In 1954, an independent group of 10 doctors from various parts of the United States made a point of investigating Hoxsey's clinic in Dallas. After the two-day inspection, which included examining hundreds of case histories and talking to patients and ex-patients, this independent group of physicians made a stunning public conclusion. They reported that the Hoxsey clinic

> . . . is successfully treating pathologically proven cases of cancer, both internal and external, without the use of surgery, radium or x-ray.
>
> Accepting the standard yardstick of cases that have remained symptom-free in excess of five to six years after treatment, established by medical authorities, we have seen sufficient cases to warrant such a conclusion. Some of those presented before us have been free of symptoms as long as twenty-four years, and the physical evidence indicates that they are all enjoying exceptional health at this time.
>
> We as a Committee feel that the Hoxsey treatment is superior to such conventional methods of treatment as x-ray, radium, and surgery. We are willing to assist this Clinic in any way possible in bringing this treatment to the American public.[6]

Here, finally, was the type of official medical endorsement that Hoxsey had been looking for to help him spread the treatment to more and more people. Unfortunately, this was not to be. The report of the 10 independent doctors was ignored by all influential parties.

Thus, Hoxsey was not only powerfully opposed by Morris Fishbein but also by others in the cancer industry. The higher-ups in the AMA may have been his most vehement opponents, but other organizations such as the NCI and FDA also helped to suppress any fair assessment of the Hoxsey therapy. Even though Hoxsey repeatedly pleaded with these groups to conduct scientific studies on his formulas, and even though thousands of patients were recovering from cancer as a result of Hoxsey's herbal mixtures, the official cancer industry's response was *not* to study it. In fact, unbelievably, official representatives from the FDA would actually "go to patients' houses, intimidate them, tell them they were being duped by a quack, and take away their Hoxsey medicines."[7]

Morris Fishbein eventually delivered a powerful blow by officially claiming Hoxsey as a hoaxer in a segment that was published in a Sunday newspaper segment and read by about 20 million people. Hoxsey sued Fishbein and the Hearst newspaper for libel and slander, and 50 of his cancer patients testified on his behalf in court. Fortunately, Harry Hoxsey won the lawsuit, although he was only awarded 2 dollars by the court.

The following excerpt from Richard Walters's book, *Options*, lays to rest any doubts that suppression of good, non-toxic cancer treatments has truly happened. Referring to Dr. Morris Fishbein after the Hoxsey lawsuit, Walters writes:

> The leader of America's "quack attack" was now on the defensive. Critics charged the AMA with being a doctor's trade union, setting national medical policy to further its own selfish interests. The United States Supreme Court agreed that the AMA had conspired in restraint of trade. Dr. Fishbein was forced to resign.
>
> In 1953, the Fitzgerald Report, commissioned by a United States Senate committee, concluded that organized medicine had "conspired" to suppress the Hoxsey therapy and at least a dozen other promising cancer treatments.[8]

But despite his legal victory over Fishbein, Harry Hoxsey's opponents eventually proved too powerful and all his cancer treatment centers were forced to shut down. The Hoxsey clinic in Dallas closed its doors in 1960, and its long-time chief nurse, Mildred Nelson, ended up moving the operation to Mexico where she faithfully administered the treatment for many more years. Thus, the Hoxsey therapy was finally pushed out of the country and effectively denied from the American public at large.

After a lifetime of fighting conventional medicine, Harry Hoxsey died in 1974. He had developed cancer of the prostate, and some sources refer to how ironic it was that he couldn't cure himself of cancer. However, Ausubel, who researched Harry's history more meticulously than anyone else, says that he *did* cure himself of his cancer using his own remedy and in fact died of other causes. Paul Peters, M.D., Harry's last doctor of record, adamantly claimed that Harry died of liver trouble and a weak heart. He vehemently said that before his death Harry was free of cancer. But Dr. Peters was out of town when Harry died, and another physician was required to sign the death certificate. This physician, not knowing the true cause of death, merely looked at Harry's medical records, saw that he had *had* prostate cancer, and wrote that down as the cause on his death certificate.[9]

Current Hoxsey Therapy

Effective cancer treatments don't die easily, however, and the Bio-Medical Center in Tijuana continues to operate and administer the Hoxsey therapy. Harry's nurse, Mildred Nelson, ran the center for 25 years after Harry's death and provided cures for many people until her own death from a stroke in 1999. The Bio-Medical Center is now being run by Mildred's sister, and information below indicates how to contact this treatment center. The Hoxsey therapy has been known to work successfully for many different types of cancer, and the center in Tijuana is currently claiming that the best responders to the treatment are those diagnosed with lymphoma, melanoma, or other types of external skin cancers. Some people find traveling to Mexico for treatment a bit daunting, but the comparatively low price of this treatment makes up for that difficulty for many. Some also find that using Laetrile along with the Hoxsey therapy is helpful. (See Chapter 6 for a discussion of Laetrile.)

People with cancer who go to the Bio-Medical Center today do not stay there as in-patients but make day visits over the border. These people are difficult to follow up on because they tend to go back home to other countries, so it is not easy to assess whether the treatment still has the same efficacy as it did when it was under Harry Hoxsey's administration. Hopefully, the United States will pass more freedom of medical choice legislation, and this amazing herbal treatment will someday be able to return to its U.S. homeland and be developed and studied further.

Resources:

Physical Address:
Bio-Medical Center
3170 General Ferreira
Colonia Juarez
Tijuana, Baja
22150 Mexico

Mailing Address:
Bio-Medical Center
Col. Madero Sur P.O. Box 433654
San Isidro, CA 92143
California

Phone: (01152664) 684-9011
FAX: (01152664) 684-9744

Email:
BioMedicalCenter@prodigy.net.mx

Treatment at Bio-Medical Center: The total cost of treatment is about $3,500. Patients pay a set "lifetime" rate that is the same for everyone and covers as many visits and as much treatment as is needed. Patients are asked to arrive by 9 A.M., Monday through Friday, and will be done by 4 P.M. No appointments are necessary.

For a consultation with the Bio-Medical Center: Consultations are extremely inexpensive. Bring any X-rays, blood test results, and so forth that are less than one-month old. If you don't have these with you, you may be charged to have them done there.

Books

Kenny Ausubel. *When Healing Becomes a Crime: The Amazing Story of the Hoxsey Cancer Clinics and the Return of Alternative Therapies*. Rochester, Vermont: Healing Arts Press, 2000.

Richard Walters. *Options: The Alternative Cancer Therapy Book*. New York: Avery Penguin Putnam, 1993.

Video

Hoxsey: How Healing Becomes a Crime can be ordered by calling (505) 989-8575.

Websites

www.alkalizeforhealth.net/Lhoxsey.htm

www.yesyoucansayno.com/history.htm

www.whale.to/c/hoxsey.html

www.mnwelldir.org/docs/cancer1/altthrpy2.htm#Hoxsey%20Formula

4

Essiac Tea

No book on alternative cancer treatments would be complete without a discussion of the herbal tea treatment called "Essiac." Like the Hoxsey therapy, Essiac has been used since the early 1900s and also has a colorful history. One of the Essiac herbs, burdock root, is also part of the Hoxsey herbal therapy. While the Hoxsey herbal formula came to America from a horse rancher, the Essiac herbal tea came to Canada as a gift from Native America.

The history of Essiac begins in the late 1800s with a Canadian woman who was suffering from advanced breast cancer. She happened to meet an Ojibwa Indian medicine man, who told her he could cure her of her illness. She didn't want to have the surgery her doctors recommended, so she decided to accept the medicine man's offer instead. He showed the woman four herbs that grew naturally in her area and told her how to pick them and brew them into a tea. He instructed her to drink the tea every day. The Canadian woman did as she was told and subsequently completely recovered from her advanced breast cancer.

Thirty years later, in 1922, this same woman was a patient in a Canadian hospital in northern Ontario. Rene Caisse, the head nurse, was bathing the now elderly woman one day and noticed a great deal of scar tissue on the woman's breast. When she inquired about it, the woman told her about how she had been dying from breast cancer 30 years earlier and was cured by an Indian herbal formula. Caisse was extremely interested, especially since the elderly woman had not had a recurrence of her cancer in 30 years. According to one account, Caisse wrote down the names of the herbs from her patient in the hospital. According to another account, she visited the medicine man herself and was given the herbal remedy directly.

However it occurred, Nurse Caisse found that the four herbs were sheep sorrel, burdock root, slippery elm bark, and turkey rhubarb root. There may have been other herbs she was originally told about, too, but these are the four she ended up using. Nurse Caisse was told that when blended and brewed together in a certain way, these herbs had more curative power than any of the four herbs individually had.

About a year after receiving the herbal formula, Rene Caisse's aunt was diagnosed with stomach cancer that had metastasized to her liver. The doctors had given up on her aunt, so Caisse brewed the herbal tea and administered it to her. The tea worked and her aunt lived another 21 years.

Caisse then started collecting the wild herbs on a regular basis and preparing larger and larger portions of the remedy in her kitchen. She got permission from one doctor to administer the remedy to some terminally ill cancer patients the Canadian medical profession had no cure for. Soon, she was treating more and more cancer patients. When she wanted to pick a name for her concoction, Caisse decided to spell the letters of her last name backwards. That is how she came to name the herbal tea "Essiac."

With the supervision of some doctors who supported her work, she was able to leave the hospital and start up her own cancer clinic in Bracebridge, Canada. She was 33 years old at the time. From 1934 to 1942, Rene Caisse treated thousands of cancer patients who had no other hope. Though she never claimed her treatment was a cure, it turned out to be just that for many people. Caisse's own mother developed liver cancer at one point and Rene put her on Essiac. Her mother recovered and went on to live another 18 years.

Most people who tried Essiac came to it as a last resort. Because so many of these people were in very late stages or had already sustained damage to their vital organs, not everyone was able to fully recover. For many, Essiac was only able to "control" the cancer, and for still others it was successful only at alleviating pain. But literally thousands of people reported complete cures from their cancer. Nurse Caisse never required payment for administration of her cancer therapy. She did, however, accept donations from anyone who could afford to give them, and her clinic was supported by these donations alone.

According to Dr. Gary Glum, an expert on Essiac who wrote the book *Calling of an Angel*, the Royal Cancer Commission of Canada held hearings in 1937 and came to the conclusion that Essiac *was* a cure for cancer.[1] Finally, the Canadian Ministry of Health and Welfare and the Canadian Parliament became involved. Around 1938, grateful former patients and friends of Rene Caisse petitioned the Parliament to give Caisse the legal right to administer her remedy to anyone who asked for it. The petition was submitted to the Parliament of Ontario with an incredible 55,000 signatures on it. This action initiated a bill in the Ontario Parliament. If passed, the bill would allow Rene Caisse to legally treat cancer patients without the constant threat of arrest. It would also give credibility to Essiac as a recognized treatment for terminally ill cancer patients. Unfortunately, this unprecedented measure fell just three votes short of being passed, and Essiac was not given the legitimacy it deserved.

Charles A. Brusch, M.D., was a well-known and highly esteemed doctor in the United States who had been the personal physician to John F. Kennedy. Dr. Brusch heard about Essiac and became very interested in it. Between 1959 and 1962, Dr. Brusch worked closely with Rene Caisse and together they treated thousands of cancer patients out of Brusch's clinic in Massachusetts. Dr. Brusch spent about 10 years studying Essiac in depth and using it clinically. After these 10 years, he concluded that "Essiac is a cure for cancer, period. All studies done at laboratories in the United States and Canada support this conclusion."[2] He even developed cancer himself and used Essiac to bring about his own complete recovery.

According to Dr. Glum, the Memorial Sloan-Kettering Cancer Center in New York also studied Essiac. However, some sources state that Rene Caisse was very protective of her formula and would not reveal all of the ingredients or methods of preparing it. These sources state that Caisse only allowed Memorial Sloan-Kettering to study one of the herbal ingredients—the sheep's sorrel. Dr. Glum states that Dr. Chester Stock at MSK did the research and discovered that the sheep's sorrel did have powerful anti-cancer properties. Glum also claims that this information was *withheld* from the American public, but was given to the Canadian Ministry of Health and Welfare. After receiving this information, rather than supporting the use of Essiac for cancer, the Canadian government immediately *banned* the sale and distribution of the sheep sorrel herb.[3]

(It is not banned in the United States or other countries, however.) One can only guess at their reasons for doing this.

During the 1960s and 1970s, Rene Caisse tried to get various pharmaceutical companies interested in producing her formula for widespread use. The only stipulation she gave them was "that Essiac be put to immediate use with cancer patients."[4] But Caisse would not give her formula to the pharmaceutical companies for testing unless they signed the agreement she requested, and without being able to test the formula first, the pharmaceutical companies would not sign the agreement.

Finally, in 1977, just before her death, Rene Caisse sold her formula to the Resperin Corporation of Toronto for a dollar. She also reportedly gave her formula to two of her friends, Mary Macpherson and Gilbert Blondin.

Rene Caisse had treated cancer patients with Essiac for almost 60 years before she died in 1978 at the age of 90. Immediately after her death, the Canadian Ministry of Health and Welfare went to her house and destroyed all of her paperwork on the Essiac formula. They burned her records in 55-gallon drums behind her house. Again, one can only guess at their reasons for doing this.

The Resperin Corporation took years to run tests on Essiac, and people in Canada could then only obtain Essiac by having a doctor's note saying they had terminal cancer and needed Essiac on an emergency basis. Eventually, however, Resperin Corporation produced the Essiac formula for widespread use. This version of it is now sold commercially out of many health food stores as well as from many sites on the Internet. Resperin's Essiac comes in dry powdered form in a box with instructions on how to brew it up as a tea at home.

But because of the delay by Resperin Corporation to market Caisse's herbal tea, another form of Essiac began to develop for commercial sale in the 1980s. This version of Essiac was backed by Dr. Brusch and was based on his clinical work with Caisse and her herbal remedy. It came to be called "Flor-Essence."

The development of Flor-Essence started out with a radio talk show host in Canada named Elaine Alexander. Alexander had become interested in Essiac and had already interviewed many people who testified to her that they had recovered from their cancer using Essiac alone. In 1984, she phoned Dr. Brusch and told him she was interested in doing a series of radio shows about Essiac and told him she would like to interview him "on the air." He agreed to do this and the first radio interview lasted two hours.

In that first radio show, Dr. Brusch told the public in no uncertain terms that Essiac was, indeed, a cure for cancer. The response from the public was unlike anything Alexander had ever seen in her 20 years in radio. All the phone lines into the station were jammed for hours with people calling in. Before the first show was over, several people had even driven to the radio station and were waiting outside in the hopes that they could get their questions answered!

Elaine did more on air interviews with Brusch and had terminal cancer patients who had been cured by Essiac as guests as well. Her radio shows on Essiac became a phenomenon and she was soon overwhelmed with people needing her help as to what they could do and how they could get Essiac. Some cancer patients got her address and began camping out at her house to get advice and help.

For several years, Alexander and Dr. Brusch did their best to help the people with cancer who were coming to them. Finally, in 1988, Alexander proposed to Dr. Brusch that the two of them become partners and produce their own Essiac product. They both agreed at this point that it would be best to circumvent the medical establishment, which up to this point was not responding to Essiac in any helpful way. They decided to drop the Essiac name because it was too closely associated with "a cure for cancer," and thus too controversial, and they decided to simply sell it as an herbal detoxifying tea.

Brusch and Alexander looked for a manufacturing company that could meet the standards required for producing a high-quality herbal preparation, and they settled on a company called Flora in British Columbia, Canada. The herbal tea was produced and sold in bottled liquid form, and named "Flor-Essence." Flor-Essence can be bought today at many health food stores as well as over the Internet.

Currently there are two main versions of the Essiac herbal tea being marketed. One is Essiac from Resperin Corporation, and the other is Flor-Essence from the Flora company. Besides these two, there are countless smaller herbal companies and private herbalists that produce and sell Essiac herbs to be brewed into tea at home. They all seem to have curative effects. Although the various forms of Essiac have never been fully accepted as formal cancer treatments, they are still being used by many people to help them recover from cancer. Right now, this herbal formula is used in some form in every state of the United States, Canada, Mexico, Australia, Europe, Asia, and Africa.

There is still some controversy, however, as to the details of the original formula Rene Caisse used. The Resperin Corporation claims they have the *true* original formula containing just four herbs. Dr. Charles Brusch and Elaine Alexander, however, assert that Brusch was given the *true* original formula from Rene Caisse and that it contained the four herbs Resperin uses, but also contains four additional herbs: blessed thistle, red clover, watercress, and kelp. These herbs are added to their bottled version of Essiac called Flor-Essence.

It seems impossible at this time to know who has the original formula Rene Caisse used on so many thousands of patients. Other sources of Essiac are sometimes referred to as "Ojibwa Tea," "Ojibwa Tea of Life," or "4-Herb Tea."

It is difficult to know which form of Essiac tea is best to recommend. I have read about and heard of some people with cancer getting well through the use of pretty much all the versions available. However, I have also heard of people for whom Essiac was not powerful enough to achieve full recovery from. One experienced herbalist told me that the quality of the herbs used is critical. There may be a big difference between the potency of herbs picked from good "wild" soil as opposed to chemically fertilized soil. And exactly how and when the herbs are picked and brewed is possibly even more important. Many factors seem to contribute to how potent or effective any herbal treatment will be. Also, Rene Caisse *injected* the sheep sorrel into her patients and none of the herbal remedies today use that approach.

There can be no debate that herbal remedies such as the Hoxsey therapy and Essiac have, historically, been extremely powerful anti-cancer treatments. In today's modern world, there are still people getting well from cancer using these herbal treatments. Finding herbal sources today that use good quality herbs and prepare the herbs optimally is the biggest concern. Since it is difficult to be sure of the efficacy of any particular version of Essiac, it might be best to use it *in conjunction* with another recovery approach with which Essiac tea is compatible. The only approach I know of that is definitely *not* compatible with Essiac, is Protocel®. But for all other alternative cancer approaches, Essiac tea can be of great supportive value. Many people even claim that the side effects of chemotherapy are greatly reduced when Essiac tea is used at the same time.

Resources:

Books

Richard Thomas. *The Essiac Report.* Los Angeles: ATIN, 1993.

Dr. Gary L. Glum. *Calling of an Angel.* Los Angeles: Silent Walker Publishing, 1988.

Sheila Snow and Mali Klein. *Essiac Essentials: The Remarkable Herbal Cancer Fighter.* New York: Kensington Books, 1999.

Cynthia Olsen. Essiac: *A Native Herbal Cancer Remedy.* Pagosa Springs, Colorado: Kali Press, 1996.

James Percival. *The Essiac Handbook.*

Websites

www.herbalhealer.com (Order 4-Herb Tea)

www.Essiac-resperin.com/en/history.html (Order Resperin's Essiac)

www.Essiacinfo.org

www.billybest.net

www.cancer-solutions.net/Homepage.html (Order Dr. Glum's book from this site, or read it for free online.)

www.ojibwatea.com (Order Ojibwa Tea)

5

The Gerson Therapy

While the Hoxsey therapy and Essiac are two of the best-known herbal approaches to cancer recovery, the Gerson Method is perhaps the best-known nutritional diet-oriented approach. Widely used since the 1940s, it is a natural, holistic approach with a long track record. It is also the method that started the trend of avid carrot juicing and coffee enemas so many people have heard about. Over the past 60 years, thousands of cancer patients have benefited from, or completely recovered, using this method. And many cases of other serious health conditions such as tuberculosis, adult-onset diabetes, lupus, and heart disease have been cured as well with the Gerson approach.

History

The founder of this famous approach was Max Gerson, M.D., a German physician of high acclaim who emigrated to the United States in 1936 and set up a medical practice in New York. But the history of his treatment started in Germany. Dr. Gerson had set up his first medical practice in Germany in 1919 and developed an effective dietary method for treating his own migraine headaches that had plagued him for years. In 1920, he began to treat other patients with migraines and, in the process, discovered that his dietary technique was also able to cure the dreaded disease lupus vulgaris. Lupus is a disfiguring type of tuberculosis of the skin that was considered incurable at the time, and Dr. Gerson was the first physician in Europe to bring about total cures for people with this disease.

After moving to the U.S., Dr. Gerson also successfully treated the famous humanitarian and Nobel Prize-winning physician, Albert Schweitzer, M.D. Dr. Schweitzer had been forced to retire from his beloved work because of adult-onset diabetes. Using a strict dietary regimen, Dr. Gerson was able to get Schweitzer off all insulin in just one month. With his health restored, Dr. Schweitzer was then able to go back to the humanitarian medical work he loved in Africa, which he continued into his eighties. Schweitzer credited his ability to keep working to Dr. Gerson and once said, "I see in him one of the most eminent medical geniuses in the history of medicine."[1]

But, most importantly, Dr. Gerson dared to treat advanced cancer patients for whom expert cancer treatment of that day was not working. One aspect of his treatment involved having his patients drink hourly glasses of freshly prepared fruit and vegetable juices. His reasoning was that these juices would supply abundant oxidative enzymes and a potassium-rich array of minerals to aid in the re-balancing and rejuvenation of the body. He began seeing success with his dietary protocols, but also began observing that some cancer patients did not have a healthy enough liver to handle the detoxification process required to recover from their cancer. So, he began to prescribe coffee enemas to help stimulate the liver functioning of his patients.

Contrary to what may be popular belief, the main purpose of coffee enemas is *not* to cleanse the colon. Dr. Gerson understood that coffee enemas were actually a way to cleanse and heal the liver. The way the coffee enema detoxifies the liver is that when this type of enema is taken into and held in the intestines for about 15 minutes, the caffeine and other chemicals in the coffee go directly through the intestinal wall and surrounding blood vessels into the liver. These substances then stimulate the clogged bile ducts of the liver and cause them to dilate and release their buildup of toxic material.

There is also evidence that these stimulating substances affect the gallbladder and cause its bile ducts to dilate and release toxins as well. Cleansing the liver and gallbladder so they can function more efficiently is important to the process of recovering from many conditions, and cancer in particular. Dr. Gerson also found that an unexpected but welcome side effect of coffee enemas was that they were often able to quickly relieve or reduce pain. One company developed a special form of coffee to be particularly good for use in coffee enemas. Called S.A. Wilson's Therapy Blend Coffee, it has been cultivated for higher levels of caffeine and palmitic acid than commercial coffee brands. To order or find out more about this type of coffee and coffee enemas, go to www.sawilsons. com. (They can also be reached by calling 866/266-4066.)

Another way Dr. Gerson began stimulating his patients' livers was by giving them liver extract injections. Dr. Gerson theorized that a combination of toxins and nutritional imbalances was at the heart of cancer, and he was the first practitioner to focus on the liver as a key organ in cancer recovery. His innovative work also focused on some very important electrolyte imbalances within the cells such as the potassium-sodium balance. To restore this type of balance, Dr. Gerson required his patients to stay strictly away from *all* table salt or salt added to foods and would also supplement his patients with extra potassium. Added to this regimen were other supplements as well, including vitamin C, digestive enzymes, niacin, a particular type of iodine, and relatively high doses of thyroid extract.

Besides nutritional supplementation, Dr. Gerson required his patients to go through rigorous changes in their diet. Besides staying away from all added salt, they had to severely restrict their intake of fat and animal protein. Gerson felt that low protein intake increased T-lymphocyte activity and promoted the release of sodium from cells. Patients had to eat primarily organic foods and prepare about a dozen fresh juices each day. They were also required to perform numerous coffee enemas every day.

Dr. Gerson was one of the first medical experts to understand, even back in the 1930s, that people's diets were nutritionally deficient and pollutants in the environment were causing toxic buildup in their bodies. He may have been the first to point out that the foods of the day were being grown in soil that has been damaged (e.g., by overcropping and chemical fertilizers) thereby causing imbalances of minerals in the foods themselves. And he pointed out the deleterious effects of commercially refined foods. He was known to have said, "Stay close to nature and its eternal laws will protect you."[2]

Dr. Gerson's focus on unprocessed foods and nutritional balance was virtually unheard of in the 1930s and 1940s since nutritional science had not become fully developed or accepted yet. In 1936, his innovative ideas for treating serious illnesses with nutrition were *not* enthusiastically received. Although Dr. Gerson cured desperate cancer patients at an amazing rate in his New York treatment center, he was shunned and ridiculed by America's mainstream medical establishment. This was at a time when the all-powerful American Medical Association was labeling the idea that diet and nutrition can affect cancer as a "false notion."

Dr. Gerson's ideas were proven to be right, however, by the incredible successes he was able to achieve with advanced diseases. In fact, he soon became known as someone who could cure "incurables," and many desperate people flocked to his clinic in New York. But Dr. Gerson's impeccable credentials as a top-notch physician and incredible record of success with cancer patients were not enough to keep him from being persecuted and harassed for his unorthodox treatment. He was treated as a quack and eventually expelled from the New York Medical Society.

In 1958, S. J. Haught, a New York newspaper reporter, received a letter from a woman who had been given two to six months to live by her cancer specialists, but had been later cured of her advanced cancer by Dr. Gerson. This reporter then decided to look into the doctor who was being called a quack by the accepted cancer authorities. Haught was told by the AMA that Dr. Gerson "had failed or refused to acquaint the medical profession with the details of his treatment."[3]

Haught found out through his journalistic research, however, that the AMA's claim was completely untrue. Dr. Gerson had been anything but reluctant to reveal his methods. In fact, Gerson had published 50 medical papers and three books, including the very detailed book, *A Cancer Therapy*, in which he described his cancer treatment methods in depth. Haught learned that many of Dr. Gerson's scientific papers had been *rejected* by leading medical journals for no reason. Thus, his medical discoveries for treating cancer had been actively blocked from exposure to other doctors.

Haught found out that the Medical Society of the County of New York had already investigated Gerson's treatment center five times, where they had examined patients, looked at X-rays, and explored other aspects of Gerson's clinic and cancer treatment. According to Haught, the findings of this Medical Society investigation were never published or otherwise made available to the public. When Haught requested that the Society's findings on Gerson's treatment be released, his request was refused. Even though Dr. Gerson tried to get his treatment officially evaluated, the medical establishment did not want to do this.

Besides having great successes with "incurable" cancer patients, Dr. Gerson was also very outspoken against the tobacco industry. This did not put him in good stead with the AMA when their biggest source of advertising revenue from the *Journal of the American Medical Association* came from the Philip Morris cigarette company! As we learned with the Hoxsey therapy, the AMA had a very powerful influence in the 1940s and 1950s over what was accepted by the medical community and what was not.

In 1946, Gerson testified in a U.S. Senate hearing in support of a proposed bill to Congress that would authorize the president to "wage war on cancer."[4] It was the first bill of its kind and if passed, would appropriate $100 million to coordinate research and collaboration by the world's top cancer experts to find a way to prevent and/or cure cancer. Senator Claude Pepper was head of the sub-committee for hearings related to this bill. Dr. Gerson was only one of the experts to testify before this sub-committee, which would go down in history as the "Pepper Commission." Dr. Gerson spent three days presenting documented evidence of recoveries he had achieved in patients who were unable to recover from treatments given by leading cancer clinics and hospitals.

Another expert who testified was George Miley, M.D., the medical director of a hospital where Dr. Gerson had treated many patients. Dr. Miley not only strongly supported Gerson's approach and testimony, he also presented a disturbing study to the sub-committee. According to Dr. Miley, a long-term survey by a well-respected physician had shown that cancer patients who received *no* conventional treatment at all actually survived *longer* than patients who were treated with surgery, radiation, or X-ray![5] James P. Carter, M.D., author of *Racketeering in Medicine: The Suppression of Alternatives*, wrote that this senate bill was ultimately defeated by intense congressional lobbying paid for by big business groups that had interests in the multi-million dollar industries of surgery, radiation, and chemotherapy.[6] Tragically, the bill that could have directed unprecedented funding toward research into other than "established" cancer treatments was defeated by only four votes.

It was just a few months after Dr. Gerson's senate testimony that Morris Fishbein began to attack and ridicule Gerson and his cancer treatment approach. Fishbein used the *Journal of the American Medical Association* as his vehicle. In his book, *Racketeering in Medicine*, Dr. Carter explains that Dr. Gerson was subjected at this point to:

> ... systematic harassment on the part of the New York State Medical Society and the New York State Licensing Board. Dr. Gerson's publications were blacklisted, and none of the reputable journals would accept them. His hospital privileges at Gotham Hospital in New York City

were revoked after his impressive demonstration of success before the Pepper Sub-committee in 1946. . . . The campaign to discredit him was likely coordinated by individuals in the AMA.[7]

But Dr. Gerson did not give up. In the early 1950s, he submitted five case histories of cancer recoveries to the National Cancer Institute and requested that an official investigation into his approach be carried out. The NCI's response was to tell Dr. Gerson it would need 25 case histories instead of just five. Dr. Gerson promptly supplied them with the requested 25 along with complete documentation. Then, after more than a year later, the NCI responded again to Dr. Gerson saying that 25 case histories would not be enough to justify an investigation, and they would need 125.[8] It appears that the NCI believed it had time and power on its side and could afford to play a cat-and-mouse game. The Gerson therapy was never fairly evaluated.

Even though Dr. Gerson was not able to see his effective cancer treatment accepted by mainstream medicine, he tirelessly continued to treat patients until his death in 1959. His cancer therapy is still being offered today at a facility in San Diego called the Gerson Institute. This nonprofit organization is run by Gerson's daughter, Charlotte Gerson. Charlotte Gerson is extremely knowledgeable and experienced in her father's treatment approach, and cancer patients flock from different parts of the world to her facility.

An overview of the Gerson method highlights two basic aspects of the treatment: (1) cleansing the body (primarily with coffee enemas), and (2) flooding it with rejuvenating nutrients, primarily from fresh organic juices. But the details of the Gerson therapy are a lot more complex than that and require careful attention in order for the treatment to be successful. A brief description of the approach is listed below, however to understand it fully one should read the books by Dr. Max Gerson or Charlotte Gerson. And the Gerson Institute highly recommends that for best results patients start treatment at either the Institute in San Diego or at another licensed treatment center. It is common for patients to spend three weeks at the Gerson Institute to ensure that they understand the full extent of the therapy, as well as to receive unique instructions for their own case, before going home and continuing it on their own.

A Brief Overview of the Current Standard Gerson Therapy

- *Thirteen fresh juices a day* from organically grown vegetables and fruits. This is to flood the body with healing nutrients and live enzymes, which help balance, detoxify, and heal all bodily systems.

- *About five coffee enemas each day.* This is primarily to heal the liver.

- *Very strict diet.* This includes, among other restrictions: no salt, no sugar, and little fat or meat.

- *Nutritional supplementation.* This includes, among other things: potassium (liquid compound solution), potassium iodide (Lugol's solution), vitamin C, digestive enzymes, thyroid, flaxseed oil, niacin, liver/B_{12} injections, CoQ_{10}, brewer's yeast, and castor oil (both orally and rectally). The Gerson Institute now also recommends Laetrile supplementation for some cases. (Laetrile will be discussed in the next chapter.)

The Gerson approach is not an easy one to do. Some people have had to hire help in order to carry out all aspects of the program required. Juicing fresh fruits and vegetables 13 times a day in itself is a full-time job. In fact, the Gerson therapy might be the most difficult alternative cancer approach available, and even the Gerson Institute does not recommend it to those who do not think they can follow the program carefully and completely. This is one reason attending the Gerson Institute in San Diego as an in-patient first is a good idea. There, patients can learn how to correctly carry out the protocol while 13 juices each day are conveniently made for them. And initial supervision is especially recommended by the Gerson Institute for those who have already been through chemotherapy or have diabetes, brain metastases, severe kidney damage, or foreign bodies such as pacemakers, breast implants, steel plates, or screws.

Dr. Max Gerson had a broad impact on the field of non-toxic cancer treatments. Because he was the first pioneer to create a widely successful nutritional approach, many of Gerson's protocols have been incorporated into other alternative methods over the years, especially the concepts of daily fresh juices, coffee enemas, enzymes, and mineral supplementation. Many people with cancer are still achieving recoveries using his approach. It is a rigorous method to follow, but for those who are able to do it successfully, the reward is great.

Resources:

The Gerson Institute   (888) 443-7766 or (619) 685-5353
3844 Adams Ave.   www.gerson.org
San Diego, CA 92116

S.A. Wilson's Therapy Blend Coffee
Bowmanville, Ontario, Canada
www.sawilsons.com
(866) 266-4066 or (905) 263-2344

Treatment at the Gerson Institute: Treatment generally involves first being an in-house patient for either one week, two weeks, three weeks, or four weeks at the cost of approximately $5,000 per week. For most people, a minimum of three weeks is recommended. The initial in-house stay is to learn the protocol. The Institute also offers a Gerson Therapy Home Package, which gives you the information needed to undertake the treatment protocol on your own, and can refer patients to clinics in other locations that are licensed to provide this therapy.

Books

S. J. Haught. *Censured for Curing Cancer: The American Experience of Dr. Max Gerson*. San Diego: The Gerson Institute, 1991.

Max Gerson, M.D. *A Cancer Therapy: Results of Fifty Cases*. San Diego: The Gerson Institute, 1958/1999.

Charlotte Gerson and Morton Walker, D.P.M. *The Gerson Therapy*. New York: Kensington Publishing, 2001.

Richard Walters. *Options: The Alternative Cancer Therapy Book*. New York: Avery Penguin Putnam, 1993.

James P. Carter, M.D. *Racketeering in Medicine: The Suppression of Alternatives*. Hampton Roads, 1993.

Ross Pelton and Lee Overholser. *Alternatives in Cancer Therapy*. New York: Simon and Schuster, 1994.

6

Laetrile

With the Gerson therapy being considered the first widely used nutritional approach to cancer, the use of Laetrile should probably be considered the second. Most of us have heard about Laetrile, but unfortunately, the public in general was given the impression that it was some kind of "bogus" or "fad" cancer treatment that fizzled out a few decades ago. Anyone looking into the true history of Laetrile, however, will find the reality to be just the opposite. Laetrile is a concentrated and purified version of B_{17}—a vitamin that tends to be high in the diets of those people around the world who rarely get cancer—and, when used correctly it proved to be the most effective cancer treatment that numerous rigorous scientists and physicians around the world had ever seen. In this chapter, you will find out how this purified version of B_{17} has been used therapeutically to help countless people overcome their cancers.

History

Laetrile treatments were promoted under the "Nutritional Deficiency Theory of Cancer," which was the first theory about cancer development to focus on a specific dietary nutritional deficiency. The specific nutrient, vitamin B_{17}, is a natural vitamin found in hundreds of foods commonly eaten by humans. These foods include lima beans, bean sprouts, most berries, yams, many seeds, cashews, macadamia nuts, millet, and buckwheat, to name just a few. In its natural state, vitamin B_{17} is also known as "amygdalin" and is part of a family of natural compounds called "nitrilosides." Almost all wild fruits and most seeds have some form of nitriloside in them.

The connection between vitamin B_{17} deficiency and cancer was first discovered by Dr. Ernst T. Krebs, Sr., a prominent physician and medical researcher. Dr. Krebs took an early interest in cancer. Soon his son, Dr. Ernst T. Krebs, Jr., who had specialized as a biochemist, joined his father in this research. By 1952, the father and son team had discovered a definite connection between vitamin B_{17} and cancer, and had developed the theory that cancer was, at least in part, a result of nutritional deficiency.

This unusual vitamin actually works like a tiny "smart bomb." On a molecular level, vitamin B_{17} is composed of four units: two units of glucose, one unit of benzaldehyde, and one unit of cyanide. The cyanide unit is tightly locked together with the other three units so that its toxic characteristics are completely inert under most circumstances. What the two doctors discovered is that there is only one situation in the human body that can cause the cyanide in vitamin B_{17} to be *unlocked* and released as a toxic substance. That situation occurs when the B_{17} molecule comes in contact with an enzyme called "beta-glucosidase." If this happens, then the unit of cyanide is released and is toxic, and the unit of benzaldehyde in the B_{17} is also released and is toxic. Moreover, these two substances working together are about a hundred times more toxic than either one is by itself!

Amazingly, it just so happens that the cyanide-unlocking enzyme, beta-glucosidase, *only* occurs to any significant degree in just one place in the body. It is only significantly present in cancer cells. Thus the toxic cyanide and benzaldehyde are released from vitamin B_{17} in the body *only when the vitamin comes in contact with cancer cells*. Apparently, nature has provided us with an ingenious defense against cancer—and it is a common dietary nutrient!

But that's not all. Nature even provided normal cells with a back-up *protecting* enzyme called "rhodanese." Rhodanese has the ability to neutralize cyanide on contact. In fact, rhodanese actually converts cyanide into other components that are beneficial to the body. By now, it should be no surprise to learn that the enzyme rhodanese is prevalent in great quantities throughout the body *except where there is cancer*. Thus, if any amount of cyanide from B_{17} does get unlocked near normal cells, the enzyme rhodanese will immediately detoxify the cyanide and convert it into non-toxic components.

Vitamin B_{17} is an all-natural, smart chemical bomb that fights cancer. And it is found in so many food sources that all we have to do is eat a varied healthy diet consisting primarily of fruits, vegetables, grains, nuts, and seeds to get plenty of it. G. Edward Griffin wrote *World Without Cancer*, the most comprehensive book about B_{17} and Laetrile. In it, he points out that the groups of people around the world who regularly ingest high amounts of B_{17} from their diets are the same groups that show extremely low incidences of cancer.

One of these groups of people are the "Hunzakuts," or "Hunza," people of the Himalayas. The Hunza people have become very famous over the years because they are some of the longest-lived people in the world. It is quite common for a Hunzakut to live to be over 100 years old, and not too uncommon for them to live to the age of 120. And this longevity goes along with a very high quality of health and vitality. Cancer, in particular, was unknown to the Hunzakuts before being introduced to modern civilization. Because of their unusual good health and long life, scientists from around the world have studied their habits and diet in great detail.

There are many healthy aspects of the Hunzakut lifestyle and diet, including clean glacial water, fresh air, fresh vegetables and fruits, and so forth, so it would be wrong to attribute their good health *solely* to just one thing. However, a very interesting fact is that the Hunzakut diet has historically been high in vitamin B_{17}—possibly the highest in B_{17} of any human diet in the world. This is because apricot trees have always been the Hunza's main crop, and traditionally, the wealth of a Hunzakut man was measured by how many apricot trees he had. And the *most* prized food of all in their culture is the soft inner pit, or seed, of the apricot, which they dry in the sun and eat as a significant part of their diet. It just so happens that dried apricot seeds are one of the highest sources of B_{17} found on earth.

Apricot seeds are like little almonds, and though quite bitter, it would be common, Griffin says, for a Hunzakut to eat 30 to 50 of them daily as a mid-afternoon snack. It has been estimated that, largely because of their apricot seed ingestion, the traditional Hunza diet may have had at least 200 times the amount of B_{17} as the average American diet. Thus, it is no wonder they never experienced cancer.

Evidence that the Hunzakuts are not just genetically wired to resist cancer has been shown by the fact that many Hunzakuts who partake in the lifestyles and eating habits of western industrialized countries often fall prey to degenerative diseases, including cancer.

Another group of people found to be traditionally free from cancer are the Eskimos. At first reflection, this seems unlikely since one would think that an Eskimo's diet would be very poor in fresh vegetables, fruits, or seeds. The secret lies in the fact that the traditional Eskimo diet is very high in meat from caribou, reindeer, and other grazing animals. Grasses around the world are typically very good sources of B_{17}, and the fresh arctic tundra grasses are even higher than most grasses in their B_{17} content. This means that the meat from the arctic grazing animals is itself very high in vitamin B_{17}. There are also certain berries in the arctic summertime that are rich in B_{17}, which the Eskimos would eat large amounts of during the spring and summer. Thus the Eskimo diet has traditionally been *extremely* rich in vitamin B_{17}. And like the Hunzas, whenever Eskimos take on modern diets, they too succumb to degenerative diseases, including cancer.

Researchers over the years have shown similar correlations between diets high in B_{17} and a low incidence of cancer among other native populations of the world as well. These include many of the native North American tribes and native peoples of South America and Africa. One very rich source of B_{17} in the tropics, for instance, is the native cassava fruit. Cassava is such a staple of many southern indigenous diets that it has been called the "bread of the tropics." It also provides protection for these people against cancer.

Philip E. Binzel, M.D., an American physician who specialized in fighting cancer with nutrition, made an interesting point in his book, *Alive and Well*. He stated that millet used to be a common staple grain for humans. Millet is one of the few grains that is very high in vitamin B_{17}. Nowadays, the most common grain people eat is wheat, and wheat has very little or no B_{17} content.

Interestingly, Dr. Krebs, Sr., has stated that in the Old Testament of the Bible there is a specification for how to prepare grains to be used in the making of bread. The formula is presented in Ezekiel 4:9 and discusses six ingredients. Five of these ingredients are rich in nitriloside content and are barley, beans, lentils, millet, and chickpeas (garbanzo beans).[1]

In *Alive and Well*, Dr. Binzel also makes the point that human beings the world over have traditionally eaten meat from animals that grazed on natural grasses, and thus the meat was almost always high in B_{17}. Today, we eat meat from animals that are primarily grain fed. Unfortunately, the type of grain most commonly used has no B_{17} content. Thus, we in modernized countries today are not only eating grains that have no B_{17} content, but we are also eating meat that in the past would have naturally supplied us with B_{17}, but now is virtually devoid of this important cancer-fighting nutrient.

Although B_{17} may be one of the most important single nutrients used by the body to fight cancer, research has shown that the mineral zinc is an important transportation mechanism for B_{17}. In other words, without zinc, dietary B_{17} does not get into the tissues of the body. Dr. Binzel states that research has also proven vitamin C, vitamin A, manganese, magnesium, and selenium are all important nutritional factors for the health of the immune system in general. Thus, many factors in the total diet of humans can be critically interlinked to support the immune system and the body's natural cancer-fighting "control mechanisms."

For their research purposes, the Krebses were able to produce a purified, synthesized version of B_{17}, and they called this "Laetrile." The Krebses were able to get Laetrile introduced into widespread experimentation in numerous laboratories around the country. In the 1950s and 1960s, countless studies on animals showed Laetrile to be a perfectly safe substance *and* effective in treating various forms of cancer. After seeing the promising laboratory results, a number of physicians decided to see if it could help their human cancer patients as well. G. Edward Griffin reported in *World Without Cancer* that "As early as 1974, there were at least twenty-six published papers written by well-known physicians who had used Laetrile in the treatment of their own patients and had concluded that Laetrile is both safe and effective in the treatment of cancer."[2]

Drs. Nieper, Navarro, and Contreras

Laetrile for cancer was not just studied in the United States, it was studied and used around the world. Hans Nieper, M.D., of Germany, Ernesto Contreras, M.D., of Mexico, and Manuel Navarro, M.D., of the Philippines were three of the early prominent practitioners and researchers of Laetrile. They were some of the first physicians to pioneer what at that time was called "nutritional therapy" for cancer. Like Dr. Gerson, these practitioners were considered *unconventional* because they looked at cancer tumors as merely the symptom of the disease at a time when conventional doctors were treating tumors with surgery, radiation, and/ or chemotherapy as if the tumor *was* the disease itself.

All three of these internationally famous physicians were dedicated to the development of this new type of treatment and to the publication of their findings. And all three achieved *astounding* results, which other physicians began to read about and duplicate as well.

Dr. Binzel

As already mentioned, Philip E. Binzel, Jr., M.D., was one of the American physicians who, in 1973, found out about the work done by Nieper, Navarro, and Contreras. He was so impressed that he started practicing nutritional therapy with his own cancer patients. After about 20 years of treating cancer with Laetrile, he wrote a book about his experiences using Laetrile along with other supportive nutritional therapies for cancer. (There were also other prominent American physicians who successfully treated cancer with Laetrile, such as John A. Richardson, M.D., of California and W. Douglas Brodie, M.D., of Nevada.)

No Laetrile practitioner ever claimed that the use of Laetrile alone was enough to cure cancer. In other words, it was never meant to be used alone like a drug. Although the use of high doses of intravenous Laetrile was key to the nutritional therapy approach to cancer, other nutritional supplements, enzymes and diet changes were also part of the program. Then, after patients were done with the intensive part of their treatment involving intravenous Laetrile, they were instructed to continue at home indefinitely with certain diet restrictions and generally continued taking Laetrile supplements.

With Laetrile, supplements, and diet changes, an uncommon number of cancer patients became cancer-free and remained cancer-free until their death from other causes. And this treatment, like most alternative cancer approaches, was not restricted to just certain types of cancer—it was effective for all types. For example, following are three cases from Dr. Binzel's book, *Alive and Well*:

Case No. 1: Polly Todd

This 59-year-old woman was seen by me for the first time on 1/10/75 with the history that she had her left breast removed one month previously because of carcinoma. Three positive nodes had been found. I will let the patient tell you the rest of her history in her own words:

"It was recommended by a prominent physician that I be a part of an experiment in a (then) new chemotherapy program. For a second opinion I went to another city where I had a personal contact with the head of a large hospital. There they told me that my odds of survival were slim, and that I should be treated with strong doses of chemotherapy and radiation. At this point, a friend told me about the Laetrile-nutritional program, which I chose."

The lady was placed on a nutritional program at that time and she has remained on it ever since. She is now 79 years old, in good health, and she has had no recurrence of her disease.

In a recent letter the patient said, "None of the above people on the chemotherapy program lived beyond 1½ years. Friends who scoffed at our choice then have much more respect now because others choosing the conventional treatment are gone, while I survive!"[3]

Case No. 9: Rex Perry

This 42-year-old man that I first saw on 6/27/79 with a history of having malignant lymphoma, which was originally diagnosed in August 1978. He had 8 months of chemotherapy, which he tolerated very well. His doctors felt, however, that there was a significant amount of disease still present. They wanted to do several more months of chemotherapy and follow this with total body radiation. The patient did not want to do this because of his concern about what it would do to his immune system. He chose, instead, to use the nutritional approach.

It has now been almost 15 years since he started his nutritional therapy. The most satisfying part of such a case history is that this patient has had no further problem with his disease. He is well and very active.[4]

Case No. 18: B. W.

This 44-year-old woman was seen for the first time on 2/6/81. She had been found one month prior to have carcinoma of the descending colon with 7 positive lymph nodes. A colostomy was not required. She received no radiation or chemotherapy.

She was started on a nutritional program. Now, some 13 years later, she has had no recurrence of her disease and leads a normal, active life.

What is so unusual about this patient? She had cancer of the colon with metastases. The odds of her surviving 5 years were one in one-thousand. Yet, she lives a normal life with no recurrence of her disease after 13 years.[5]

After many years of working with cancer patients using Laetrile (nutritional therapy), Dr. Binzel analyzed the success of his treatment. He separated all of the patients he had treated into two groups, those with primary cancer, and those with metastatic cancer. In the primary cancer group, there were 180 patients with 30 different types of cancer. After 18 years, 87.3 percent of these patients *did not die* of their cancer. When he subtracted the seven patients who died of unknown causes to conservatively concede they *may* have died from cancer, he still showed an amazing 83.3 percent long-term recovery![6]

According to Dr. Binzel at the time he published the above results, the American Cancer Society was officially claiming that with conventional treatment involving *early detection* and treatment of primary cancer that *had not yet metastasized*, ". . . eighty-five percent of the patients *will die* from their disease within five years."[7] Thus, nutritional therapy using Laetrile was clinically shown to be *by far* more effective than conventional cancer treatments.

Successful treatment of metastatic cancer is always more difficult to achieve because of the damage already done to the body, but even Dr. Binzel's rate of recovery for the metastatic group was impressive when compared to conventional treatment methods. His group of metastasized cancer patients consisted of 108 patients treated with nutritional therapy. After 18 years, 70.4 percent did *not* die from their cancer, and when he conservatively subtracted the 9 patients who had died of unknown causes, he still had a whopping 62.1 percent who did not die from their cancer in 18 years! This is truly incredible when compared to the American Cancer Society's official statistics on modern conventional cancer treatment. Recent ACS statistics show that *only 0.1 percent (or only one person out of every thousand) of patients with metastasized cancer who are treated with conventional treatments will survive five years.*[8]

Thus, Dr. Binzel could keep an average of 62 patients out of every 100 with metastasized cancer alive for a minimum of 18 years, while the conventional doctors could only keep about one in every 1,000 patients with metastasized cancer alive for five years. And Dr. Binzel's treatment success with nutritional therapy was similar to most of the other pioneering physicians using Laetrile, such as Dr. Hans Nieper, Dr. Ernesto Contreras, Dr. Manuel Navarro, and Dr. John A. Richardson. So his was not an isolated record.

But once again, the fight with the established cancer industry was a big one. Despite the fact that prominent physicians and researchers all around the world were showing positive results using Laetrile for cancer, the president of the American Cancer Society of California wrote a condemning article at the end of 1973, claiming that "Laetrile is goddamned quackery!"[9]

The Suppression

Unfortunately, nutritional therapy involving Laetrile was the recipient of one of the worst onslaughts of suppressive tactics ever used by the cancer establishment. These tactics involved outright harassment of physicians who administered it as well as intentional dissemination of disinformation (outright lies to the public as to its effectiveness). *Every* physician in the United States who attempted to help their patients with Laetrile was harassed by various agents of the cancer industry. This included physicians being arrested, hauled into court for no good reason, sometimes thrown in jail, and eventually having their medical licenses taken away. To go into the details of these physicians' ordeals would be beyond the scope of this book, but simply researching the history of any American practitioner of Laetrile will show this to be true.

The disinformation put out about Laetrile was focused around two general issues: (1) that Laetrile is too toxic for people to use because it contains cyanide; and (2) that it is simply not effective in treating cancer. The "toxic" argument is laughable. How can something be called toxic when it is ingested whenever a person eats lima beans, bean sprouts, almost any seed or nut, berries, millet, and other foods; when animals thrive on natural foods high in it; and when the healthiest people on earth eat diets extremely rich in it? Also, if it is so toxic, then why is vitamin B_{12} allowed to be sold as a health supplement? Most people don't know that vitamin B_{12} *also* contains the same type of cyanide molecule that is in vitamin B_{17}.

Moreover, according to G. Edward Griffin, "aspirin tablets are twenty times more toxic than the equivalent amount of Laetrile."[10] Yet aspirin is a highly touted and promoted product. Of course, when compared to the radiation and chemotherapy treatments that are routinely approved by the FDA, the subject of Laetrile being toxic moves into the realm of the absurd. Unlike most drugs that *may* have toxic side effects, when it comes to chemotherapy and radiation, toxicity *is the goal*. Chemotherapy and radiation treatments routinely involve toxicity that is simply off the scales, and many deaths have been documented as a *direct* result of these treatments. Apparently, the FDA and the cancer industry believe that the side effect of "death" is tolerable, as long as it comes from treatments they endorse!

As to the claim that Laetrile is simply *not effective*, this long ago moved out of the realm of the "absurd" and into the realm of the "criminal." Powerful people at Memorial Sloan-Kettering, the American Medical Association, the American Cancer Society, the National Cancer Institute, and even the FDA *lied* to the public and press about Laetrile. And they did it effectively enough to get Laetrile suppressed almost completely. For the most complete exposé of the suppression of Laetrile, there is no better source than the well-documented book *World Without Cancer* by G Edward Griffin. Let's look at some of the information presented by Griffin to get an idea of how the public has largely been denied an effective non-toxic cancer treatment.

According to Griffin, one of the first dramas of deception occurred at the Mayo Clinic around 1978. Studies on Laetrile there were *not* conducted according to the correct protocol given by the physicians who had been using it, and there have been serious doubts that the Laetrile used in the Mayo Clinic study was even of good quality or purity. As a result of their improperly done studies, the Mayo Clinic researchers concluded that they found no effectiveness of Laetrile on cancer. Many practitioners who had already witnessed great success using Laetrile on their own cancer patients believed that the Mayo Clinic clinical trials had been deliberately designed to fail.

The next drama, and possibly the most criminal story of deception, occurred at Memorial Sloan-Kettering Cancer Center in New York. Between the years 1972 and 1977, Laetrile had been tested on animals with cancer under the direction of one of the country's most respected scientists, Dr. Kanematsu Sugiura. Dr. Sugiura was Memorial Sloan-Kettering's senior laboratory researcher, and he found Laetrile to be *highly effective* against cancers of all types. Yet most medical professionals never knew about his findings because the higher-ups at Sloan-Kettering found ways to get around his results. According to Griffin,

> Dr. Kanematsu Sugiura . . . reported that, in his experiments with mice, Laetrile was more effective in the control of cancer than any substance he had ever tested. This was not acceptable to his superiors. Instead of being pleased at the possibility of a breakthrough, they brought in other researchers to duplicate Sugiura's experiments and to prove they were faulty. Instead, the follow-up studies confirmed Sugiura's. Undaunted, his superiors called for new experiments over and over again, following

procedures designed to make the tests fail. Eventually they did fail, and it was that failure that was announced to the world.[11]

Support for the above facts can also be found in Ralph W. Moss's book, *The Cancer Industry*. Ralph Moss was a Ph.D. science writer when he was hired to work at Memorial Sloan-Kettering Cancer Center in 1974, and he went on to become its assistant director of public affairs. He claims he was fired in 1977 for "opposing their cover-up of positive data on the drug Laetrile."[12] But Moss was not a writer to simply curl up his tail and run. He went on to write several books in which he presented in-depth exposés of the cancer industry's outright opposition to and suppression of non-toxic, alternative treatments.

Even though Memorial Sloan-Kettering claimed Laetrile was ineffective against cancer, other respected laboratories around the world came up with positive results in carefully controlled studies on mice. Some of these were Scind Laboratories of San Francisco in 1968, the Pasteur Institute of Paris in 1971, and the Institute von Ardenne of Dresden, Germany, in 1973.[13] There were also numerous prominent physicians around the world who found Laetrile to be effective with their human cancer patients. One of these physicians, Dr. Shigeaki Sakai of Tokyo, published an article in 1963 in the *Asian Medical Journal*, in which he stated:

> Administered to cancer patients, Laetrile has proven to be quite free from any harmful side effects, and I would say that no anti-cancer drug could make a cancerous patient improve faster than Laetrile. It goes without saying that Laetrile controls cancer and is quite effective wherever it is located.[14]

And in 1972, Dr. Hans Nieper of West Germany told U.S. reporters:

> After more than 20 years of such specialized work, I have found the nontoxic Nitrilosides—that is, Laetrile—far superior to any other known cancer treatment or preventative. In my opinion it is the only existing possibility for the ultimate control of cancer.[15]

One piece of "misinformation" that was publicized in the early 1980s may have been the final straw in breaking down public acceptance of Laetrile. It was widely reported that actor Steve McQueen died as a result of going to Mexico in 1980 for treatments of Laetrile in an attempt to treat his cancer. What the presses around the country *failed* to report was that McQueen actually *was* cured of his cancer over about four months as a result of Laetrile and other alternative treatments. However, a benign, non-cancerous tumor remained in his abdomen, which he chose to have removed for cosmetic reasons. It was because of complications from this surgery that he died, not from the cancer.[16]

The Steve McQueen case is just one example of how incorrect media reporting caused millions of Americans to believe that Laetrile was just another hoax.

With so much evidence of Laetrile's effectiveness, not only through laboratory controlled studies, but also through patient use around the world, it is hard to believe that the cancer industry was able to suppress it so effectively in the United States. And it is just as hard to understand why. The only possible answer appears to be "money." According to Griffin,

> The trail of corruption leads all the way to the FDA itself. A study conducted by *USA Today* revealed that more than half of the experts hired to advise the government on the safety and effectiveness of medicine have financial relationships with the pharmaceutical companies that are affected by their advice.[17]

The lengths the cancer industry has gone to in order to make sure that Laetrile does not pose a threat to their profits have been truly amazing. Unbelievably, even *the sale of apricot seeds*, one of the richest natural sources of B_{17}, is greatly restricted. It is almost impossible to find apricot seeds in stores anywhere, including health food stores, and the only way to obtain apricot seeds now is by ordering them from a few sites on the Internet. I was not too surprised to find out that these sites are not allowed, by law, to list any benefits for cancer along with the product, and it appears that even these few sites are getting pressured to shut down.

Current Laetrile Therapy

Like the Hoxsey therapy, the use of Laetrile for cancer was largely pushed out of this country and into Mexico. Some physicians in the United States still administer it intravenously, but they rarely advertise that they do for legal reasons. The best way to ascertain who is administering this is just by asking the different alternative cancer treatment clinics that one comes across. There are many clinics in Mexico that anyone can go to for treatment and their websites often do advertize the administration of either Laetrile or B_{17}. As with any other type of treatment, be sure to look into the credibility of the doctor or clinic you are considering, and try to talk with some patients who have been successfully treated by that practitioner to make sure the treatment is being administered effectively.

One cautionary note: Laetrile stands for "*laevo*-rotatory mandeloni*trile* beta-diglucoside." The "laevo" part refers to a purified form of B_{17} that turns polarized light in a left-turning direction. In his book, *The Cancer Industry*, Ralph Moss states that the original form of Laetrile, patented by the Krebses, was purified to only contain this left-turning, or laevo, form. However, many of the commercial versions of Laetrile in use today are mixed (or racemic), meaning they contain both the left-turning and right-turning forms of B_{17}. According to Moss, Dr. Krebs, Jr., believed that only the left-turning form was effective against cancer and that the commercial racemic versions were much less effective than the pure Laetrile he and his father had patented.[18] Thus, it is a good idea to double-check the purity of the Laetrile in use by any practitioner with whom you are considering working.

Resources:

Some clinics offering intravenous Laetrile or B_{17} therapy:

Reno Integrative Medical Center (775) 829-1009
6110 Plumas, Suite B www.renointegrative.com
Reno, NV 89509

Oasis of Hope Clinic (888) 500-4673
Tijuana, Mexico www.oasisofhope.com
(Dr. Ernesto Contreras's Clinic)

Issels Treatment Center (888) 447-7357
Tijuana, Mexico www.issels.com

(See also section on Mexican Cancer Clinics in Chapter 17.)

Websites

www.laetrile-info.com

www.apricotpower.com (866) GOT-PITS (866/468-7487)

www.apricotsfromgod.com

www.laetrile.com.au

www.czlonkamediagroup.com

http://alternativecancer.us/laetrile.htm

Books

G. Edward Griffin. *World Without Cancer: The Story of Vitamin B₁₇*, revised edition. Westlake Village, California: American Media, 1997.

Dr. Philip E. Binzel. *Alive and Well: One Doctor's Experience With Nutrition in the Treatment of Cancer Patients*. Westlake Village, California: American Media, 1994.

W. Douglas Brodie, M.D. *Cancer and Common Sense: Combining Science and Nature to Control Cancer*. White Bear Lake, Minnesota: Winning Publications, 1997.

Ralph W. Moss. *The Cancer Industry*. Equinox Press, New York, 1999.

Dr. Kelley's Enzyme Therapy

Enzyme therapy, or "Metabolic Therapy," is another very impressive natural approach to cancer recovery that was developed and popularized by Dr. William Donald Kelley in the 1960s and 1970s. This approach revolves around the primary factor of high-dose supplementation with pancreatic enzymes and is based on a scientific explanation of cancer called "The Trophoblast Theory."

History

The trophoblast theory of cancer was first put forth in 1902 by John Beard, Ph.D., a Scottish embryologist. Dr. Beard presented evidence that cancer cells are virtually indistinguishable from certain pre-embryonic cells. These cells of early pregnancy are called "trophoblast" cells. During the early stages of every human pregnancy, trophoblast cells are those cells that grow very quickly to produce the umbilical cord and placenta.

One of the characteristics common to both cancer cells and early fetal trophoblast cells is that both types of cells produce a detectable hormone known as CGH, or chorionic gonadotrophic hormone. Luckily, CGH can be readily detected in urine. What is so fascinating is that no other cells in the human body produce CGH other than cancer cells and trophoblast cells of early pregnancy. This means that anyone who takes a CGH urine test and gets a *positive* result, is either a woman who is pregnant, or a man or woman with cancer.

In fact, common over-the-counter early pregnancy tests are designed to detect CGH to tell whether a woman is pregnant or not. However, the levels of CGH put out by cancer are not nearly as high as the levels put out during pregnancy and EPT tests are not sensitive enough to detect the lower levels of CGH present when a person has cancer. So, do *not* expect to be able to use an early pregnancy test to accurately tell whether you have cancer or not. Also, over the decades, researchers more commonly refer to CGH now as "HCG," which is the same thing and stands for human chorionic gonadotropin. But for the purposes of this discussion, we will continue to refer to it as CGH.

One of the early Laetrile doctors, Manuel Navarro, M.D., working at a university in Manila in the 1960s and 1970s, actually *proved* a particular CGH urine test to be 95 percent effective at detecting cancer of all types. And it turned out that the 5 percent assumed to be inaccurate test results were always false positives, as opposed to false negatives. In other words, the 5 percent supposedly inaccurate test results were only with people who didn't *appear* to have cancer, but over time, hindsight revealed that many of those people did in fact later develop cancer. Thus, the CGH test accuracy was very probably much better than 95 percent, and the test could detect cancer even before the disease was otherwise diagnosable.

Unfortunately, this test is not used by conventional medicine today. However, there is still a way to get this urine test done for early cancer detection. Various sources of instructions for how to collect your own urine sample and send it to the Philippines for just $50 can be found online by searching "Navarro HCG Test." But keep in mind that test results should not be relied upon solely for determining cancer status. Cigarette smoking, the use of steroids or other hormones, or even the use of vitamin D, may cause false positive results.

There is also a modified blood test that was developed by Dr. Schandl of Florida which checks for two forms of the HCG hormone and can be used for early cancer detection. It can be obtained as part of the "Cancer Profile" blood panel offered through Schandl's laboratory in Florida. (For more information on this test, go to www.CAProfile.net.)

Trophoblast cells of early fetal development are vital to the life of all humans. They are the cells that quickly produce a protective environment (placenta) and source of nourishment (umbilical cord) to the developing fetus. Since trophoblast cells perform such an important job during early fetal development, nature has provided them with a brilliant way to remain unaffected by the mother's immune system, which would normally attack them as foreign. This effective defense mechanism turns out to be a special protein coating that surrounds every trophoblast cell. The protective coating carries a negative electrostatic charge that allows the trophoblast cell to resist attack by the mother's immune system because all of the attacking white blood cells *also* happen to carry a negative electrostatic charge. Since "like polarities" repel each other, trophoblast cells are able to *electrostatically repel* any white blood cells that would normally attack them.

An example of this type of repelling process that has been observed by most of us in everyday life occurs when we notice static electricity causing our hair to stand up on our arms or head. What is really going on when this happens is that, for a short period of time, all of the hairs and the skin on a person's body happen to contain a predominance of the same polarity of electrostatic charge. Thus, since like polarities repel each other, each hair is electrostatically repelled away from the skin and at the same time is repelled away from the other hairs around it. This is the same mechanism by which trophoblast cells repel white blood cells of the immune system.

Cancer cells *also* carry this particular type of protective protein coating with a negative electrostatic charge. This protein coating does *not* occur around normal healthy cells of the body. Therefore, cancer cells and trophoblast cells of early pregnancy have the same built-in protection from white blood cells, and this is one reason cancer can be so difficult for a person's immune system to get rid of.

During early pregnancy, trophoblast cells create the umbilical cord and placenta, and they do this very quickly by rapid cell division and invasive growth into the uterine wall of the mother. This rapid invasive growth pattern is very much like the pattern of invasive cancer. The obvious advantage of the rapid growth is that the protective environment and food supply mechanism for the fetus are rapidly formed.

So, why do trophoblast cells and cancer cells have so much in common? Dr. Beard of Scotland published a detailed explanation in 1911 in his book, *The Enzyme Treatment of Cancer and its Scientific Basis*. But to explain the trophoblast cell/cancer cell connection in a simpler way here, I will present ideas from cancer treatment pioneer William Donald Kelley, D.D.S. and Kathy P. Fairbanks, Ph.D. (www.drkelley.info/articles/archive.php?artid=283), as well as other investigators.

In short, during early pregnancy, within the first five days after fertilization, human embryonic cells divide into two basic types: (1) embryo-blasts, which develop into the embryo, and (2) trophoblasts, which form the placenta and umbilical cord. While the trophoblast cells are doing their job to create the placenta and umbilical cord, the embryoblasts are differentiating into the three primary germ layers (ectoderm, endoderm and mesoderm). The ectoderm cells develop into the skin, brain, and nerves of the fetus. The endoderm cells develop into the linings of the lungs, intestines, liver, pancreas, and other areas. The mesoderm cells develop into the muscles, blood, bone, and reproductive organs.

According to Drs. Kelley and Fairbanks, the mesoderm cells develop into the vast majority of cells in the body and eventually make up almost all the different cell types. Because the mesoderm cells can potentially develop into so many different types of body cells, they are referred to as "pleuripotent." Many different complicated factors go into the designation of what type of body cell a mesoderm germ cell will become, and some of the cues come from the germ cell's immediate surroundings and local tissue that it has migrated into. Drs. Kelley and Fairbanks claim that it is normal for every human adult to have a certain number of these mesoderm pleuripotent germ cells still scattered throughout the body in a "sleeping" sort of state. These sleeping germ cells have not yet differentiated and are still very similar to the trophoblast cells of early pregnancy. Under certain conditions, they can turn into malignant cancer cells.

One recent confirmation of this concept is reported by the previously mentioned cancer researcher, Ralph W. Moss. According to Dr. Moss, modern-day scientists have now confirmed a "stem cell"-cancer link. He writes:

> In 1998, mainstream scientists made a huge leap in understanding cancer when they discovered (and patented) embryonic stem cells (ESC). They did not reference Beard in their paper, but they used the term "toti-potent" that had often been applied to describe germ cells, meaning that they were capable of developing into any other tissue.[1]

Author G. Edward Griffin claims that there is a normal and healthy function for these trophoblast-like germ cells in the adult body. He says these cells may get triggered into action wherever *healing* in the body needs to occur. They are the perfect cells to do the job because they are trophoblast-like, therefore fast-growing, and they are also able to develop into almost any type of body cell. The body naturally triggers them into action at any site that requires healing, and this is done with the help of certain hormones, such as estrogen and other steroid hormones. These hormones occur in both men and women and are well known to be found in high concentrations around areas of tissue damage.

Thus, according to Griffin and the trophoblast theory, cancer is the result of a completely normal process in the human body (i.e., the healing process) that has not been effectively kept under control. It might be said that it is *only when the healing process gets out of control* that detectable cancer can occur.

One-time damage to cells that is temporary, like a laceration, deep bruise, or broken bone, will generate trophoblast activity at the site of the wound that will usually be controllable. In other words, once the healing process is complete, the trophoblast-like healing activity is turned off. But where this healing process can get *out of control* is with cell damage that is of the "chronic" type. A common example of this would be when a person's cells in his or her lungs are damaged *chronically* through smoke inhalation from cigarettes day in and day out. In this type of situation, there is a constant activation of trophoblast healing activity.

Chronic cell damage can occur from many sources, including exposure to certain chemicals, toxins, radiation, or even as a result of poor diet that does not supply cells of the body with the building blocks they need. The bottom line is that chronic cell damage constantly triggers trophoblast-like germ cells for healing, and these cells multiply very fast and have a way of protecting themselves from the immune system. Under *normal* circumstances, there are natural control mechanisms in the human body that are designed to keep the trophoblast-like cells from multiplying too much, just as there are during early pregnancy and fetal development. So what are these natural control mechanisms?

The discovery of the primary control mechanism first came to light when researchers studied embryonic development. They discovered that the trophoblast cells of early pregnancy multiplied rapidly to form the placenta and umbilical cord *up until the eighth week of pregnancy*. But then the trophoblast cell proliferation stopped abruptly. For a long time, no one understood how or why this happened.

The answer came when researchers realized that it is during the eighth week of fetal development that the baby's pancreas first begins to function. One of the main jobs of the pancreas is to create a variety of pancreatic enzymes. Many of these enzymes go into the digestive tract and help us digest our foods. Breaking down proteins and other nutritional compounds is what they're good at. But others circulate via the bloodstream throughout all parts of the body. When certain pancreatic enzymes come across a trophoblast-like cell, they break down (or digest) the negatively charged protein coating. Once this coating is broken down, white blood cells of the immune system are no longer electrostatically repelled and are then able to attack and destroy the trophoblast cell. Thus, in the case of pregnancy, the fetus's pancreatic development is perfectly timed to occur just when the placenta and umbilical cord development should be stopped.

Critical for understanding cancer is the concept that pancreatic enzymes *continue* throughout our lifetime to attack and destroy the negatively charged protective coating around trophoblast-like cells that are triggered for healing purposes. If a person's supply of pancreatic enzymes is low or chronically stressed and depleted for some reason, and if other factors in the immune system are also stressed, then trophoblast cell growth *can* get out of control during healing processes and possibly turn into cancer.

It is interesting to note that cancer is almost *never* found in the first segment of the small intestine, or duodenum. This is the area of the intestine that the pancreas transfers its enzymes into first. The duodenum is therefore literally "bathed" in pancreatic enzymes, and cancer of the remaining intestinal tract increases in frequency in direct proportion to the distance from this area.[2]

You might well ask at this point, "If pancreatic enzymes unmask cancer cells, then why does cancer of the pancreas occur?" The answer is that, in the pancreas itself, pancreatic enzymes are in an *inactive* state. They are converted to an *active* state only after they reach the small intestine, and they are circulated into the bloodstream from the intestinal tract after that.

A damaged or underperforming pancreas may not produce optimum levels of enzymes and can thereby contribute to cancer as a deficient control mechanism. This brings up another interesting observation, which is that people who are diabetic and have a malfunctioning pancreas are actually three times more likely to develop cancer than non-diabetics.[3]

One last point about trophoblast cells is warranted here and has to do with "malignant" versus "benign" tumor cells. In *World Without Cancer*, G. Edward Griffin makes the point that when cancer is in its very early stages, the body sometimes tries to "seal off" the cancer by surrounding it with non-cancerous cells of that area of the body. This can then result in a benign lump or polyp. Griffin explains:

Under microscopic examination, many of these tumors are found to resemble a mixture or hybrid of both trophoblast and surrounding cells; a fact which has led some researchers to the premature conclusion that there are many different types of cancer. But the degree to which tumors appear to be different is the same degree to which they are benign; which means that it is the degree to which there are *non-cancerous* cells within it.

The greater the malignancy, the more these tumors begin to resemble each other, and the more clearly they begin to take on the classic characteristics of pregnancy trophoblast. And the most malignant of all cancers—the chorionepitheliomas—are almost indistinguishable from trophoblast cells.[4]

Many years after the Scottish embryologist, Dr. John Beard, proposed the trophoblast theory of cancer cell development, a retired Yale University professor named Dr. Howard Beard (who was, strangely enough, *not* related to Dr. Beard of Scotland), further advanced the understanding of how pancreatic enzymes affect cancer by discovering that the two most important cancer-controlling enzymes of pancreatin are "trypsin" and "chymotrypsin." But it wasn't until the 1960s that any medical practitioner really put these ideas to the test, and actually began *treating* cancer patients with high doses of pancreatic enzymes. The first pioneering practitioner to do so was an American dentist named Dr. William Donald Kelley, and his method of treating cancer began with curing himself of his own advanced, metastasized cancer.

Dr. Kelley had the misfortune of being diagnosed in 1963 with cancer in his pancreas, liver, and intestine. The pancreas and liver have historically been considered very "deadly" places for cancer to be, and the survival rates remain dismally low with conventional treatment even today. For localized pancreatic cancer *caught early*, modern surgery can still only offer a five-year survival rate of about 5 percent. And for *metastasized* pancreatic cancer, the long-term survival rate with current conventional treatment is about zero. (Approximately 30,000 Americans are diagnosed with pancreatic cancer each year and most of them die within a year of their diagnosis.)

It is no wonder that when Dr. Kelley was diagnosed with cancer in *both* his pancreas and liver, as well as in his intestine, his doctors only gave him a few weeks to live. Yet, Dr. Kelley found a way to naturally overcome his metastasized, late-stage cancer by developing and following his own personal program. And he remained cancer-free for about 40 years after his diagnosis.

After attaining his own cure, Dr. Kelley went on to help thousands of other people overcome their cancers, attaining one of the highest cure rates of any practitioner. His treatment protocol is estimated to have benefited approximately 33,000 people over a 30-year period, and the cancer patients who diligently stuck to the program had a very high rate of complete recovery.

Dr. Kelley named his form of treatment "Metabolic Therapy." He saw cancer as a result of faulty metabolic functioning and felt it was of key importance to tailor the treatment to each patient and their metabolic type. To this end, he developed a system to classify each of his patients into one of ten basic metabolic categories. In general, the five basic components of Kelley's metabolic program were:

1. Supplementation of high doses of pancreatic enzymes (following an on/off cycle) along with other nutritional supplements

2. Detoxification of the body primarily through coffee enemas

3. Nutritionally adequate and balanced diet

4. Neurological stimulation (chiropractic adjustments, physical therapy, craniosacral therapy)

5. Spiritual attitude

Dr. Kelley incorporated many of Max Gerson's concepts into his treatment approach, such as fresh juices and coffee enemas, but his approach differed in numerous details from Dr. Gerson's as well. Probably the contribution that Dr. Kelley is best known for is his promotion of the understanding that pancreatic enzymes are of *key* importance to natural cancer recovery. He did this by being the first practitioner to prove the role of pancreatic enzymes in cancer recovery over three decades of clinical practice and thousands of patients.

As early as 1969, Dr. Kelley published a book about his method of treating cancer. Called *One Answer to Cancer*, the book soon became very popular in underground nutritional circles. However, like Hoxsey and Gerson, Dr. Kelley was harassed by the establishment. Amazingly, even Dr. Kelley's freedom to write a book about his methods was denied when, in a 1970s federal court trial, he was ordered to never speak or write about cancer again!

Dr. Kelley was repeatedly attacked for not focusing strictly on dental medicine, and in 1976 his dental license was suspended for five years. In 1986, after many years of harassment, Dr. Kelley finally gave up his practice of metabolic counseling and stopped treating cancer altogether. He claimed in his last book, *Cancer: Curing the Incurable Without Surgery, Chemotherapy, or Radiation* (published in 2000), that there were numerous sinister attempts to suppress his innovative cancer therapy. Unfortunately, these attempts were successful enough to keep his treatment approach out of mainstream medicine, even though he had been achieving unheard-of successes with metastasized cancer cases the medical establishment had little hope of curing.

Since Dr. Kelley passed away, other practitioners around the country have been administering forms of his treatment to cancer patients with success. Two of these practitioners work together in a New York practice: Nicholas Gonzalez, M.D., and Linda Isaacs, M.D.

Dr. Nicholas Gonzalez

Before Dr. Kelley closed down his metabolic counseling practice, Nicholas Gonzalez, a medical student at Cornell University, decided to look into Dr. Kelley's method of treating cancer. When he approached Dr. Kelley about this in 1981, Kelley freely allowed Gonzalez to review the records of more than 10,000 cancer patients he had treated and to contact the patients. Gonzalez was astonished to find that so many accurately diagnosed cases of metastasized cancer had been cured. Many of these people were thriving 10 or 15 years after their diagnosis.

Gonzalez interviewed and evaluated over 500 cases in detail, and also performed a rigorous independent study of Kelley's pancreatic cancer patients. Gonzalez chose pancreatic cancer for his detailed report because of its extremely low cure rate among conventional approaches. He focused on 22 pancreatic cancer cases in Kelley's files, each of which had been diagnosed through biopsy at a major medical institution. The results of his study were extremely impressive:

- Ten of the 22 patients *never* followed Kelley's protocol. They lived an average of 67 days.

- Seven of the 22 patients followed Kelley's protocol *partially*. They lived an average of 233 days.

- Five of the 22 patients followed Kelley's protocol *completely*. They experienced total, long-term recovery.

Because Gonzalez only focused on the 22 cases that rigorously met his high research standards (such as being diagnosed through biopsy at a major medical institution), the results of his study boldly refuted the common myth that most people who recover from cancer using alternative approaches were misdiagnosed and never had cancer in the first place. Yet, even though Gonzalez used rigorous standards for his study and wrote up his results with careful documentation, he was scorned and ridiculed when he tried to publish his findings. Unbelievably, even in the 1980s, the academic medical world could not accept that a nutritionally based treatment approach to cancer could bring about such incredible recoveries in advanced cases.

Current Treatment

Many of the basic aspects of Dr. Kelley's method are continued by Dr. Nicholas Gonzales and Dr. Linda Isaacs in New York City. They currently treat people using their own modified Kelley approach. Although the Gonzalez-Isaacs program is best known for the treatment of pancreatic cancer, they also treat *all* other types of cancer, as well as other debilitating diseases such as multiple sclerosis, chronic fatigue, and lupus.

Typical treatment involves patients taking up to 45 grams of pancreatic enzymes each day (five to seven capsules six times a day). These specially developed enzymes are unique to the Gonzalez-Isaacs program and cannot be purchased commercially elsewhere. Including other supplements, each cancer patient may consume a total of 130 to 160 capsules a day. Also included in the program are digestive aids such as pepsin and hydrochloric acid, and supplemental concentrates (in pill form) of raw beef organs and glands. Patients must generally prepare three fresh juices each day and, for detoxification, most are required to perform two coffee enemas a day. Both the supplementation protocol and the dietary regimen for each patient are individualized according to the patient's metabolic type and disease state.

In an article about the Gonzalez-Isaacs program published in a 1996 issue of *Life Extension* magazine, writer Terri Mitchell sums up Gonzalez's theory about metabolic typing in the following way:

> Dr. Gonzalez believes that the physiology of patients with cancer invariably turns up as either too acid or too alkaline. Patients who have too much acidity have a predominance of sympathetic nervous system activity. Those who are too alkaline lean towards parasympathetic activity. The sympathetic nervous system is the part of the brain involved in 'fight or flight' activity. This primitive survival mechanism gears up the heart and lungs at the expense of other organs such as the pancreas and stomach. People who are born with a propensity towards sympathetic activity have hyper-vigilant stress responses, but low parasympathetic activity such as digestion.
>
> People who lean towards the parasympathetic are the opposite. Their pancreas, intestines and other organs are working overtime, but their stress response organs are asleep. Dr. Gonzalez' goal with these patients is to augment their sympathetic activity. The idea is to balance sympathetic and parasympathetic physiology.[5]

Like Dr. Kelley, Gonzalez believes that personal psychological and spiritual changes also need to be part of a cancer patient's program. He has been quoted as saying, "I've had patients whose cancer didn't get better no matter how perfectly they did my program, until they resolved serious emotional issues in their lives."[6]

Interestingly, Dr. Gonzalez doesn't worry about the *size* of a person's tumor, and actually prefers to see the tumor enlarge during treatment. In his thinking, this means that the body is causing a natural healing inflammation response. He also does not believe that it is always necessary to destroy a tumor in order for a patient to heal. In other words, Gonzalez says that ". . . sometimes the body will wall off a tumor and just keep it there like an old bird's nest."[7] Dr. Gonzalez's concepts are supported by the many long-term recoveries of his patients. He claims to be able to achieve a 70 to 75 percent success rate with those patients who comply with their individualized program.

Case Stories

A number of different journal articles about the Gonzalez-Isaacs program have been written and published. The following case stories 1 and 2 were published in the October 1996 issue of *Life Extension* magazine and are paraphrased here:

Case Story #1 — Lung Cancer Metastasized to Liver, Pancreas, and Adrenals

In 1991, a 70-year old man named Mort was diagnosed after X-ray and surgery with lung cancer. CT scans then showed that his cancer had already spread to his liver, pancreas and adrenals. His oncologist recommended *no treatment*, indicating that there was none available that could help Mort. Within 2 months, Mort's wife found out about Dr. Gonzalez and Mort started on the Gonzalez-Isaacs program. In four months, Mort's tests indicated he was improving. Five years after his diagnosis, Mort was still alive and doing well.[8]

Case Story #2—Breast Cancer

A woman named Henri-Etta had gone through traditional treatment for breast cancer, including surgery and six months of chemotherapy. She went into remission, but about four and one-half years later the breast cancer came back. Her oncologist offered chemotherapy again, but this time she refused. Henri-Etta found out about the Gonzalez-Isaacs approach and, after an evaluation, started on that program instead. About nine years after her cancer diagnosis, in 2003, Henri-Etta was still alive and feeling great.[9]

The following story is paraphrased from the October 2000 issue of *Total Health* magazine (vol. 22, no. 5).

Case Story #3—Metastasized Melanoma

In 1983, a man named Bill began having chronic sinus problems. An ENT specialist prescribed various treatments that didn't help. Finally, surgery was performed and some polyps were removed. Lab reports on the polyps indicated melanoma. A CT scan was performed which revealed a small tumor behind Bill's left eye. In 1984, a lengthy neurosurgery was done to remove the tumor along with a small piece of bone. Bill's oncologist thought they had successfully removed all of the tumor.

But in 1987, Bill started having abdominal pains. Another CT scan showed a large abdominal tumor which a needle biopsy indicated was, once again, melanoma. Surgery was performed at Sloan-Kettering to remove the tumor, but this time all of the cancer could *not* be removed due to risk of damaging some vital organs. At this point, Bill chose to decline follow-up chemotherapy or other conventional treatment. Instead, he searched around for alternatives.

Bill finally started seeing Dr. Gonzalez and Dr. Isaacs in May of 1988. By December of that year, his tumor had stabilized. In the summer of 1992, four years later, his tumor began to grow again. After discussing his situation with Dr. Gonzalez, Bill again went to Sloan-Kettering to have the tumor surgically removed. The surgery was very successful and revealed that his tumor was completely encapsulated, and there was no evidence that the cancer had spread anywhere else. Three years later, when his testimony was taken in 1995, Bill was still happily thriving, and still doing the Gonzalez-Isaacs program.[10]

It is evident from these case stories, as well as from the accounts of many other cancer patients, that the Gonzalez-Isaacs approach to treating cancer is effective. Although it is well-known for treating pancreatic cancer, it can also bring about long-term recovery for a variety of other cancers, and includes cases of metastasized or late-stage cancer. Much of the credit for this approach must go to Dr. Kelley, but since Dr. Kelley has passed away Dr. Gonzalez and Dr. Isaacs in New York have contributed to the effectiveness of this method. From all accounts, they are excellent practitioners who can be sought out currently by people wishing to pursue this effective approach as a way to *outsmart their cancer.*

Resources:

Nicholas J. Gonzalez, M.D., P.C.   (212) 213-3337
Linda L. Isaacs, M.D.   www.dr-gonzalez.com
36A East 36th Street, Suite 204
New York, NY 10016

[Lecture tapes are available that give a detailed explanation of the program, and can be ordered from the above website.]

For Evaluation and Consultation: If possible, prospective patients should review the requirements for evaluation that are listed on the above website before applying for treatment. Along with one's application, prospective patients should send any relevant biopsy and blood work results along with their CT or MRI written reports. (But don't send the actual film.) Pre-appointment evaluation of this material will be done, then a two-session "in-person" evaluation meeting in the New York office will be scheduled over two consecutive days.

Treatment: The overall cost of the Gonzalez-Isaacs treatment program will vary with each patient, but generally is about $600 a month, or $5,000 to $6,000 per year (as of this printing). About three-quarters of this cost is for the supplements. Every patient is required to return at certain intervals for a repeat physical exam and assessment of their dietary and nutritional needs, as these may change over the course of treatment. These follow-up evaluations will be an extra charge.

Pamela McDougle   (208) 424-7600
Nutritional Consultant
Boise, Idaho

For Evaluation: Call the phone number listed above. Pamela McDougle was the last person that Dr. Kelley himself trained. She is a foremost expert on Dr. Kelley's original Metabolic Therapy and is a nutritional consultant for those wanting to use his approach.

Program Fees: The overall cost for in-depth consultation is approximately $2,500 for the first six months, not counting supplements. Supplements, including Dr. Kelley's original formulation of enzymes, cost about $800 to $1300 per month for the first year, then usually less after that.

For Training: Pamela McDougle also trains healthcare practitioners (doctors, naturopaths, chiropractors, nurses) who are interested in learning Dr. Kelley's Metabolic Nutritional approach. Call for more information about small group or individual trainings.

Books

William Donald Kelley, D.D.S., M.S. *Cancer: Curing the Incurable Without Surgery, Chemotherapy, or Radiation.* Baltimore: College of Metabolic Medicine, 2000.

Richard Walters. *Options: The Alternative Cancer Therapy Book*. New York: Avery Penguin Putnam Publishing, 1993.

Websites

www.dr-gonzalez.com

www.drkelley.com

www.drkelley.info/articles/archive.php?artid=283

8

Burzynski's Antineoplastons

A truly different approach to treating cancer came to the United States in 1970 when physician and medical researcher Stanislaw Burzynski emigrated from Poland. Dr. Burzynski's unique method is *not* based on healing the body with herbs, diet, nutrition, cleansing, or enzymes, as are the methods presented in previous chapters. Yet his approach is heralded as one of the most promising cancer treatments ever developed. Though expensive, it is non-toxic and has brought about countless complete cures. Those suffering from lymphomas and brain cancers, including pediatric brain cancers, do particularly well. For those who can afford it or who qualify for trials, Burzynski's approach is currently being offered at his clinic in Houston, Texas, where patients are treated by a large staff of qualified doctors.

History

Like Dr. Gerson, Dr. Burzynski came to this country with an impressive academic medical background. Born in Poland in 1943, he showed remarkable abilities in chemistry at an early age. He studied medicine and, at the age of 24, graduated first in his class of 250 students at his medical academy. One year after obtaining his M.D., he also obtained a Ph.D. in biochemistry. Stanislaw Burzynski gained recognition as one of the youngest people in the history of Poland to receive *both* an M.D. and Ph.D. diploma.[1]

101

Growing up in Poland during and after World War II was not easy for Stanislaw. His father, a teacher, was imprisoned for two years by the Nazis because he continued to teach Jewish students after the Nazis had segregated Jews into walled ghettos. In the late 1940s, when Poland was overrun and controlled by communist Soviet Union, life became difficult in other ways. The Burzynski family property was taken away from Stanislaw's family, and his brother began to fight in the anti-communist underground, risking his life on a daily basis. Stanislaw's brother was eventually killed in 1948 while fighting in the resistance movement. While still a boy, Stanislaw often had to defend himself in physical fights that were triggered by prejudices during this class-conscious era of Poland. As a result of his own physical fights, and after watching his brother and father stand up to oppression, Burzynski turned into a person who knew the meaning of fighting for what one believed in.

When Burzynski started medical school, he quickly became involved in research. During his years as a medical student, he studied amino acids and peptides and published papers about his work. He first started analyzing amino acids in wild mushrooms to see if he could turn some of the toxic chains of amino acids that were present in the mushrooms into new antibiotics. Then, he moved on to studying other organic substances, including blood and urine, that contained peptides. (Peptides are short chains of amino acids.) He began finding peptides in human blood and urine that no one had ever known about before. According to Burzynski, "Nobody had bothered to identify them. Nobody cared what they were."[2]

Dr. Burzynski decided to see if the unidentified amino acid compounds he was finding might be related to kidney disease, and he prepared his doctoral thesis on this subject. The work of identifying these compounds was difficult and required very modern chromatographic equipment as well as hard-to-get chemicals.

After a while, Dr. Burzynski began to wonder if the peptides he had discovered might be linked, not only to kidney disease, but also to cancer. He suspected this as a possibility because people with primary kidney disease (PKD) appeared to have an overabundance of some of these peptides, and he knew that another researcher in Poland had discovered that people with PKD rarely suffered from cancer. Dr. Burzynski began to wonder if the peptides themselves were able to inhibit cancer in some way.

Just as Dr. Burzynski was beginning to look into this, he began to have problems with the communist regime controlling Poland. Dr. Burzynski had already refused to join the communist party and this had branded him as a dissenter and independent thinker. One way the Polish authorities dealt with free thinkers was to draft them into the army. Thus, in 1970, Dr. Burzynski received orders to report for military duty. If he complied, he would be sent to North Vietnam to fight with the Viet Cong. Because of how the Polish military worked, this could mean it might be decades before he would be able to return to Poland and his scientific research.

Instead of reporting for military duty, Dr. Burzynski quickly obtained a passport and immediately left Poland for New York. When he arrived in the United States, he only had a few dollars in his pocket and his paperwork documenting the 39 peptides he had identified. Soon, Dr. Burzynski received a message from Poland that he would never be allowed to work in any medical school of that country again. He knew then that he would never be able to go back to his home country.

Luckily, shortly after arriving in the United States, Dr. Burzynski got a job at Baylor College of Medicine in Houston. In the university's department of anesthesiology, a scientist named Georges Ungar was studying brain peptides and how those peptides impacted the transmission of memories. Dr. Burzynski's own work on peptides fit right in.

When Stanislaw Burzynski started work at the Baylor College of Medicine in Texas, he had already identified naturally occurring peptides (small chains of amino acids) that could be found in the blood of healthy persons, but not in the blood of people with cancer. Since he thought that the types of peptides he had discovered might have an *inhibitory* effect on cancer, he chose to name them "anti-neoplastons." The term "anti" means opposing, or against, and a common medical term for cancer is "neoplasm" from the Greek word that means "new growth." The term "antineoplaston" was coined by Dr. Burzynski, though conventional medicine has used the word "antineoplastic" before.

At Baylor, Dr. Burzynski was able to move forward with his research and to formulate his own theory that certain types of peptides, or antineoplastons, were actually part of a *biochemical communication system* that complimented the rest of the immune system and could regulate the out-of-control division of cancer cells to eventually bring them back to a normal state. He also discovered that not all the peptides he isolated had an impact on cancer cell cultures. In fact, most of them did not show any anti-cancer activity.

As he continued his research, Dr. Burzynski began to identify specific antineoplastons that had anticancer properties against certain types of cancers. Then, he found one special antineoplaston that actually showed anti-cancer activity against a *broad spectrum* of cancer types. This discovery was huge. Dr. Burzynski called the broad spectrum antineoplaston "Antineoplaston A" and began to concentrate his cancer research on it.[3]

Also while doing research at Baylor, Dr. Burzynski met his future wife Barbara. Barbara was an M.D. and Polish immigrant as well. Barbara Burzynski soon joined Stanislaw in his research, and over the next 15 years or so they worked together, isolating antineoplastons, breaking down Antineoplaston A into smaller fractions, and learning how to produce the most effective antineoplastons synthetically. In 1974, Dr. Burzynski was granted research funding and support from both the National Cancer Institute and the University of Texas M.D. Anderson Cancer Center.

After a while, the use of antineoplastons in a laboratory setting on cancer cell lines was going so well that it was time to start using them in animal studies. However, what Dr. Burzynski found was that, while the antineoplastons he had isolated could shut down human cancer cell lines, they had very little or no effect on similar cancers in animals. In other words, he discovered that the antineoplastons were "species-specific" in their chemical communication traits.[4]

Since Dr. Burzynski's antineoplastons were ineffective on animal cancers, he decided in 1976 that it was time to go straight to their use on people. He chose to start with terminal cancer patients who were considered untreatable, or for whom all other treatment had failed. Since he had passed the Texas medical licensing exams in 1973, Dr. Burzynski felt he was qualified to do this. But the Baylor College of Medicine would not allow him to perform human clinical trials unless he had an investigational new drug (IND) permit from the FDA. Dr. Burzynski spent months filing paperwork to get the IND, a process that generally only takes a matter of weeks for pharmaceutical companies with promising new drugs. Apparently, the FDA was *not* interested in complying with Burzynski and kept asking for more and more documentation. Burzynski kept supplying it until, eventually, his IND application comprised thousands of pages—and when stacked on the floor was over 6 feet tall.[5]

Dr. Burzynski was never given the IND permit by the FDA. However, he finally got permission by one independent hospital to test his antineoplaston compounds at their facility—as long as he only used his protocol on people for whom all other treatment had failed. These early antineoplaston treatments on humans showed great promise. He began to see people recover who'd been given only a short time to live by the medical establishment. With more and more refinement of his technique, Dr. Burzynski's treatment approach began to show an overall effectiveness that was *better* than traditional cancer treatment methods.

In 1977, Dr. Burzynski opened up his own private practice in Houston, Texas, which he called the Burzynski Clinic. This became the place where he could legally administer antineoplastons to desperate patients. In the early years, the production of antineoplastons was laborious because the peptides had to be isolated from human urine. Eventually, however, Burzynski perfected a way to synthesize the antineoplaston compounds he needed from chemicals. He developed a large manufacturing plant in Houston and made sure that it met every FDA standard for manufacture of pharmaceuticals. The Burzynski Clinic in Houston is now a large treatment center that employs about 20 physicians and a large staff of other medical personnel.

Over the past 25 years, thousands of patients have been treated at the Burzynski Clinic with antineoplaston therapy for terminal cancer and other types of devastating diseases. Dr. Burzynski has authored and co-authored 184 scientific publications and has presented scientific papers at international conventions. He also holds over 160 patents for his treatments in 35 countries around the world. Antineoplaston therapy is non-toxic and has brought about long-term recovery for countless cancer patients.

Julian Whitaker, M.D., of southern California has looked into Dr. Burzynski's approach in detail. He explains how Burzynski's treatment works against cancer in this excerpt from one of his newsletters:

> Antineoplastons consist of small peptides, components of protein, and peptide metabolites that are given by mouth or intravenously. They work by entering the cell and altering specific functions of the genes: Some activate the tumor suppressor genes that prevent cancer, while others turn off the oncogenes that force the cancer cell to divide uncontrollably. Like rifle shots to the heart of the malignant process, the antineoplastons cause cancerous cells to either revert to normal or die without dividing.[6]

In a 1996 special supplement of his popular monthly newsletter, Dr. Whitaker reported numerous cases of people who had recovered from cancer using antineoplaston therapy, three of which are reported below as case stories 1 through 3. Case stories 4 and 5 were testimonials I recorded from Burzynski patients I spoke with myself.

Case Stories

Case Story #1—Adult Malignant Brain Tumor

A 35-year-old school psychologist named Pamela began experiencing double vision in 1987 and, after going through tests, was diagnosed with a tumor in her brain stem. It was classified as an "anaplastic astrocytoma," grade 3. She underwent surgery and two months of radiation, but these treatments did not get her cancer under control. The highly malignant tumor in her brain just kept growing. She was offered chemotherapy, but refused it because her doctors told her there wasn't much chance the chemo would do any good anyway.

In April 1988, Pamela had a follow-up MRI which showed that her tumor was about the size of a quarter, about twice as large as when she was first diagnosed. At this point, a resident at the University of California, San Francisco hospital told her to get her affairs in order because she only had 6 weeks to 6 months to live.[7] Luckily for Pamela, she then found out about the Burzynski Clinic. By July 1988, she had started on antineoplaston therapy.

To Pamela's sheer joy, an MRI in September 1988 showed her tumor had decreased 30 to 40 percent in volume. By the following January, there was no sign of the tumor in her brain at all.[8] She continued on antineoplastons for about two years and her tumor never showed up again. When she was re-checked in 2003, Pamela was still doing fine and had not received any treatment of any kind for 13 years![9]

Case Story #2—Breast Cancer Metastasized to the Bones

In 1990, a woman named Carol underwent a mastectomy and received chemotherapy for "infiltrative and intraductal cancer of the breast."[10] Four years later, she found out that her cancer was still growing and had spread to her bones. First discovered in her spine, she now had cancer in her hip, clavicle, and ribs as well.

It was at this point that Carol began antineoplaston therapy from the Burzynski Clinic. The antineoplaston treatment first halted the spread of her cancer and then began to reverse it. About a year and a half later, the cancer in Carol's clavicle, hips, and ribs was completely gone and she only had a slight involvement of the lumbar spine which was, in fact, reducing. She also claimed to be feeling better than she had in 10 years.

Case Story #3—*Prostate Cancer Metastasized to the Bones*

A 61-year old business man named Ernesto was diagnosed with metastatic prostate cancer in 1995. The diagnosis was confirmed by biopsy. A bone scan showed that his entire skeleton, legs, ribs, spine, and skull were full of cancer as well. At the time of Ernesto's diagnosis, his PSA count was 960. (A normal PSA count would normally be below 4.) He refused most conventional treatment, and only went on a testosterone blocker called Lupron which his doctor hoped would help but did not expect it to stop Ernesto's cancer.

Within just a couple of weeks of his diagnosis, Ernesto started on antineoplaston therapy. After only three weeks of treatment, his bone pain subsided. Six months later, his PSA reading was down to 1.4. Remarkably, each time he received a scan he could see his cancer receding more and more from his bones.[11] The last anyone heard from him, Ernesto was doing fine and living a normal life.

Case Story #4—*Prostate Cancer*

Prostate cancer appears to respond well to antineoplaston therapy, and here is one more case story from a man I was able to contact personally. His name is John.

In January 1990, when John was 64 years old, he was diagnosed with prostate cancer. His prostate gland was completely encircled with tumors which, when biopsies were taken, were found to be malignant. (At the time, the Gleason scale and PSA test had not yet been developed for more detailed diagnosing.)

John got an appointment with Dr. Burzynski later that same month. According to John, Dr. Burzynski wanted to be absolutely sure of his diagnosis and sent him to another hospital in Houston for a second opinion. This hospital gave John the same diagnosis as the first one. At this point, Dr. Burzynski put John on antineoplastons in capsule form and sent him home with a three-month supply.

In May 1990, after about three months on the capsules, John returned to Houston for an examination. X-rays showed that John's tumors were "healed," but Dr. Burzynski wanted him to continue on the capsules for a few more months. In August 1990, John went back to Houston once again. This time, X-rays showed that John's tumors were all gone.

The PSA test had just become available, so Dr. Burzynski sent John home with a prescription to get this test done. John had several PSA tests performed over the next three to four months. All showed very low readings, so his doctor finally said he didn't need to keep getting them. He now only gets his PSA level checked whenever he goes in for a general health check-up.

John is currently 77 years old and it has been 13 years since he was diagnosed with cancer. He lives a normal, happy life. John has not experienced any recurrence of his cancer and his PSA test results have remained completely normal.

Case Story #5—Non-Hodgkin's Lymphoma

Mary Jo is a woman whose cancer recovery story has been written up in numerous publications. In 1991, when Mary Jo was only 40 years old, she was diagnosed with low grade non-Hodgkin's lymphoma. It was 100 percent follicular lymphoma, and she consulted with physicians at USC, UCLA, Stanford Medical Center in California, and the Dana-Farber Cancer Institute in Boston. They all told her that there was no conventional treatment that could cure her cancer. The Dana-Farber Institute offered Mary Jo an autologous bone marrow transplant with high-dose radiation as her best chance for recovery. This treatment procedure is extremely risky and can cause serious side effects, including death. Mary Jo decided to turn it down.

Not wanting to give up, Mary Jo and her husband researched other options that might be available and eventually found out about Burzynski's treatment. In 1992, Mary Jo flew to Houston and started on antineoplaston therapy. For about the first two months she took the antineoplastons in capsule form. This involved 60 capsules a day. But the capsule regimen did not seem to be working effectively enough on her cancer, so she then switched to using an "infusion pump." This is the most effective way to administer antineoplaston therapy, and involves carrying around a small pump that is attached to a catheter surgically inserted into the chest. The pump releases a constant slow drip of antineoplastons into the body for about 10 hours a day. Mary Jo says that this pump was not difficult to deal with, and that she could basically do everything she would normally do without any problem. She also says there were no side effects from the treatment.

After 9 months of treatment on the infusion pump, Mary Jo was pronounced in remission by both her oncologist at UCLA and by

Dr. Burzynski. She remained in remission for about two years, when two swollen lymph nodes indicated a possible recurrence. It was never determined whether her enlarged nodes were really the cancer recurring or just a reaction to a cold or infection. But just to be safe, Burzynski put her back on treatment immediately. After only three months on capsule treatment, a follow-up CT scan showed Mary Jo in remission again. She has been cancer free ever since, which, at the time of this writing has been for the past 11 years!

Case Story #6—Childhood Brain Tumor

Paul was a five-year-old boy in 1986 when he was diagnosed with a large slow-growing tumor in his brain. Doctors told Paul's family that the tumor was inoperable and he would not live to see his tenth birthday. Paul's parents sent his scans to the head of the pediatric neurosurgery department at the Mayo Clinic. At that time, this was Dr. Patrick Kelly. Dr. Kelly reviewed the scans then wrote to Paul's parents: "I have reviewed the MRI scans on your five-year-old son Paul . . . it is the largest tumor I have ever seen in this area in anybody ever referred to me for surgery. I showed your scans to a number of my colleagues here who feel that it is inoperable . . . . Without surgery, your boy will die."[12]

Because of the serious risks involved in attempting surgery or radiation, Paul's family elected *not* to pursue those treatments. By 1988, they finally found out about and started Paul on Burzynski's antineoplastons. By the time he started antineoplaston therapy, Paul's tumor had grown to the size of an orange. On antineoplastons, the tumor gradually shrank down until it was no longer visible and, over the next 17 years, Paul grew to be a healthy young man with no more signs of cancer.

NOTE: More personal cancer recovery stories from people who used antineoplaston therapy can be viewed at the website www.burzynski patientgroup.org. Just click on "Our Stories." These recovery stories include a wide variety of cancer cases.

Theory and Efficacy

Dr. Burzynski and his colleagues at the clinic are now quite specific about how antineoplastons work. They explain that

> . . . antineoplastons work on cancer cells to interrupt the signal transduction in the ras oncogene pathway, which causes cells to divide endlessly.

At the same time, antineoplastons activate the p53 tumor suppressor gene, which tells the cells to undergo programmed cell death. Healthy cells remain unaffected under these processes.[13]

Antineoplaston treatment is completely safe and non-toxic to the individual and could be seen as the first successful form of gene therapy for cancer. At one point, Dr. Burzynski presented the FDA with details on 74 clinical trials using antineoplastons to treat cancer. In one of these trials, the antineoplaston therapy was *seven times* more effective than surgery, radiation, and chemotherapy.[14]

By comparison, chemotherapy looks like a barbaric practice from the middle ages. It indiscriminately poisons healthy cells along with cancerous ones and is extremely toxic to the body as a whole. Chemotherapy is based on the concept that, though chemotherapy kills all cells in the body indiscriminately, the fast-growing cells of the body are killed the quickest. Cancer cells tend to grow and replicate faster than other cells in the body, and thus are most hard hit by cytotoxic drugs (chemotherapy). Hair cells are also fast-growing compared to most normal cells of the body, and that is why chemo patients often lose their hair. Chemotherapy is, more or less, a shotgun approach that kills as many of the fast-growing cells of the body as possible in a relatively short period of time.

But chemotherapeutic drugs can rarely be effectively used to kill *all* the cancer cells in a person's body. This is because, to ensure that all the cancer cells are killed, one would probably have to use enough chemotherapy that would also kill the patient. Thus, when a patient is said to be "in remission" as a result of chemotherapy, that does *not* mean the patient is cancer-free. At best, chemotherapy treatment may kill on the order of 90 percent of the cancer cells in the body. This leaves around 10 percent of the cancer cells still surviving, which could be millions of cancer cells. Those cancer cells that are left just begin again doing what they are good at, which is multiplying quickly. And since the cancer patient's immune system has generally been devastatingly weakened by the chemo, these multiplying cancer survivor cells have very little opposition.

On the other hand, because Dr. Burzynski's treatment involves the administration of antineoplastons which specifically turn off the activity of the "oncogenes" of the cancer cells, they interrupt the signal that causes rapid cell division. At the same time, the antineoplastons activate the tumor suppressor genes which stimulate normal cell death. Thus, antineoplastons simply encourage abnormal cancer cells to become normal or die off, and don't adversely affect normal healthy cells at all. Patients can be *deluged* with this treatment for many months until, gradually, all of the cancer cells are controlled. Also, unlike chemotherapy, Burzynski's antineoplastons work on a broad range of cancers. These include brain cancer, lymph cancer, lung cancer, bladder cancer, prostate cancer, and breast cancer, among others.

Brain cancer (which chemotherapy does *not* work well on) responds particularly well to antineoplastons. This is important because the other form of conventional treatment for brain cancer, which is radiation, is also limited in efficacy. In fact, because brain cancer responds so well to antineoplastons and typically so poorly to chemotherapy, a highly respected Seattle oncologist and faculty member of the University of Washington Medical School carried out his own independent review of 17 of Dr. Burzynski's brain tumor cases. This oncologist, Robert E. Burdick, M.D., carefully examined the 17 patients' medical records and wrote a detailed report. On page 2 of Dr. Burdick's report, he states:

> The following is a summary of the 17 cases that I have reviewed. Of the 17 patients there were 7 complete remissions, one patient having had a second complete remission after he discontinued antineoplaston therapy which resulted in his tumor regrowing. There were 9 partial remissions, 2 cases of stable disease and no disqualifications. The average duration of therapy with antineoplastons necessary to obtain a complete remission was 10 months with a range of 2 to 20 months. The average duration of antineoplaston therapy necessary to obtain a partial response was 8 months with a range of 1 to 14 months. The average duration of complete remissions is 16+ months with all 6 complete remissions continuing to remain in remission to the best of my knowledge through January 1, 1997. The duration of complete remissions ranged from 3+ months to 40+ months with the duration of partial remissions averaging 18+ months and ranging from 5 to 78+ months.[15]

In discussing the above results, Dr. Burdick remarks,

> The response rate here is an astounding 81 percent, with an equally astounding 35 percent complete remission rate. Such remission rates are far in excess of anything I or anyone else has seen since research work on brain tumors began.[16]

Dr. Burdick also comments,

> It is very rare, currently, to ever get a complete remission or cure in a patient who has a malignant brain tumor using our standard modalities

of surgery, radiation, and chemotherapy. . . . As a rough estimate, neurosurgeons do well to cure one in every 1,000 brain-cancer patients they operate on. Radiation therapy slows the growth of adult tumors, gaining perhaps one month of life, and again may result in a cure in only one in 500–1,000 patients, those cures being in the pediatric age group. Similarly, chemotherapy research, despite 30 years of clinical trials, has not resulted in the development of a single drug or drug combination that elicits more than an occasional transient response in primary brain tumors.[17]

Dr. Burzynski has tirelessly continued to seek official evaluation and investigation into his antineoplaston therapy. In his book, *The Burzynski Breakthrough*, Thomas D. Elias quotes Burzynski as saying, "I began asking in 1981 for the NCI and the American Cancer Society to review our patient records, but for years, neither would do it."[18] Finally, in 1991, an NCI team of doctors paid a site visit to Houston to investigate antineoplaston therapy. Elias quotes Burzynski commenting on the NCI investigation in the following words:

> I have no idea why, but they spent only one day here. We had prepared 20 brain tumor cases for them, but they had time to examine only seven. They reviewed all the medical records in each case, including MRI and CT scan films and pathology slides. They also inspected our chemical plant. When I asked them to stay longer and look at more cases, they told me that seven would be more than enough to prove the point.[19]

Even though they stayed only one day, the NCI site investigators were able to confirm the anticancer activity of antineoplastons. They also verified five complete remissions of the seven cases they evaluated. Later on, the NCI would minimize Dr. Burzynski's work by implying that he had only presented them with seven of his best cases. In saying this, the NCI was ignoring the 13 other cases Dr. Burzynski had prepared for their evaluation.

In the late 1990s, clinical trials of Dr. Burzynski's antineoplaston therapy produced very positive results in patients with malignant brain tumors and non-Hodgkin's lymphoma. In particular, the trials included 81 patients with astrocytoma brain tumors. Of these brain cancer patients, 73 percent benefited from the treatment; 32 percent achieved either complete remission or more than a 50 percent decrease in tumor size, and 41 percent of the brain cancer patients showed less than 50 percent decrease in tumor size but had no disease progression.[20]

Researchers in Japan have also carried out clinical trials on antineoplaston treatment with very promising results. Japanese doctors treated patients with advanced colon cancer with liver involvement using a combination of antineoplastons and low-dose chemotherapy. Since the dose of chemotherapy was below the threshold of toxicity, they did not identify any significant side effects. In randomized controlled clinical trials they found over five years survival in 91 percent of patients compared to 39 percent in the control group treated with chemotherapy alone! The same center found that antineoplaston AS2-1 capsules given to patients with liver cancer increased time to recurrence after standard treatment to 16 months compared with five months in the control group.[21]

Dr. Burzynski has never claimed that his antineoplaston therapy is a cure for all cancers. However, his clinical practice has proven without a doubt that antineoplaston therapy is able to turn many cancers into manageable diseases with long-term survival and often *does* bring about complete, long-term recoveries.

Attempts at Suppression

Even though antineoplaston therapy has been proven without a doubt to work better than conventional treatments for cancer, Stanislaw Burzynski has been the recipient of repeated attacks from the cancer industry. Refusing to give Dr. Burzynski an IND permit for clinical trials was the FDA's first overt resistance to his work. Then, in 1985, agents of the FDA barged into his Houston clinic accompanied by an armed marshal and confiscated the medical files of over a thousand cancer patients being treated there. Dr. Burzynski's 11 file cabinets of patient records and other medical documents were never given back to him. Eventually, Dr. Burzynski acquired a court order that allowed him to set up a copy machine in the FDA building 20 miles from his office. Here, he and his staff were permitted to copy medical records as they were needed.[22] This was done of course at Burzynski's own expense.

In 1995, the Burzynski Clinic was raided a second time by the FDA and thousands of documents *again* confiscated. Many legal battles ensued with hearings before grand juries. Finally, the FDA indicted Burzynski on 75 counts of mail fraud, contempt, and violation of FDA laws. If convicted, he could face up to 300 years in prison for practicing his proven non-toxic, life-saving techniques. There were a series of congressional hearings, and many of Burzynski's cancer patients testified or wrote letters to Congress in his defense.

In January 1997, Burzynski's court trial began. The FDA had three basic charges against him:[23]

1. Violation of an injunction

2. Mail fraud

3. Selling an unapproved drug in interstate commerce

All of the above charges proved to be bogus, and the FDA could not substantiate their claims that Dr. Burzynski was doing anything illegal. On March 3, 1997, the judge declared a mistrial and dismissed all charges against the doctor. The FDA could not come up with a single patient who would say anything bad about Dr. Burzynski. To the contrary, many of his patients were picketing and chanting outside the courthouse in support of Burzynski throughout the entire trial. Their picket signs read "Save the doctor who saves lives," and "I was cured by Dr. B."[24]

It is interesting to note that the issue of whether antineoplastons *actually worked* for cancer patients was never allowed to be a subject throughout the trial. Apparently, that was the one issue the FDA wanted to avoid. In fact, when the trial began to look like it was *not* going in the FDA's favor, chief prosecutor Clark complained, "The defense got the best of all worlds. They got to bring in the patients and imply that the stuff works, but we could not bring in experts to question its effects."[25] According to Dr. Julian Whitaker, Congressman Richard M. Burr proclaimed that the government's treatment of Dr. Burzynski was "one of the worst abuses of the criminal justice system [he had] ever witnessed."[26]

Today, Stanislaw Burzynski is still fighting to get antineoplastons accepted by the cancer industry and available to every patient who needs them. He finally got permission to conduct phase II clinical trials at his clinic in Houston using antineoplastons to treat cancer, HIV infection, and other autoimmune diseases. These trials have been overseen by the FDA and have had to conform to FDA regulations. Unfortunately, this means that only *certain* patients could meet the requirements to qualify for treatment in the trials. In many cases, these requirements involved the stipulation that only patients who had already gone through chemotherapy or radiation with unsuccessful results could be admitted to antineoplaston trials.

Because the Burzynski Clinic has had to comply with FDA regulations for trials, the doctors there have sadly been forced to turn away as many as 90 percent of the cancer patients who came to them for help. The greatest tragedy is that many of the cancer sufferers turned away were children with brain tumors.

The other tragedy is that, until antineoplaston therapy for cancer is fully approved by the FDA, it is still being considered an experimental treatment and not being covered by health insurance companies. Although Dr. Burzynski's treatment is not as expensive as typical chemotherapy, the difference is that most people can get their insurance companies to pay for most of their chemotherapy treatment costs. Without insurance coverage, the cost of antineoplaston treatment is too high for many people to afford. Treatment costs vary for different patients, but intravenous antineoplaston therapy for cancer typically runs about $7,000 per month. Antineoplaston therapy via capsules is less expensive.

For those patients who get a consultation but don't qualify for antineoplastons, the Burzynski Clinic has other options that have also shown success with cancer. For instance, "sodium phenylbutyrate" is an oral compound that has been found to be transformed by the liver into antineoplastons. Sodium phenylbutyrate from the Burzynski Clinic generally costs about $4,500 per month.

The high cost of treatment has been one of the things for which Dr. Burzynski has been criticized. Some critics have accused him of taking advantage of his patients. However, with just the smallest amount of research, anyone can see that just the opposite is true. Both Dr. Burzynski and his wife make much *lower* salaries than the average oncologist in the United States. Also, discussion with some of Dr. Burzynski's patients reveals that there have been many people who could not ultimately pay all their bills to the clinic and were not pursued.

Rather, it appears that the high cost of treatment is a direct result of three factors: (1) Dr. Burzynski must meet the salaries of a large staff of doctors and highly skilled technicians; (2) the expense of running his large plant to manufacture antineoplastons to FDA standards is very high; and (3) he constantly has to pay legal fees to defend his life-saving practice.

It is a shame that people with cancer who carry health insurance can get their medical bills covered if they undergo mutilating surgery, damaging radiation, or toxic chemotherapy, but *not* if they choose to undergo a treatment that is more efficacious and at the same time is totally safe to their bodies. But for many people with incurable cancer, it has been well worth it to come up with the money they needed for antineoplaston treatment.

To find out whether you or your loved one would qualify for antine-oplaston therapy and to find out what the cost would be, call the Burzynski Clinic and set up an in-person consultation immediately. There are many types of malignant cancers being treated at the clinic. The treatment protocol and length of treatment varies from patient to patient. Many patients are administered treatment via capsules or tablets and undergo no intravenous treatments. Others receive treatment intravenously via catheter attached to an infusion pump. (The dosage and dosing schedule depend on the type of cancer.) The infusion pump and therapy bags are small and light enough to be carried around by a young child.

Treatment generally requires an initial stay in Houston for one to three weeks. The Burzynski Clinic is an outpatient facility, but daily visits for the first few weeks help to assess how well the patient is responding to treatment and what dosage is optimum for them. After the initial few weeks, patients can then continue their treatment at home with follow-up visits to the clinic about every two months. When patients achieve a complete response of long duration, the intensive therapy may then be discontinued and the patient will continue with less intensive therapy in capsule form for another eight to twelve months.

There may be some insurance companies that will pay for antine-oplaston therapy, so if you are interested in this form of treatment, it is worth checking with your insurance group about it. As stated before, many people have found it worthwhile to come up with the cost of this treatment on their own, when their insurance company did not pay for it. This non-toxic form of cancer treatment is simply remarkable in its effectiveness and definitely something to look into for anyone with a cancer diagnosis.

Resources:

The Burzynski Clinic   (713) 335-5697
9432 Old Katy Road, Suite 200   www.burzynskiclinic.com
Houston, TX 77055

(To request a general information packet through the mail, call the above number or email your request to info@burzynskiclinic.com.)

For Consultation: In-depth consultation appointments at the Burzynski Clinic can be scheduled and generally run two to four hours long.

Cost of Treatment: Treatment costs vary greatly due the treatment protocols being tailored to each patient. A general ball-park figure would be around $4,500 to $7,500 per month (as of this printing). Depending on how many months treatment is required, the total cost could run around $100,000 or more.

Books

Thomas D. Elias. *The Burzynski Breakthrough*. Nevada City, California: Lexikos, 2001.

Richard Walters. *Options: The Alternative Cancer Therapy Book*. New York: Avery Penguin Putnam, 1993.

Ralph W. Moss. *The Cancer Industry*. Equinox Press, New York, 1999.

Newsletter

Dr. Julian Whitaker's Health and Healing Newsletter, Mid-February 1996 Supplement.

Websites

www.burzynskiclinic.com

www.burzynskipatientgroup.org

www.burzynskipatientgroup.org/burdickreport.htm

9

Protocel®
History and Theory

As much as I was amazed by the effectiveness of other alternative non-toxic approaches to cancer, I was stunned by the effectiveness of a brown liquid formula called Protocel®. Because there are few other sources of in-depth information published about this remarkable product, four chapters of this book are devoted to the Protocel® formula alone.

Protocel® is a unique single-product approach that does *not* rely on herbs or vitamins or minerals for their anti-cancer activity and does *not* rely on boosting the immune system. It was designed to specifically target cancer cells in a way that makes them eventually fall apart and die, leaving normal healthy cells unharmed. And it does this by targeting the *anaerobic* aspect of cancer cells.

The brilliant Nobel prize-winning scientist, Dr. Otto Warburg, argued that all cancer cells are primarily anaerobic. Dr. Warburg lectured extensively on his discovery that, in the human body, cancer cells primarily use the fermentation of glucose to obtain most of their energy rather than primarily using oxygen to help them "burn" energy from various substances like all normal healthy cells do. He fervently argued that the prime difference between cancer cells and normal healthy cells is that healthy cells are aerobic and cancer cells are anaerobic in how they produce energy for themselves.

Protocel® targets *anaerobic* cells by interfering with their cell respiration (energy production). Since all the healthy cells of the body are *aerobic*, they are not harmed. (More details on this will be presented later.) By only negatively impacting the anaerobic cells of the body, Protocel® effectively targets cancer cells and other unhealthy cells without harming any of a person's normal healthy cells.

Protocel® is currently being sold as a general health-enhancing product. It is marketed as a "cell cleanser" because of its powerful ability to rid the body of non-productive, damaged cells that have converted to anaerobic functioning to survive. Because anaerobic cells are involved in so many chronic illnesses (such as arthritis, chronic fatigue, high blood pressure, diabetes, multiple sclerosis, viral infections, and others), Protocel® can be effective in improving a variety of health problems. It is important to understand that Protocel® is *not* currently being sold or advertised as a treatment for cancer and is being marketed with no claims as to its effectiveness against cancer or any other disease.

However, this formula *was* originally created as a cancer treatment by the chemist who developed it, and for those people who *choose* to use Protocel® for their cancer, it can be extremely effective. And it is one of the cheapest and easiest approaches available. A person can simply order Protocel® over the phone and have it delivered to their home in a few days. They don't have to go through the rigors of difficult diet changes, frequent juicing, intravenous treatments, mountains of supplements, or enemas. They merely drink a small amount of the formula in water four or five times a day. Protocel® is completely non-toxic and only costs about $100 to $120 a month.

History

Protocel® has a very interesting history, particularly regarding how the product was originally conceived. It was developed by an American chemist named Jim Sheridan who first called his formula Entelev®. Later, it was renamed Cancell® and then finally Protocel®. Today, Protocel® is the only true duplication of Jim Sheridan's original Entelev®/Cancell® formula according to the Sheridan family. The following is a brief history of how this product came into being.

Jim Sheridan was born in 1912 in a Pennsylvania mining town. His father and both his grandfathers were coal miners. To help support his family, he had to work side jobs while he was going to high school. Finally,

Sheridan was fortunate enough to win a scholarship to Carnegie Tech in Pittsburgh. He initially had aspirations of being a mining engineer and Carnegie Tech had the best program in the country at the time. In his freshman year, however, Sheridan realized he was really destined to be a chemist and switched to chemistry as his field of study instead.

What is important to understand about Jim Sheridan is that, even as a young man, he was devoutly spiritual. He knew he had a good mind and in his early teens he would pray to God that he be able to use his intellect to help mankind. Unlike most other boys in high school, he also prayed to be able to someday help find a cure for cancer. For Sheridan, it wasn't his ego at play here. He truly wanted to be of service to his fellow man. Soon, he would experience a series of auspicious events that would lead him in that direction.

These events started in late high school when Sheridan started having a series of recurring dreams. They were unusual in that he kept seeing a chemical formula over and over again. This formula meant nothing to him and he could find no one else who understood it either. However, after Sheridan started college, he came face to face with the chemical formula of his recurring dreams. It was listed in print in the title of an article he came across by accident. The article was printed in a huge source book, and Sheridan just happened to have opened the book to that page. It was an article related to cancer and known carcinogens.

The next important event that led to the development of Sheridan's unique formula occurred in April 1931, while he was demonstrating some chemistry concepts at a Carnegie Tech open-house meeting. A high school boy asked Sheridan if the bright yellow color of a liquid in one beaker was caused by something called "chromate." Sheridan said that it was, and one of the students then wanted to know how that color could be changed to a different color. To this, Sheridan answered that any change in the oxidation state of the sample would result in a color change. He then went to a shelf and picked an acid at random and proceeded to add the acid to the solution in the beaker to demonstrate. To Sheridan's complete surprise, the liquid in the beaker turned all the colors of the rainbow in perfectly defined layers! He and the high school boys stood there dumbfounded, looking at six layers of color in the beaker in the very order they would occur in a rainbow—red, orange, yellow, green, blue, and violet.

This unusual result even astonished the professors who were there, and everyone gathered around to see the amazing sight. One professor stated that it looked like a case of "rhythmic banding," and if it were, then each band of color would be 2.7 times the width of the band above it. Upon measuring the bands of color in the beaker, they found this was indeed the case, though none of the professors or students understood the significance of this rhythmic banding phenomenon.

Shortly after this episode, and unconnected with the incident involving the beaker, Sheridan was given a long-term project by his advisor that involved studying the effects of changes in dielectric constant on reactions between positive and negative ions. This work was related to a recently published theory called the "Debye-Hückel Theory." For several years after the odd incident with the rainbow colors in the beaker, Sheridan worked on testing the validity of the Debye-Hückel Theory. In order to be competent enough to do this, he had to take two years of physical chemistry. He was also forced by his advisor to take an advanced course called "Theory and Thermodynamics of Solutions" *three times* (despite the fact that he received an "A" each time he took the class).

Once Sheridan started studying the Debye-Hückel Theory, he also realized that the chemical formula he had dreamed about in high school, and then had found by accident after starting college, was in fact associated with the Debye-Hückel Theory! Looking back, it certainly seemed that events were leading Sheridan in a very specific direction.

The final important event in the development of Sheridan's formula occurred on September 6, 1936. It happened in the afternoon while he was taking a nap. During this nap, Sheridan had an unusual dream. He explained it in these words:

> The dream brought together the event of the rainbow in the beaker and the work on the Debye Theory. In the 1936 dream, the layers of the rainbow represented the respiratory enzymes. Each color represented an enzyme at a specific redox level. The electrons from the Debye Theory represented the energy units in the respiration moving from glucose to oxygen via that respiratory system. Somehow, the dream suggested the possibility of controlled altering of the pathway of energy flow and energy production in the respiratory system to: (a) cause a cancer, or (b) cure a cancer.[1]

Jim Sheridan was profoundly affected by the guidance he felt he had received in this dream. He wrote:

> When I woke up, I felt that I had received my *marching orders*. Three years later I bought my first mice and I was on my way in my basement lab. The suggested cure was to make the cancer cell even more primitive—to the point where the cancer cell would lyse.[2]

(The terms "redox," "lyse" and "respiratory enzymes" will be explained shortly.) Jim Sheridan dedicated himself to pursuing the goal put forth in his afternoon dream of 1936. It took him many years of hard work and trial and error to develop his formula fully. In fact, he actually worked on the formula from the 1930s until the 1990s. Most of that time, Sheridan worked on "the project," as he called it, at home after hours or whenever he had some spare time. He made his living by being employed full-time doing other work. At first, Sheridan was employed as a chemist at Dow Chemical Company. While working there, he studied law and passed his bar exam, eventually becoming a patent attorney. In 1946, Sheridan left Dow Chemical to practice law.

At this point, Sheridan was able to fully stock his laboratory at home where he continued to develop his formula and use mice for testing. He never stopped working on his "project." By the early 1950s, he obtained a private grant to work at the Detroit Cancer Institute, where he further improved his formula in a more formal laboratory environment. After a while, Sheridan began getting 70 to 80 percent positive results on the mice cancers he was treating. He kept working on his material and improving it, and by 1983, he felt he finally had a formula that could consistently cure about 80 percent of the mice.

Sheridan originally named his product Entelev®, which stems from the classical Greek phrase "Entelechy" (pronounced enteleekee). Sheridan's understanding was that "Entelechy" translated as "that part of man known only to God," and he added the letters EV to represent "electro-valence." Thus, he created the name "Entelev" to mean the *electrovalence of man known only to God*. The electrovalence part will be explained in the next section as we look at the theory behind Sheridan's formula.

Theory

To understand the theory behind Jim Sheridan's formula, we start with the concept that all cancer cells are primarily anaerobic. Cancer cells are not the *only* type of anaerobic cell found in the body, however. In other words, we can have *other* types of anaerobic cells in our bodies that are not necessarily cancer cells. But any human cell that is anaerobic is unhealthy or abnormal, and these unhealthy anaerobic cells tend to be involved in illnesses of various sorts.

In a nutshell, this is how Protocel® works: When a person takes Protocel® regularly every day, the formula biochemically lowers the voltage of every cell in the body *just a little bit*. (Actually, for those with technical backgrounds, the more accurate term is "capacitance" rather than voltage, but most people understand the term voltage better.) This results in an approximate voltage reduction of about 10 to 15 percent and Protocel® accomplishes this by interfering with the production of ATP (adenosine triphosphate) in the cell. Because anaerobic cells obtain their energy by the fermentation of glucose, or "glycolysis," instead of by oxidation like normal cells, they operate on a minimum energy level and sustain a lower voltage than normal cells. The slight reduction in voltage caused by Protocel® shifts the cancer cells downward to a point below the minimum that cancer cells need to remain intact. When this happens, the cancer cells (as well as other anaerobic cells of the body) break down, or "lyse," into harmless protein. In other words, they cannot hold themselves together anymore and they simply fall apart!

Normal healthy cells of the body, on the other hand, sustain such a high voltage level that the slight reduction in voltage caused by Protocel® does not hurt them. This is why Protocel® is deadly to cancer cells but harmless to the rest of the body. The details of how this happens are somewhat complicated, but the following is a simplified explanation of how Protocel® works, using an analogy to car batteries.

One could say that all the cells of the human body are somewhat like little car batteries in the sense that they must manufacture and deliver energy throughout the cell so that the cell can perform its important functions. This process of producing and distributing energy in each cell is called "cell respiration." (Most of us think of respiration as the process of breathing oxygen through our lungs, but on a cellular level, the term "respiration" refers to the acquiring and distributing of energy for the cell, not to breathing oxygen.) Every cell in the body can only grow, divide and carry out its specific functions as long as the cell can continue to get sufficient energy to support those functions. This could be likened to how the battery in a car can continue to do its job only as long as the engine is kept running to resupply the battery with the energy that continually gets used up. If the supply of energy to the car battery is cut off while the energy from the battery is still outgoing, as when a person turns the engine off but leaves the lights on, then the battery energy reserves will be used up and the car battery will eventually "die."

Although human cells are somewhat like car batteries, they are also infinitely more sophisticated. So, when *more* energy is being used up than is getting supplied to the cell through respiration, the cell doesn't immediately die. Instead, it tries to compensate by transforming itself to need less energy. It does this by making changes in its respiration.

To understand this process, we need to know that, central to the respiratory system of each cell, there is something called the "oxidation reduction system." Scientists often refer to this as the "redox system." Although every cell in the body has a redox system, there are gradations of how advanced, or efficient, this redox system is in various types of cells. These gradations could be looked at as the steps on a ladder. Different types of cells in the body could then be represented as different points on this ladder. In Sheridan's own words,

> The oxidation reduction system can be thought of as a ladder, with a different chemical reaction taking place on each step. The respiratory reaction which takes place on each step of this ladder is the same as on every other step in what it produces (i.e. energy for the cell to do its work), but each step is also different from every other step in the sense of how effective the reaction is.
>
> The bottom steps of the ladder involve relatively simple or 'primitive' respiratory reactions. An example of a primitive reaction would be yeast while it is fermenting. Keep in mind that this is still an amazingly complex reaction. It is only 'simple' or 'primitive' compared to the other reactions in the oxidation-reduction system.
>
> The higher steps involve more complex respiratory reactions. The primitive reactions at the bottom of the ladder take place without oxygen being present. The higher respiratory reactions require the presence of oxygen. Generally, for 'reduction' you are moving down the ladder. For 'oxidation' you are moving up the ladder.
>
> Each 'step' on this ladder has a different 'potential'. 'Potential' means a measurable *electrical voltage*, like a small battery would have. Primitive yeast cells which are fermenting will give off a certain amount of electrical energy, i.e. movement of electrons. (We are talking about very *small* amounts of electrical energy.) As you move up toward the top of the ladder you will get increased potential energy. Thus, the potential electrical energy at the top of the ladder is greater than at the bottom. The top of the ladder has a potential of about +0.4 volts while the bottom is about −0.2 volts.[3]

Thus, a normal, healthy aerobic cell would be represented high on the ladder, and anaerobic and primitive cells would be represented lower on the ladder.

According to Sheridan's theory, a healthy cell will maintain a balance of ingoing and outgoing energy and will remain over time in its same position on the redox ladder hierarchy. Short-term drains of energy on cells are usually no problem, and cells can normally regain their balance without serious difficulty. But just like a car battery, if there is a *long-term*, severe drain on the energy of a cell, then there can be a serious problem. In a chronic energy drain situation, the balance point of the cell's respiration system will eventually be affected to where the point of balance *will be forced to occur at a lower oxidation reduction level for the cell to survive.*

When this energy balance point is forced to go lower, the cell could be said to move down the redox ladder. And it can continue to move down the ladder until it hits what Sheridan called a "critical point." According to his theory, this critical point is the lowest point the cell can go on the redox ladder and still retain its primary similarities to a normal cell. However, at this critical point, the cell is also now on the highest point of the ladder that could be said to apply to primitive cells. In other words, the cell that is forced to move down the redox ladder to survive can get to a point where it is, essentially, straddling the fence between being "normal" and being "primitive."

According to Sheridan, this is a very interesting point for a cell to be at. At this straddling point, the cell actually becomes quite stable because it is not enough like a normal cell to be differentiated and to function normally, but it is also not enough like a fully primitive cell for the body to know how to get rid of it. It is also at this critical point where the cell *may* become an anaerobic cancer cell.

Sheridan concluded that it would be difficult to move a cancer cell *back up* the redox ladder and make it normal again. He devised his formula to work by taking advantage of the fact that the cancer cell sits on the critical point of the ladder, or right on the dividing line between normal cells and primitive cells. By reducing the voltage (or potential) of every cell in the body just a tiny bit, those cells that are sitting on the fence are the most affected. The reduction of potential caused by Protocel® effectively reduces their respiration ability just enough to push them *down* the redox ladder to where they are fully in the primitive zone, or even past it. At this point, the cancer cells are not able to produce enough energy to survive, and they subsequently die off through the process of lysing. In one article, Sheridan wrote that the way his formula affects cell respiration is

> . . . by shunting off 'energy units' of the cell as it is working, so the energy is not going through the respiratory system. (An 'energy unit' is two electrons and a proton). Thus, work is being done by the cell, but not respiration . . . If work is being done, but not respiration, the cell is forced

further down the oxidation-reduction ladder. Thus, once respiration is reduced, the cell is forced down completely into the primitive state.

One of the chemicals which reduces respiration is catechol. The natural catechols have many different oxidation-reduction potentials (i.e. the level on the oxidation-reduction ladder where the particular catechol will work or operate.) The trick is to find one that works at the same level as a cancer cell, i.e. at that 'critical point' level.

Entelev/Cancell was developed to act like a catechol, i.e. to inhibit respiration at the critical point.[4]

(**NOTE:** "Catechol" here refers to a *type* of chemical, the way "acid" or "enzyme" does.) By following guidance that came to him in a dream, Sheridan was able to develop a truly ingenious way to cause cancer cells, as well as other anaerobic cells of the body, to self-destruct.

Tony Bell, Ph.D., is a chemist who understands on a detailed, technical level how Sheridan's formula works. To put it in simple terms that most of us can understand, Dr. Bell explains that for each cell in the body, the voltage of the cell operates as the cement or glue that holds the cell together. Healthy aerobic cells operate on a much higher energy level or voltage than unhealthy anaerobic cells. So, in terms of energy voltage, healthy cells have plenty of energy to spare. But according to Dr. Bell, cancer cells sit right on the edge of the cliff in terms of voltage, and have very little to spare. When the voltage of a cancer cell is reduced by 10 to 15 percent the cell subsequently loses the "cement" that holds it together, and it breaks down into harmless protein that the body can then easily dispose of.

This process of the cancer cells breaking down is called "lysing," and it involves the bursting of the cancer cell membrane. This particular way of cancer cells falling apart often results in a clear or somewhat yellowish, egg white-like substance. The body then processes this substance out (which is really just dead cancer cell parts) through various elimination systems. In other words, when cancer patients use Protocel®, this egg white-like material *may* come out of them through any avenue that the body uses to get rid of waste. Thus, people using Protocel® for cancer will often see mucousy material in their feces and/or urine, or experience a runny nose or crusty eyes in the morning. Sometimes, people will even cough or vomit up mucousy whitish stuff. If any of this happens, it can generally be taken as a good sign that dead cancer cell parts are being ejected out of the body.

Many people looking into the Protocel® formula first want to know what is in it. This is perfectly understandable. However, some of the ingredients are quite common, such as potassium and sodium, while others in a proprietary blend are so unusual they would mean little to most people. What is clear is that Protocel® is not an herbal formula, it is not a vitamin or mineral supplement, it is not homeopathic, and none of its ingredients are particularly known for their anti-cancer activity by themselves.

The most important thing to remember about this formula is that it is only when all the parts are put together in just the right way that they work as a whole against cancer. Thus, the ingredients should not be evaluated individually, since putting them together with just the right process produces a unique end result—a powerful formula that is able to inhibit respiration at the critical point in cancer cells.

Side benefits of the Protocel® formula are that it is less toxic than an aspirin a day, it is somewhat of an immune system booster, and it is an extremely powerful antioxidant. Testing done at the Brunswick Laboratories in Massachusetts showed Protocel® to have an ORAC antioxidant value of approximately 1.4 million (μmole TE/L). This means it may be the *most* powerful antioxidant ever tested in this way. But remember, Protocel® does not get rid of cancer by being an antioxidant or by boosting the immune system. It gets rid of cancer by interfering with the production of ATP in anaerobic cells to the point where they can no longer hold themselves together and they fall apart. Thus, Protocel® directly kills cancer in this way, though technically there are no whole dead cancer cells left over when Protocel® is done with them. (Only broken down cancer cell parts.)

In the next chapter, we will look at some remarkable testimonials from people who have used Jim Sheridan's unique formula to *outsmart* their cancer.

10

Protocel®
Case Stories

This chapter highlights 15 real-life case stories of people who used Jim Sheridan's formula for their cancer recovery. To show how long this formula has been working for people, I have included some cases that go back to the early days when the formula was called Entelev® and Cancell®. Back then, it was always *given* away to cancer patients for free. (More on that and another man named Ed Sopcak, who donated his time and money to produce tens of thousands of bottles of it will be discussed in the next chapter.) It wasn't until the year 2000 that Jim Sheridan's formula was finally produced as a dietary supplement for sale and re-named Protocel®.

Thus, people have only been *purchasing* this formula as an official product since the year 2000—but many were able to use it for free at least as far back as the 1980s. When Protocel® finally became available, the original Entelev® was reproduced and named "Protocel® Formula 23" and the original Cancell® was reproduced and named "Protocel® Formula 50."

(**NOTE:** Anyone who is impressed with the following case stories and interested in using Protocel® for their cancer should read Chapter 12 carefully for how to use it effectively. There are "do's" and "don'ts" to using this approach that can make the difference between achieving full recovery or not.)

Dr. Bell, who was mentioned in the previous chapter, became interested in this formula when one of his own family members came down with cancer, and we'll start with the story of his brother first.

Case Story #1—Lung Cancer Metastasized to Brain

Dr. Tony Bell first became acquainted with Sheridan's formula (then called Cancell®) when his brother, Frank, was diagnosed with cancer in 1989. Frank's cancer was non-small cell lung cancer. His doctors proceeded with treatment by first surgically removing one of Frank's lungs. Then, in 1990, they found out that the cancer was in Frank's other lung as well and had also metastasized to his brain. Frank's doctors directed radiation at the brain tumors, but it had little effect and the tumors remained.

Shortly after the radiation treatments, Frank had a heart attack because his lung cancer had seriously stressed his heart. He survived the attack, but was too ill to undergo chemotherapy at this point. Frank's doctors sent him home and gave him about two months to live. They told the family not to worry about the cancer, because at this point it was probably Frank's heart that would kill him.

Frank then heard about Cancell® and asked his brother, Dr. Bell, to look into it for him. Dr. Bell looked into it and didn't think it would work, but told his brother he might as well try it because it wouldn't hurt him. After taking Cancell® for a while, Frank told Dr. Bell, "I don't know if the Cancell® is working on the cancer or not, but it sure is a lot better than morphine because I'm not in pain anymore!"

After seven months on Cancell®, more tests and scans were done and the doctors couldn't find any evidence of cancer in Frank's lungs or brain, or anywhere else in his body! Luckily for Frank, his heart was somehow strong enough for him to play golf on an almost daily basis for six more years, during which time he remained cancer-free. When Frank finally passed away, it was due to heart failure—*not* cancer.

Case Story #2—Kidney Cancer

Another amazing testimonial comes from an 86-year-old man named Gunther. In early 1997, when Gunther was 80, he started feeling lousy.

He went in for a general checkup and renal cell cancer was found in his left kidney. Gunther's doctor told him that chemotherapy does not work very well for kidney cancer, and he recommended that Gunther have his kidney entirely removed.

While Gunther was thinking about this, he searched the Internet for more information. Incredibly, he found four other people who had been in a similar situation to him. They all four had renal cell cancer in one kidney, and they all four had had their kidneys removed. Unfortunately, they all four said that the kidney cancer had then metastasized to other parts of their bodies. The good news, however, was that all four of these people had then recovered from their metastasized kidney cancer by using Cancell®. Gunther talked with some of these people and decided not to have the surgery. Instead, he found someone who had a few extra bottles of the formula, and in mid-April 1997 Gunther started taking Cancell®.

Toward the end of April, Gunther traveled to Germany. Someone there convinced him to seek a second opinion about his kidney cancer. He agreed to do this and had a consultation with a cancer specialist there. The German specialist came to the same conclusion as Gunther's American doctor, and told him he should have his kidney taken out.

At this point, Gunther decided to have his kidney removed and made an appointment with the German doctor for the surgery. But before the surgery was performed, Gunther heard that a doctor back in the United States at the Cleveland Clinic was one of the world's best specialists on kidney cancer. He immediately called from Hamburg to make an appointment at the Cleveland Clinic, cancelled his surgery, and flew back to the United States to consult with this top kidney cancer specialist instead.

In Cleveland, another CT scan was performed and the specialist pronounced again that Gunther had a dangerous renal cell tumor on his left kidney. His right kidney looked fine with just a benign cyst on it. This doctor said the same thing as the other two had. He suggested Gunther have his kidney removed. Gunther finally scheduled the recommended surgery with this specialist and it was set for mid-July 1997. (He was also still taking the Cancell® he had started in mid-April.)

Three days before surgery, Gunther was back at the Cleveland Clinic to have his pre-surgery exam. But he was by this time feeling so good that his doctor thought it would be alright to postpone the surgery. So Gunther once again cancelled his appointment to have his kidney removed. He just kept taking the Cancell® and visiting his doctor for checkups.

In December of that year, Gunther underwent another CT scan. It showed no change in the size of the tumor, and Gunther was still feeling good. So the doctor said, "Let's just continue to watch it." In another six months, another CT scan was performed that also showed no tumor growth. At this point, Gunther got lazy about getting his cancer checked and went a while without another scan. He kept taking the Cancell® for about two years (from April 1997 to mid-1999), then stopped the Cancell® and didn't worry about it anymore.

In September 2000, however, Gunther became ill and developed a high fever. After hearing about his history of cancer, the doctor did an ultrasound on his kidney and surrounding areas. The result was that the doctor could not find any tumor at all.

At the time of this writing, Gunther is now almost 87 years old and more active than many young people. He swims laps every morning for 45 minutes, he is still active in business, and he travels around the world quite a lot for pleasure. No one would guess that he'd been diagnosed with kidney cancer six years earlier. And no one would guess that he had *never* gone through any surgery, chemotherapy, or radiation. The only thing he ever did was to take Cancell®.

Case Story #3—Pancreatic Cancer

Pancreatic cancer is well known as one of the most deadly types of cancer. So it was truly exciting to speak with a 69-year-old man who had recovered from this type of cancer through the use of Cancell® alone. His name is Bill.

In March of 1988, Bill was diagnosed with pancreatic cancer and his doctor didn't think he would live more than six months. He chose not to do conventional treatment of any kind, and instead immediately started taking Cancell®. Bill took Cancell® for two and a half years, between 1988 and 1991. After doing so, he was pronounced cancer-free. His doctors were astonished.

Bill told his story in a very simple, matter-of-fact way. He didn't take any vitamins, minerals, herbs, enzymes, or supplements of any kind while he was on Cancell®. All he did was take ¼ teaspoonful of the formula every six hours (3 times during the day and once in the middle of the night), along with going off sugar and cutting back on his intake of red meat. He has remained healthy and completely free of cancer for over 15 years!

Case Story #4—Breast Cancer Metastasized to Bones

A story of breast cancer that had metastasized to the bones was told to me by a woman named Roberta. Roberta was 65 years old when I spoke with her, but when she was only 41, she was diagnosed with breast cancer. That was in October 1979. Back in those days, doctors didn't do lumpectomies, they just went straight to mastectomy. So she underwent a mastectomy immediately after her diagnosis and, during the surgery, five of her lymph nodes were removed to see if the cancer had already metastasized. Unfortunately, it had. After the surgery, Roberta was treated for about six months with chemotherapy and toward the end of that period she also went through a three-week round of radiation.

Roberta went through the full treatment regimen that her doctor had planned for her. But after completing it, she started having some physical problems as a result of the chemotherapy and radiation. One of the problems was that, as a result of the radiation being targeted near her throat, Roberta began having serious difficulty swallowing. The other problem was that she suddenly developed insulin-dependent diabetes. This last development was quite a surprise, since she had never suffered from any sort of diabetes before, nor had she shown signs that she was starting to develop it.

After receiving the mastectomy, chemo, and radiation, Roberta was given a bone scan. But the results showed that the cancer was *not* gone and had, instead, metastasized to her bones with spots on her clavicle and ribs. Luckily for Roberta, she had heard about Entelev® and had already started taking it. Her doctor didn't think the Entelev® would do her any good but didn't discourage her from taking it.

A couple of months after her first bone scan, Roberta was given a second scan. This time, the suspicious spots had reduced in size considerably. For a number of months more, Roberta did nothing in terms of treatment except take Entelev®. In those days, there wasn't as much known about the effects of diet or supplements on cancer, and so she didn't take any other nutritional supplements or do anything different with her diet at all. She stayed on the Entelev® until all of her scans and blood tests were completely normal, and the doctors couldn't find evidence of any cancer whatsoever. Then she continued to take the formula for a few months more just to be sure. She hasn't had a recurrence of her cancer since. Roberta has been monitored regularly by a cancer specialist for the past 23 years, and all her tests have continued to be normal.

Case Story #5 — Central Nervous System Cancer (Glioblastoma Multiforme, Stage IV)

The following case of a woman named Elonna is considered one of the most celebrated of all Cancell® recoveries. That is partly because Elonna was diagnosed with a very rare form of nervous system cancer called Glioblastoma Multiforme, stage IV. (According to conventional medicine, malignant glios are virtually always fatal.) Her case was also somewhat famous because when she was diagnosed with cancer she had just given birth to quintuplets. One baby unfortunately did not survive, but the other four did. According to Elonna, she was given a CT scan when the four babies were about two-and-one-half weeks old in order to diagnose some severe pain she had been having during and after the pregnancy. They found that the source of the pain was a tumor on her spinal cord in the thoracic area.

An additional MRI and a consultation with a neurosurgeon were done, then Elonna was taken into surgery to have her tumor removed. After the surgery, she was paralyzed from the waist down and told that the tumor was malignant and they were *not* able to remove all of the cancer throughout her spine. She was also told that now there would be free-floating cancer cells in her spinal fluid that would quickly travel to her brain and develop into new tumors. Her doctors said she would not live to see her four babies' first birthday.

Elonna's doctors wanted to put her through either a very aggressive bone marrow chemotherapy treatment, or 30 treatments of radiation at very high calibration. Either treatment choice would cause her body great damage and with either treatment the doctors could still not hope for her to live more than three to six months. Obviously, her conventional options were not good. But because of the media attention that Elonna received as a result of giving birth to quintuplets and receiving a rare cancer diagnosis soon afterward, many people saw her story on television or in the newspapers. As a result, she and her husband were barraged with mail containing concerned suggestions as to alternatives. One of these suggestions was to try Cancell®.

Elonna was skeptical about Cancell® at first. Her initial words to her husband were, "If there was a cure for cancer, don't you think they would be using it instead of letting thousands of people die?" But she had no other choice and her husband seemed to have faith that Cancell® would work. On November 12, 1989, Elonna started taking Cancell®.

She decided to refuse the conventional treatments of chemotherapy and radiation that had been offered to her since they could promise her no more than six months anyway. She really wanted to be able to take care of her babies and watch them grow up.

At the end of Elonna's second week on Cancell®, and into her third week, she was admitted back into a local hospital for eight days because of blood clots and a hemoglobin problem. Luckily her doctor allowed her family to come into the hospital every day and administer the Cancell® to her around the clock.

According to Elonna, after several weeks, she began to notice an improvement in her condition, though she still could not walk. However, it was only 18 hours after her first dose that she began to eliminate the cancer waste product. She says, "It literally poured out of me: I threw it up; my bowel movements were extremely loose and stringy and frequent. I lost it in my urine; my nose ran so much I had to keep a tissue with me at all times. I sweated it out profusely; and I had hot and cold flashes and night sweats. When the nurses would give me a sponge bath after a night sweat, the water would be a golden brown color with what they referred to as 'tapioca balls' floating in it."

The lysing symptoms Elonna experienced were worth it. Amazingly, by February 1990, only about three and a half months after she started on Cancell®, new scans of her brain and entire spinal cord came back negative for any signs of cancer.

Elonna stayed on Cancell® for a total of two years and three months to be sure all of her cancer was gone and to help repair a great deal of the extensive nerve damage that had been caused by the cancer and the surgery. She had to go through agonizing physical therapy to regain her ability to walk again, but she is now walking and living a normal life. Best of all, she has been able to see her children grow up and enjoy them to the fullest, thanks to Cancell®. It is now over 18 years after Elonna's bout with cancer, and she continues to remain completely cancer-free.

Case Story #6—Melanoma, Stage IV

Roma is an 80-year-old woman who also has quite a story to share. In October of 1989, when she was 66 years old, Roma was diagnosed with melanoma. A few months before, she had noticed a dark spot on the big toe of her right foot. She didn't think anything of it, but it came to the attention of a doctor she was seeing about a bone spur problem in her foot. The doctor did not suspect cancer, and he proceeded to cut into the dark spot with a knife and attempted to dig it out with tweezers. This procedure did not do any good, and the opening he created never healed.

Roma finally went to another doctor, who took some scrapings of the now oozing dark spot for biopsy. The diagnostic results came back stating it was melanoma. Her doctors then debated whether or not to surgically remove the whole foot or just part of it. They settled on removing her right big toe and a great deal of extra tissue going about halfway up her foot. But in just two weeks after the surgery, melanoma spots started showing on her second toe, the one next to the big toe that had just been removed.

At this point, Roma decided to try an alternative treatment and went down to a clinic in Mexico where she was instructed to do 13 juices and several coffee enemas each day. She stayed there for one week, which cost her $3,000, then went home and continued the juicing and enema regimen for a full three months. But although the melanoma was not spreading throughout her body, it continued to grow slowly. At this point, her melanoma cancer was now considered to be stage IV.

Then a friend told Roma about Cancell®. On May 23, 1990, she started taking Cancell®. No longer doing the juicing/enema regimen, she simply took Cancell®, eliminated sugar and cut back on red meat in her diet. Roma says that it wasn't until about the second to third month on Cancell® that she noticed the melanoma was getting smaller. Finally, it quit seeping around Christmas 1990. The spots never completely went away, but they eventually changed color to a light brown. In every other way, she felt normal.

After two-and-one-half years on Cancell®, Roma's doctors performed another biopsy and could find no indication of cancer at all. At that point, she stopped the Cancell® and has not experienced any recurrence of her melanoma since.

Case Story #7—Intestinal Cancer

In May 2001, Sarah was 83 years old and suddenly got very sick. She was experiencing a lot of vomiting and diarrhea. She was finally taken into the hospital and an ultrasound revealed a mass in her intestine which turned out to be a large malignant bowel tumor. Sarah went into surgery where the doctors removed as much as they could of the tumor, but proclaimed that they couldn't get it all. Her cancer had not yet metastasized, but the tumor was shaped like a large comma and the tail end of it, which would have been too risky to remove, still remained in her body after the surgery. Sarah spent three weeks in intensive care and then her doctors wanted to schedule her for more aggressive treatment with chemotherapy. Sarah did not want to undergo this course of treatment and flatly refused.

Toward the end of the summer, Sarah had still not done any more treatment of any kind since the surgery and was back to feeling very sick every day. But by this time her daughter had heard about Protocel® and she was able to convince her mother to try it. In August 2001, Sarah started taking Protocel® Formula 23. According to Sarah, after just one week of taking Protocel® she started to feel better. Soon, she began to notice mucousy material coming out of her body through her bowel movements.

At one point that summer Sarah's daughter, Elizabeth, was in church and met up with her mother's doctor. The doctor told Elizabeth, "Your mother's *got* to have chemotherapy." Elizabeth knew this doctor personally and liked him very much. But she replied to him, "No, she's going to go the natural route." Upon hearing that, the doctor grabbed Elizabeth's arm and marched her out of the church with him. Once outside, he adamantly said, "Your mother will be dead in a year if she doesn't do chemotherapy!"

But Sarah chose to remain steadfast in her use of Protocel® and continued to decline conventional treatments. Over the next few months, Sarah felt better and better and more than two years later, she was still feeling great. At that time, a series of comprehensive lab tests all indicated that she was in remission and as Sarah liked to say, "on Protocel® and prayer!"

Case Story #8—Prostate Cancer

Sarah's 89-year-old husband, Bernard, also had a Protocel® story to tell. At age 85, Bernard was diagnosed with prostate cancer. His doctors surgically removed a tumor on his prostate and Bernard was scheduled to get some follow-up treatments to make sure the cancer did not recur. But unfortunately, Bernard's doctor suddenly died, and as a result Bernard did not get any more treatment of any kind for eight months. Then he heard about Protocel® from his daughter and started taking it at the same time his wife Sarah did. When he started the formula, his PSA count was 19. In about eight months' time, just through using Protocel® alone, his PSA was down to 4.

Bernard never did any conventional treatment other than the surgery for his prostate cancer. At the time of this writing, he is still doing fine and considered cancer-free.

Case Story #9—Prostate Cancer

Albert is 73 years old. Five years ago, Albert was diagnosed with prostate cancer. A needle biopsy was performed that included five or six samples, and from these Albert's prostate cancer was given a "Gleason" scale rating of 4.5. (The Gleason scale is a scale from 1 to 10 that indicates how aggressive, or fast-growing, a man's prostate cancer is.) Thus, Albert's cancer was just about in the middle of this scale. His PSA level at the time was 13, and his prostate gland was enlarged.

Luckily for Albert, he already knew about Protocel® at the time he was diagnosed and he immediately went on the formula. Albert never underwent surgery, radiation or any other conventional treatment for his cancer. After six months on Protocel®, his PSA count went up to 16. But then it started to go down, eventually stabilizing at 9.7. (It is common for the PSA count to rise for a while as the cancer is lysing away.)

For many men, 9.7 would still be a high PSA count. But in Albert's case, this had been his "normal" reading for five to six years prior to his cancer diagnosis. His doctor theorized that Albert had calcification in his prostate gland, which causes irritation and inflammation, and that this raised his PSA level above what is considered normal for most men.

For a few more years, Albert's PSA count remained stable at 9.7. He continued to get tests done over the years (PSA tests, digital exams, CT and bone scans, blood work-ups, and an MRI), and his doctors have continued to pronounce him free of cancer. In early 2003, Albert's PSA reading went down to 7.0. This was the lowest PSA reading that Albert had ever had. Albert continues to feel great and to show no sign of cancer.

Case Story #10—Brain Cancer

Steve is a 41-year-old, happily married man with two sons. On Christmas Day 2000, he suffered a grand mal seizure during a nap. After being unconscious for about 30 minutes, he woke up with blood on his shirt (from biting his tongue) and his family and paramedics staring down at him in horror. A CT scan showed that Steve had an abnormality in the left frontal lobe of his brain. He was given a common anti-convulsant drug called dilantin to keep his seizures under control. A few weeks later after a biopsy, Steve was told that he had a malignant tumor, just under the skull in his speech center, which was about 80 percent the size of a golf ball. It was surgically removed and diagnosed as an "anaplastic astrocytoma, grade III." Steve's prognosis was grim. He was told he had about a 10 percent chance of living five years, but *only* if he did numerous rounds of radiation, likely to be followed by chemotherapy.

At this point, which was 35 days after his surgery, he underwent another MRI. The cancer he was dealing with was apparently *extremely* aggressive (fast-growing) because this MRI showed that the tumor had already grown back. Steve spent an arduous recovery after the surgery and opted for the recommended 35 days of radiation treatments. But he did only three days of treatments and decided he had gathered enough evidence that he believed Protocel® could take care of his cancer without any more conventional treatments.

Steve subsequently refused further radiation and went on Protocel® Formula 23 alone. After four weeks on Protocel®, another MRI was performed. This time, no change in the size of the tumor had occurred. This was a really good sign, since the cancer was so aggressive and any lack of growth at this point was positive. Steve continued on the Protocel®, and two months later another MRI was performed. This time the scan showed that the tumor had greatly reduced in size. Two months more on Protocel® and the tumor was even smaller and no longer enhancing! This meant that the MRI no longer showed "active" cancer and the remaining tumor mass could be considered benign.

Steve was told by others who had used the formula that, after about four to five weeks on Protocel®, he might go through a period of his original symptoms returning (in his case, dizziness and difficulty thinking and talking.) Steve was warned that this could occur because the tumor might be lysing enough at that point to cause a certain amount of pressure in the brain. He was also told not to worry if this happened, because this would mean that the tumor was shrinking. According to Steve, four weeks and four days after he started Protocel®, he did experience a period of dizziness and difficulty thinking. But he got through it without much trouble, and then he just started to feel better and better.

Steve continued to feel fine for more than three years after being diagnosed with his very aggressive brain cancer, and all his follow-up MRIs

continued to show no tumor activity. However, Steve had stopped taking Protocel® shortly after his tumor stopped enhancing and apparently
he stopped too soon. In December 2003, he started feeling a return of
symptoms and an MRI showed new enhancement and tumor growth
in his brain. Steve immediately went back on Protocel®, and as of this
writing in March 2004, he is continuing on Protocel® to get rid of his
new tumor growth.

(**NOTE:** In general, tumors anywhere in the body other than the brain
will eventually disappear completely over time with the use of Protocel®.
Small brain tumors will also eventually completely disappear. However,
large tumors in the brain will sometimes only shrink to a point, then stop
highlighting and stop growing. At this point, some people have chosen to
have the benign mass surgically removed, while others have been able to
easily live a normal life with the benign mass still in their brain. Steve's
experience is an important reminder that when an active tumor has become
benign, even though there is no discernable enhancement on an MRI,
there could still be some active cancer cells within the mass somewhere.
And these active cells could start growing again as soon as Protocel® is
stopped. Thus, it is probably best to stay on Protocel® indefinitely as long
as there is any mass left in the brain at all.)

Case Story #11—Childhood Leukemia

Sydney is a wonderful seven-year-old girl. In 1999, when she was only
two, she was diagnosed with "acute lymphoblastic leukemia." Two-year-
old Sydney was given chemotherapy for about a year. At that point, her
doctors and family were hoping that she would be able to transition to
"maintenance" therapy, but a bone test in October 2000 showed that
she still had cancer in her bone marrow. Sydney had relapsed, and her
doctors wanted to perform a bone marrow transplant involving aggressive chemotherapy at this point. Her family was told that even *with* the
bone marrow transplant, Sydney probably only had a 10 percent chance
of survival.

Before making a decision, Sydney's family sought a second opinion
from another prominent hospital. The doctors at this hospital told them
that Sydney would probably only have a 5 percent chance of survival
after the transplant.

In January 2001, Sydney's family chose to decline the bone marrow
transplant which offered so little hope. They also declined any further

chemotherapy or other conventional treatment. Instead, they started Sydney on Protocel®. Sydney showed mild symptoms of lysing which mostly involved loose stools that had mucous material in them. Amazingly, when Sydney went back for her next checkup, which seemed to her mom like after just a matter of weeks, there was no more evidence of leukemia!

Sydney has continued to take Protocel® and has also continued to get tested about every three months (including bone marrow tests) for the past few years. All her tests have continued to be negative for cancer. Recently, Sydney's doctor told her family they don't have to bring her in for checkups anymore, but Sydney's mother still feels more comfortable doing the testing once in a while. Sydney's last test was on January 8, 2003, and again showed her to be cancer-free. As of this writing, little Sydney continues to feel perfectly fine and is currently enjoying attending school.

Case Story #12—Kidney Cancer Metastasized to Both Lungs

Many people whose cancer has already metastasized to other organs have fully recovered through the use of Entelev®, Cancell®, or Protocel®. Like Roberta in case story #4, Kathy was another one of these people. In late 1991, Kathy became sick. She was extremely tired and achy and had lost 40 pounds. For a while, the doctors couldn't figure out what was wrong. Finally, in March 1992, they discovered that she was suffering from renal cell carcinoma in her right kidney. Later that month Kathy went into surgery and her right kidney and surrounding lymph nodes were removed. The lymph nodes were clear, but the kidney tumor was big. It measured 7 by 14 centimeters. The surgeons actually had to remove two of her ribs to get it out.

After surgery, Kathy's doctors were going to discuss follow-up chemotherapy or radiation with her, but she didn't want to do either. She had too many nurses in her family who'd seen the horrors of these treatments, and her own investigation indicated that there was no effective conventional treatment for renal cell cancer anyway, other than surgical removal of the kidney. And, with only one kidney left, this type of surgery was no longer an option.

So, Kathy declined further treatment. But in June, she was worried about her lungs and requested a chest X-ray. The X-ray indicated that something was there and the doctors then did a CT scan. The scan showed numerous nodules in both of Kathy's lungs. To diagnose these nodules more specifically, Kathy underwent a two-hour needle biopsy procedure. The biopsy result came back as "metastasized renal cell carcinoma, stage IV." The other result from the biopsy was that the procedure collapsed one of her lungs, and Kathy had to recover in the hospital for five days.

At this point, with metastasized renal cell cancer, Kathy's doctors did *not* recommend follow-up treatment. They did not say specifically, but their attitude suggested that there was no hope and they had nothing to offer her. So she went home. She had already been looking into alternatives and, fortunately for her, circumstances finally led her to Cancell®.

At the end of August 1992, Kathy started taking Cancell®. She took only one other supplement, which was Bromelain, along with it. Other than the Cancell® and Bromelain, Kathy followed a very healthy eating program she had created on her own. She stayed completely away from white sugar (though she did use honey and pure maple syrup) and drank a gallon of distilled water every day. She also drank one glass of fresh juice each day (apple, carrot, and spinach) and ate a lot of organic fruits and vegetables. She kept a healthy mix of organic almonds, sunflower seeds, and raisins around at all times for snacking and made vegetable soup with cabbage, potatoes, celery, and V-8 juice. Kathy did not restrict her intake of meat, and freely ate chicken, fish, and beef.

On January 25, 1993, five months after starting on Cancell®, Kathy got another scan of her lungs. This time, she only had two nodules left, one in each lung. This was a great improvement since the doctors had initially diagnosed her with "numerous" nodules. Then in March, Kathy went into surgery to have a swollen lymph gland in her collar bone area removed. She was worried that it might be malignant, but the biopsy showed there was no cancer in it. This was good news, but the *really* good news was that the doctors did one more chest X-ray before the lymph node surgery, and it revealed that the last two nodules in her lungs were both gone. A few months later, in June 1993, Kathy got a total body CT scan, along with a variety of blood tests. All of the results came back the same—no evidence of cancer anywhere!

Kathy's metastasized renal cell cancer was completely gone after 10 months on Cancell®. She stayed on the Cancell® another eight months to be sure that there would be no return of her cancer, after which she went to a maintenance schedule of taking Cancell® just three to six months each year. For the past 11 years she has had no recurrence of cancer.

The year that Kathy was pronounced free of cancer, 1993, she organized an informal picnic gathering for Cancell® users so that people could share their stories and learn more about it from others. She continued this as an annual tradition for many years before finally stopping it. According to Kathy, "I promised the good Lord I would do something to help more people know about this."

Case Story #13—Stomach Cancer Metastasized to Lymph and Bones

Another remarkable story of recovery from metastasized cancer belongs to Robert. In May 2000, when Robert was 54, he and his wife were vacationing in Las Vegas. One day, Robert suddenly fainted and then began vomiting blood. He was rushed to the hospital, and after scoping his stomach, the doctors told Robert he had stomach cancer, stage IV. The scope had revealed a 5.8 centimeter tumor. Also, the wall of his stomach was about 3 inches thick around the tumor instead of the normal 1-inch thickness. The doctors gave Robert 2 pints of blood to get him back home so that he could be treated by his local doctors.

Once home, Robert's doctors performed a cauterization in his stomach to stop the bleeding and administered antibiotics to him. More tests revealed, however, that Robert's stomach cancer had already metastasized. He was soon diagnosed with MALT lymphoma, which is a cancer of the stomach lining, as well as non-Hodgkin's lymphoma. (MALT stands for mycosa-associated lymphoid tissue.) As if that were not enough, a bone scan and bone marrow biopsy then showed he had cancer in his bones as well, and another scan showed two spots on his liver.

Robert's doctors recommended a chemotherapy regimen called "CHOP" along with radiation directed at the stomach tumor. (CHOP stands for three chemo drugs and a steroid: cyclophosphamide, doxorubicin, vincristine, and prednisone.) They told Robert and his wife that if he did *not* undergo this type of treatment, he would probably live no more than three months.

But Robert refused all chemotherapy and radiation and just took Protocel® every day instead. In June of 2000, he began taking Protocel® Formula 23 in distilled water. He also started taking an Ellagic Acid supplement, enzymes, and aloe vera juice for detoxing and cleansing. After a while, Robert started experiencing a lot of odd stuff coming out of his body in his bowel movements and also saw that his urine was often very "bubbly" in the toilet bowl.

Exactly two months after starting Protocel®, at the end of August

2000, Robert underwent another stomach scoping. He was thrilled to hear that his tumor had shrunk from 5.8 to 3.5 centimeters in size. They then found out that the two spots on his liver were no longer there! On his next visit two months later, his stomach tumor was again decreased in size. Finally, on December 22, 2000, after undergoing yet another scoping, a set of scans, and blood tests, Robert was told that according to all diagnostics, his cancer was gone. In just six months, his stomach, lymphatic, and bone cancer had disappeared! (The spots on his liver had disappeared as well, but it had never been definitively determined that they were cancer. They may have been a pre-cancerous or other sort of condition that also got resolved through the use of Protocel®.)

Robert continued to take Protocel® for a total of two years from the day he started to make sure that all the cancer in his body was completely taken care of. He knew that modern diagnostic tests cannot detect every last cancer cell and that even when diagnostic scans show a person to be "all-clear," there can still be many microscopic cancer cells that are not detectable. He now plans to take just one bottle of Protocel® each year, which is about a two-month supply, as a maintenance program for the rest of his life. Robert's recovery from metastasized cancer is an incredible success story.

What did Robert's doctor think of his recovery? In late December 2000, when Robert was told that all his cancer was gone, his wife asked his main doctor what he thought Robert's recovery could be attributed to. The doctor knew all along that Robert was taking Protocel® and not doing chemo, but for some reason, he couldn't believe it was the Protocel® that did it. The doctor's reply was that it was probably the strong antibiotics that had been administered to Robert for his stomach ulcerations early in the summer that brought about his remarkable cure.

Case Story #14—Cervical Cancer, Stage 3B

Janis was another person who underwent an amazing Protocel® recovery. At only 48 years old, she was diagnosed in January 2002 with "small-cell cervical cancer, stage 3B." Prior to the diagnosis, she had been quite sick for more than six months but had been misdiagnosed as having "polymyalgia rheumatica." Her doctor had placed her on a very heavy regimen of prednisone at the amount of 80 milligrams a day for five-and-one-half months. By the time they realized she had cervical cancer, the tumor was very large and had probably been stimulated to grow quickly by the high doses of prednisone which are capable of suppressing the immune system.

In January 2002, Janis started bleeding profusely. She was rushed to the hospital where she was given seven units of blood. She was told that she nearly died, but as a result of this episode, she was finally diagnosed correctly. Janis was told she had a large tumor on her cervix (about 8 centimeters, or 4 inches across) that had attached to her pelvic wall. Because her cancer was "small-cell," surgery was out of the question. Janis was told that if surgery were performed on small-cell cervical cancer, the small cancer cells would escape into the bloodstream and quickly spread to her spine and brain.

The very day after her diagnosis, Janis was started on beam radiation treatments. She continued to receive this type of radiation five days out of each week for three months. During that time, she was also treated with two lots of radiation implants. Along with the radiation, on her second week after diagnosis, Janis was started on chemotherapy as well. The chemotherapy continued throughout the entire three months of treatment.

By the end of the three months of aggressive radiation and chemotherapy, however, Janis's cancer had *not* responded to the treatment and her tumor was even *larger* than before. Moreover, she was so sick at this point she was throwing up every half hour and couldn't even keep a tiny bit of water down. Her bowels had completely seized up and stopped functioning due to the heavy amount of pain medication she had to take. Her weight had plummeted from 240 to 140 pounds, and she was very near death.

At this point, her doctors could no longer successfully rehydrate Janis, and they concluded that one more treatment of chemotherapy would kill her. Her doctor finally arranged for hospice care and told her husband that if Janis were extremely lucky, she might live three months. But realistically, he said, she probably would live only two to four more weeks.

The very day Janis was started on hospice, in April 2002, her husband Ralph began searching the Internet for another solution. He found a doctor of naturopathy who knew about and had recommended Protocel®. He advised Ralph to obtain a bottle of it for Janis to start taking immediately.

At first, it was difficult for Janis to take the formula and keep the liquid down. She was just barely able to manage the small doses throughout the day. Janis and her husband had no idea whether Protocel® could help her, but they had no other options.

As Janis tells the story, after two and a half weeks on Protocel® she threw up for the very last time. After seven and a half weeks on Protocel®, she was finally out of pain and able to stop all her pain medication. This allowed her bowels to start working again. Also, at this point, she went back to her doctor for a checkup on her cancer. Her doctor was amazed to see Janis walk into the office. Moreover, examination showed that the tumor had already reduced half in size!

When Janis went back about four months later, her tumor was measured at only 2 centimeters, which was less than one-quarter its original size, and she was back to living normally. After being on hospice with only two to four weeks to live, Janis had gotten her life back! She continued to feel better and better, and began spending much of her time helping others to recover from cancer using Protocel®.

Unfortunately, Janis felt so well that she stopped using Protocel® too soon. (As noted in case story #10, it is imperative that people do *not* stop taking Protocel® as soon as they appear to be in remission, but should stay on it much longer to be sure that every last cancer cell has lysed. See Chapter 12 for a recommendation as to how long to take Protocel® after diagnostic tests come back all clear.)

Sadly, a number of months after stopping Protocel®, Janis suffered a recurrence of her cancer in her liver. By the time it was noticed, it was too late for Protocel® to save her. But Janis's husband, Ralph, commented that when she passed, an examination showed that the cancer in her cervical area was completely gone. He was grateful for the extra time his wife had and feels that if she had just continued on Protocel® longer before stopping it, she would *not* have experienced the metastases to the liver and would be alive today.

Case Story #15—Childhood Brain Cancer

Nicki is an eight-year-old girl, currently living a completely normal life. But just over three years ago, soon after she turned four in June 2000, Nicki developed a fever and had a grand mal seizure. She was rushed to a hospital emergency room where a CT scan was taken, then transferred to the hospital, where doctors surgically inserted a "shunt" to treat the hydrocephalus condition that had developed. After that, a biopsy was performed on Nicki which showed she had a slow-growing tumor in her brain. The biopsy diagnosis came back "low-grade astrocytoma, grade 1 to 2," and was located in the basal ganglia and thalamus regions. The doctors concluded that the tumor had grown to the point where it was pressing on a ventricle in Nicki's brain, and this is what caused the seizure and the hydrocephalus.

Because Nicki's tumor was "octopus-like" and had tentacles infiltrating the rest of her brain, it was considered non-operable. She was also considered too young to undergo radiation. So, after recovering in the hospital for a few weeks, Nicki was started on chemotherapy. Nicki's mom, Vicki, was led to believe by the doctors that they would be giving Nicki some new type of chemo that had been achieving great results. The doctors also said that Nicki had a strong likelihood of living five years, which they considered to be a very good prognosis. (This, on the other hand, did not sound so good to Nicki's mom.) The chemotherapy regimen that was prescribed was procarbazine, vincristine, and CCNU.

According to Vicki, administering the chemotherapy to her daughter was a terrible ordeal. The chemo was in capsule form, but the pills were large and very difficult for Nicki to swallow. They had to hold her down and force the pills into her. Forcing these pills down at times caused little Nicki to cough up blood. Vicki hated to do it, but she wanted her daughter to live, so they continued with these pills for about 10 months. Finally, one doctor told Vicki she could open up the capsules and mix the contents into some sweet food for her daughter to eat, but this ended up a disaster. Nicki got red all over and covered with hives. Paramedics had to be called, and they gave her an injection of Benadryl.

After 10 months of chemo, Nicki's tumor was still unaffected. It had not decreased in size, although it had not increased either. After Nicki's bad reaction to the opened-up pill, the doctors decided to switch her to a different chemotherapy regimen. This time, they put her on vincristine and carboplatin. This second protocol was so devastating to Nicki that her mother had them stop it after only three treatments. Nicki's blood counts had dropped severely, she needed a blood transfusion, and her mom felt deep down that the new chemo regimen was killing her little girl.

Vicki just couldn't put her daughter through any more chemotherapy. None of the treatments had caused a reduction in the size of the tumor. The very night Vicki said "enough," and took Nicki home from the hospital, she read about Protocel® from her Internet research. She started Nicki on Protocel® Formula 23 immediately, which was on September 10, 2001. Nicki was then five years old.

Giving Nicki Protocel® was easy. Vicki just put a quarter teaspoonful of it into a little bit of juice for Nicki to drink at various intervals throughout the day. After two months of being on Protocel®, Nicki went back for another MRI. When she was first diagnosed a year before, Nicki's tumor had been measured at 7 centimeters by 3.5 centimeters by 2.5 centimeters. Now, the tumor measured 6.5 centimeters by 3.0 centimeters. It was the very first time that Nicki's tumor had reduced in size!

Nicki's next MRI three months later showed the tumor to be stable again with no visible decrease in size. But another MRI in October 2002 did show another decrease. This time the tumor measured 5.4 centimeters by 3.0 centimeters. When the neurosurgeon came out of the room where he had been looking at Nicki's scans, he said, "Keep doing what you're doing!"

Nicki's life has been perfectly normal since she's been on Protocel®. She was fortunate to not suffer any serious neurological damage or noticeable cognitive impairment from either the cancer or the chemotherapy. Whether or not Nicki sustained minor neurological damage is still pending, but she does not appear to have any significant problems. Now, in 2004, Nicki goes to school, plays, and does everything else eight-year-olds do. She experienced little in terms of visible lysing signs during her recovery. Since her MRI in June of 2003, her brain tumor has remained stable in size and it is most likely that the tumor is now completely benign. Nicki has just started second grade and is able to perform on the same level as the other children and shows no symptoms whatsoever of having cancer!

Nicki's mother, Vicki, claims that what the doctors told her when they first prescribed the chemotherapy, was not true. They told her that the chemo they wanted to put Nicki on was "new" and had been achieving very good results. Vicki's subsequent research, however, showed that the chemo they prescribed had actually been around for about 30 years and was *not* achieving great results according to everything she read. Looking back on it now, Vicki can see how much she needed to trust the doctors in the beginning. She says she understands people who hear about Protocel® but don't choose to use it. Vicki says, "If I had been told about Protocel® when Nicki was first diagnosed, I wouldn't have believed it could work either. I know I wouldn't have put her on it then. I would have still gone along with whatever the doctors said we should do." Now, she just feels grateful that she came across Protocel® when she did, and tells others about it who are dealing with cancer.

(**NOTE:** As mentioned at the end of case story #10, tumors anywhere in the body other than the brain will generally disappear completely over time with the use of Protocel® and small brain tumors will also eventually completely disappear. However, large tumors in the brain may sometimes only shrink to a point, then stop highlighting and stop growing. They may be seen as having gone dormant so-to-speak at this point. If this happens, it might be best to continue taking Protocel® indefinitely to make sure the mass does not become active and start highlighting and growing again. If the benign mass can be surgically removed, then Protocel® could be stopped after using it for 8 to 12 months *after* the surgical all-clear point to make sure every last cancer cell has lysed.)

The above case stories show how powerful this easy-to-use and inexpensive liquid formula can be for treating cancer in the elderly, middle-aged, young adults, and even small children. To read about and listen to more Protocel® recovery stories that are just as remarkable, go to www. OutsmartYourCancer.com and click on "Success Stories." There, you will even be able to read about and listen to how some people have used Protocel® successfully to treat their dogs with cancer! Plus, there are some inspirational recovery stories on the audio CD at the back of this book that are not written up in the text.

11

Protocel®
Suppression of the Formula

After reading the Protocel® case stories of the previous chapter, the first thing one would likely wonder is, "Why did this formula *not* become an accepted cancer treatment?" In other words, the obvious question is, "Why aren't all the doctors and cancer treatment centers around the country recommending it?"

Well, the answer is simple. *It was officially suppressed.* As a result of this suppression, Jim Sheridan's original Entelev®/Cancell® formula never got approved by the FDA. And if a medical treatment is not approved by the FDA and endorsed by the leading cancer organizations, doctors generally won't hear about it. If a doctor *does* hear about it, he or she will not have any accepted source to go to for more information about the treatment and would not be legally allowed to prescribe it even if he or she wanted to.

How did Jim Sheridan's formula get suppressed? As is commonly the case, it happened over a number of years and as a result of a variety of events. It was not, however, a result of Sheridan's not going through the right channels, or not working with the right organizations. In fact, Jim Sheridan worked from 1935 to 1937 in the analytical lab at Dow Chemical Company in Michigan, from 1950 to 1953 at the Detroit Institute of Cancer Research (now called the Michigan Cancer Foundation), and from 1961 to 1963 at the Battelle Institute in Columbus Ohio (an organization that commonly tested new chemo agents for the National Cancer Institute.)

One of the early suppressive events occurred when Jim Sheridan was working at the Detroit Institute of Cancer Research. At that time, the Pardee Foundation was the source of funding for the research Sheridan was doing. Also at that time, Sheridan's formula was resulting in an 80 percent cure rate in laboratory mice with cancer. According to journal writer Marcello Gallupi, who researched and wrote articles on the Entelev®/ Cancell® story in 1991 and 1992, the Detroit Institute's director decided in late 1953 that it was time to put Sheridan's formula through a clinical program. The director consulted with other experts as well, including the Dean of Medicine at Wayne University, three oncologists from nearby hospitals, and Mr. Grant Clark (a New York representative of the American Tobacco Company). These experts all reviewed the formula's results on laboratory mice and agreed that it was time to move to the next step, which was a human clinical program. The Tobacco company representative said that a check for $450,000 had been written for this effort and that any number of millions of dollars would follow, if required.[1]

The only glitch in the plan to start clinical trials occurred when the Detroit Institute's director informed the American Cancer Society of the intended clinical program. The American Cancer Society responded by saying that they did not approve of the program "because Jim Sheridan had not proved that he owned the idea."[2] This was a bizarre twist, with no apparent precedent. However, the American Cancer Society was powerful enough to immediately halt the clinical program on Entelev®, and within a few months, Jim Sheridan was suspiciously fired from the Detroit Institute of Cancer Research. Sheridan later heard that all the results of his research at the Institute had been burned!

The next event to block Sheridan's formula from being officially analyzed (and thereby kept out of mainstream medicine) occurred in 1963. He had been working for two years in the Biosciences Division of the Battelle Institute in Columbus, Ohio. At that time, Battelle Institute was a research center where many promising chemotherapeutic agents were being tested for the National Cancer Institute. Sheridan's formula was also being tested there. After 10 months of assessing the formula, which was having very good results with cancer, Dr. Davidson of the Battelle Institute requested permission from the NCI to test Entelev® in an NCI laboratory. But Dr. Davidson asked if the test could be executed over a 28-day period, rather than the five-day period chemotherapy tests at NCI were usually given. (Since Jim Sheridan's formula was not a poison like chemotherapy agents, but instead worked on blocking the respiration capabilities of cancer cells until they fell apart, his material took a little longer to work.)

The incredible answer that came back from the NCI was, "No!" In other words, the National Cancer Institute *refused* to study a cancer treatment that took 28 days rather than five days to show results. Because of this stance by the NCI, there was also no more money to continue researching the formula at Battelle. So once again, Sheridan's experiments were forced to cease.

Between 1978 and 1980, Sheridan was finally able to get the National Cancer Institute to run animal tests on his formula. As is commonly the case, the NCI requested from him any information on special requirements it should know about to do the tests on mice. He complied by writing them a letter that stated three requirements. Specifically, Sheridan wrote that the NCI: (1) should not inject the formula into mice, but should administer it orally in water; (2) should make the test period at least 28 days long; and (3) should not test the formula on mice with leukemia, because mice with leukemia *always* die within 18 or 19 days, and it takes longer than that for the formula to work effectively.

After the test was done, Sheridan got a letter back from the NCI stating that his formula had been completely ineffective. But when he looked into how they had done the tests, he found that they had *not done any of the three things he specified.* They had injected his formula into mice, instead of administering it orally in water. They had used mice with leukemia, instead of mice with any other type of cancer. And they had completed the whole test in eight days instead of giving it the full 28 days.

At this point, Sheridan called the NCI and asked someone to look into the files and see if his letter was actually there. It was, and the person he spoke to apologized and ordered the animal testing to be done again. After the test was completed a second time, Sheridan received the same type of letter as before, stating once again that his formula was completely ineffective. Upon telephoning the NCI once more, he found out that they had completely ignored his instructions *a second time* and had once more injected the formula into mice with leukemia over an eight-day period. Either the NCI was not competent at giving specific instructions to their laboratories or it just didn't want the formula to be tested correctly.

Some people who understand the workings of the National Cancer

Institute and the laboratories it farms tests out to, believe that the above failure of the NCI to correctly test Sheridan's formula on mice was not so much "deliberate" as it was the result of an "institutional blind spot." All of the procedures for testing cancer treatments have been set up to test highly toxic drugs like chemotherapy. These procedures have been in place for decades, and certain protocols are ingrained in every step. For highly toxic drugs, injecting the drug into mice with leukemia over no more than eight days works perfectly fine. However, for a non-toxic agent that requires just a little more time, the institutionalized process fails. Many people feel it was probably a deliberate attempt to thwart any good results.

It is true, however, that the current official methods for testing cancer treatments are based on "fixed assumptions" of how any cancer treatment *should* work. Sheridan believed this type of assumption could make it impossible to find solutions. He argued that an example of this folly would be if the federal government had decided to help fund the building and testing of a flying machine back in 1900, and looking around at things that fly (bugs, birds, and bats), it decided that all flying machines should have wings that flap up and down. Enter the Wright Brothers. Their flying machine would have failed all tests because it had stationary wings, rather than the anticipated wings that flapped up and down.[3]

But Sheridan did not give up. On April 9, 1982, he submitted his Notice of Claimed Investigational Exemption for a New Drug under section 505(1) to the FDA, and on May 20, 1982, the FDA issued him the IND number 20,258.[4] Apparently, the wording and implication of the IND number granted to Sheridan indicated that his product was now ready for a clinical program. However, soon after this, Sheridan received word from the FDA stating that the material known as Entelev® had been put on "clinical hold" because of lack of data assessing its toxicity. The FDA then informed Jim that he needed to have an "LD-50" test performed on his formula. The LD-50 is a toxicity test using animals that is done in various FDA-approved laboratories around the country to establish the safety level of a product.

Sheridan had already had several "minimum lethal dose" (MLD) tests using animals done on his formula *before* the FDA granted him this IND number. MLD testing is where a technician injects a group of mice with the material being tested in bigger and bigger doses. At the point where 50 percent of the mice die from the material, the minimum lethal dose amount is established. The reason Sheridan had done several of these tests was that every time he changed the formula even the slightest bit, a new toxicity test had to be done.

All of the MLD tests indicated the formula was non-toxic. In fact, it was so non-toxic that the laboratory technicians performing at least one of the tests told Sheridan they finally had to stop injecting larger and larger amounts of his formula into the mice when they got to the point that they felt the mice would literally "blow up" if they injected any more into them. Even with the massive doses they were injecting into the mice, they could *not* get 50 percent of the mice to die.

However, getting the official LD-50 test performed on his formula *after* the IND number had been issued was another matter. Sheridan tried for many years to get this toxicity test done. Three different times he had the process started at three different FDA-approved labs. But all three times, after finding out what the material was, the lab would for some reason refuse to do the test. According to Sheridan, the laboratory would either tell him that they were too busy, or keep delaying the test and never get to it. One time, Sheridan had even gotten to the point of paying a lab in full for the LD-50 test he had requested. But then this lab, too, came up with some reason as to why they could not do the toxicity test and refunded Sheridan his money.

Sheridan finally got an idea of what may have been happening when he heard through a friend that one of the labs he was trying to get a toxicity test done at was actually visited by an FDA representative who directly threatened the lab out of doing the test. This was the FDA's way of blocking Sheridan from going to the next step in his attempts to get his cancer formula officially evaluated.

Jim Sheridan witnessed other suppressive events as well. For instance, at one point a doctor he personally knew left his position at Memorial Sloan-Kettering to devote his efforts to researching Cancell®. Unfortunately, however, this doctor was from another country and before he could do the research, he found himself being threatened with deportation.

Another way that Sheridan tried to get his formula into mainstream medicine was by attempting to get pharmaceutical companies interested in it. Each time a pharmaceutical company looked into it, they would be very interested at first. But as soon as they found out that the formula was *not* something they could patent and thereby make exorbitant profits from, the pharmaceutical companies always completely lost interest.

In the early 1980s, another development occurred. However, this time it was a very fortunate one. A metallurgist and engineer named Ed Sopcak got involved with Sheridan's formula. Sopcak was already in business for himself and decided to take on the task of producing Entelev® in large quantities so that it could be available at no cost to cancer patients. Sopcak believed that Entelev® was a gift from God and should be given away to people. So he used the profits from his already established foundry business to pay for the non-toxic ingredients that went into making the formula and to pay for the postage required to ship it to people. With Jim Sheridan's agreement, Sopcak decided to rename the formula "Cancell®."

From about 1984 to 1992, Ed Sopcak *gave away* about 20,000 bottles of Cancell® to people with cancer. Agents from the FDA visited Sopcak regularly about once every six months. But there was nothing they could do to stop his activities since he was simply giving the product away and not selling it.

Incredible recovery testimonies started coming back to Sopcak and Sheridan from people using Cancell®. More and more people with cancer, many of whom were in late stages, were getting well. At one point, the two men were invited to speak at a meeting in southern Michigan that would be attended by a number of people who had successfully used Cancell® to treat their cancer. According to Sopcak, four local TV stations had been invited to film the event and air it on the news. But, unfortunately, none of the TV crews showed up. One station claimed it was too short-staffed, and the three others that had been invited claimed that the FDA had threatened to have their licenses revoked if they covered the event. Thus, the media coverage was controlled and effectively blocked by the FDA. (Whatever happened to freedom of the press and fearless journalism?)

Finally, on November 13, 1990, the National Cancer Institute agreed to test the formula once again, this time "in vitro," which meant they would administer it to various cancer cell lines in petri dishes. Even though this was just a 48-hour test *not* using animals, it is still a valid test often used for early evaluation of a new treatment. The Cancell® formula proved to be *highly effective* against all the strains of cancer that the NCI tested it on. Jim Sheridan now felt renewed hope that it would finally be approved. But he was shocked when he received a letter from the NCI stating that they were *not* planning to pursue his formula as a medical treatment.

At this point Jim Sheridan's son, James, was amazed and decided to get involved. James Sheridan is currently, and was also at that time, a district court judge for the State of Michigan. Judge Sheridan called the NCI directly for an explanation and spoke to Dr. Ven Narayanan, who was the head of drug testing for the NCI at that time. When asked why his father's formula was considered a failure, Dr. Narayanan agreed that the tests showed the formula to be effective at killing cancer. But he then went on to tell Judge Sheridan, "I could also obtain these results with chemotherapy, if I wanted to, but anything that would get results *this good* would be too toxic to humans!"[5] Judge Sheridan then suggested to Dr. Narayanan that he, for a moment, hypothetically assume the formula is *not* toxic to humans at therapeutic levels. At that point, Dr. Narayanan made it clear he would not even be willing to consider assuming such a thing. Then, he pointed out to Judge Sheridan that his father, Jim Sheridan, had not yet proved his formula was non-toxic. In other words, he had not had an LD-50 toxicity test run on it yet.

Jim Sheridan and his family were stumped. They were caught in a classic "double bind." The FDA would not pursue his formula without an LD-50 toxicity test that was done *after* the issuance of the IND number. But the only labs able to do the test would not do it because of pressure from the FDA. And the NCI and FDA both chose to ignore the fact that all the Minimum Lethal Dose tests Jim Sheridan had done before the IND number was issued had all shown the formula to be non-toxic. In fact, it is probable that the NCI knew the formula was non-toxic. With the NCI ignoring all previous toxicity tests and not allowing any new ones to be performed, they could then brush off the phenomenal in vitro test results by claiming that any formula that worked *that* well must be too toxic to humans!

Following are nine graphs showing the official NCI in vitro test results. The first eight graphs show the results of different dosages of Cancell® on eight different types of cancer. The ninth graph shows a superposition of all the eight previous graphs. The original data was requested by Dr. John Zimmerman, director of the Bio-Electro-Magnetics Institute of Reno Nevada, through the Freedom of Information Act. The National Cancer Institute supplied Dr. Zimmerman with the test results for these graphs and the NCI cover letter along with the original NCI data can be found in the *BEMI Currents* Journal, Volume 3: Number 4 of March 1993. An article written by Jim Sheridan and edited by Dr. Zimmerman, which explains the 9 graphs, is also printed in that same issue.

A brief explanation of these graphs is warranted here. The vertical axis on the left of each graph represents the percentage of growth in the cancer cells tested. On this left axis, 0 means "no growth," 30 means 30 percent growth, −30 means 30 percent death of cells, and −100 means that virtually all the cancer cells in the petri dish are dead at this point.

The horizontal axis on the bottom of each graph represents the dosage of Cancell® administered. It presents the dosage of Cancell® used in micrograms per milliliter (μg/ml), and in a Log_{10} scale. This means that the "1," "2," "3," and "4" on the bottom horizontal line are powers of 10. (Thus, 1 actually means 10 μg/ml, 2 means 100 μg/ml, 3 means 1,000 μg/ml, and 4 means 10,000 μg/ml.)

The different types of solid, dotted and dashed lines on each graph represent different specific cell lines for each type of cancer tested. These cell lines are defined underneath each graph.

To anyone looking at these graphs, two main characteristics jump out. The first characteristic is that, except for the leukemia cell lines, all other types of cancer tested (non-small cell lung cancer, small cell lung cancer, colon cancer, central nervous system cancer, melanoma, ovarian cancer, and renal cancer) proved to respond with either 100 percent cell death, or very near to 100 percent cell death within a certain dose range over a very short period of time. In the case of a devastating disease such as cancer, a substance that can simply bring cancer growth to zero is quite an accomplishment. One that can cause almost 100 percent cell death in a 48-hour period is a *remarkably* good result and definitely worth looking into!

The second characteristic that jumps out is that the optimum dose range on all the graphs was approximately between 100 and 1,000 μg/ml. After that, as the dose amount is increased by factors of ten, the amount of cell death decreases. This means that at much higher doses, the Cancell® formula was actually *less* effective at causing cancer cell death. What is evident from this characteristic is that Cancell® was *not toxic*. No toxic substance would become *less* able to kill cells at higher concentrations. This characteristic was probably an artifact of the tests being done in petri dishes, rather than in the human body. People using Sheridan's formula in real life have found higher doses to cause *more* cancer cell death—but it is not always desirable to kill cancer too fast.

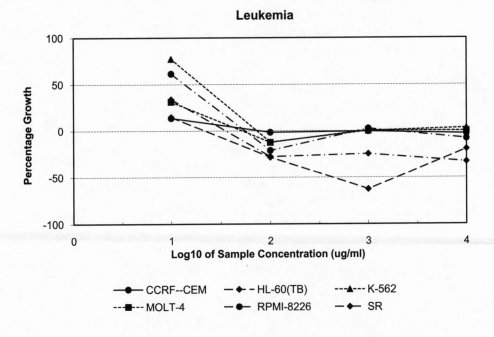

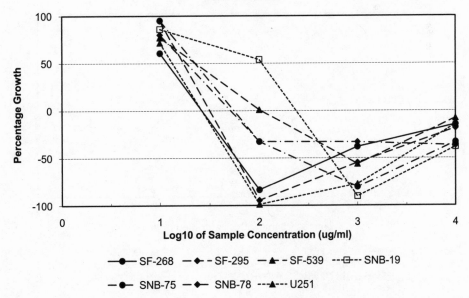

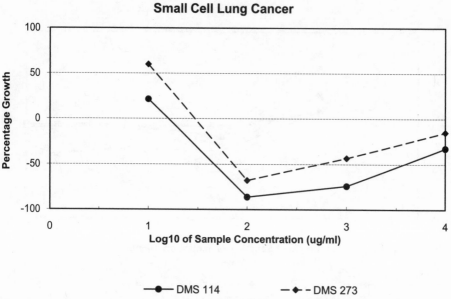

Small Cell Lung Cancer

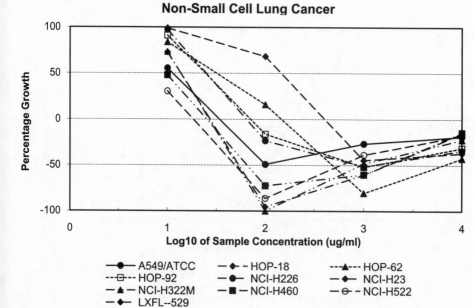

Non-Small Cell Lung Cancer

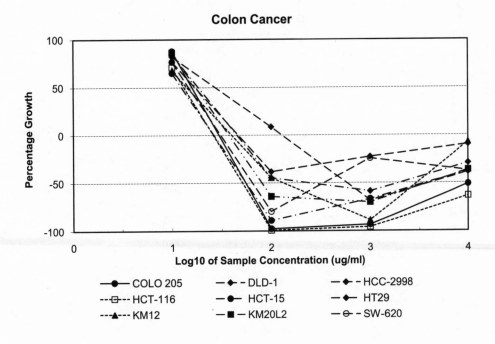

Colon Cancer

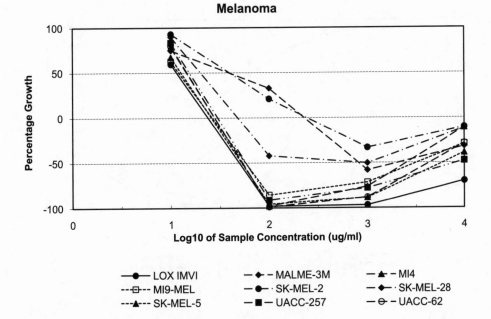

Melanoma

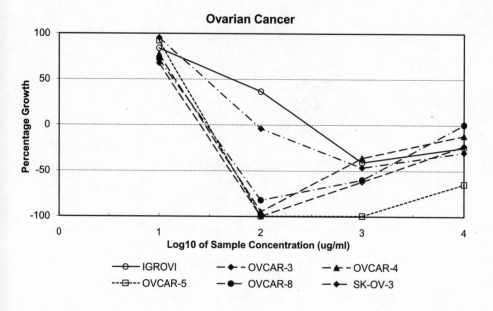

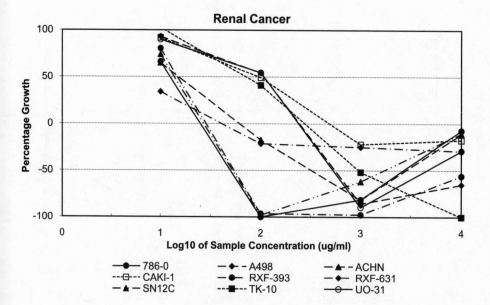

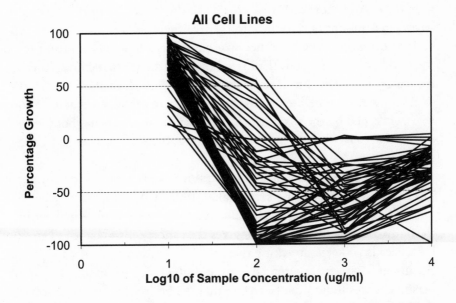

The above official National Cancer Institute testing was done on Cancell® over a mere 48-hour time period. If continued over a longer period of time, it is likely that ALL of the graph results would have fully reached –100, meaning 100 percent cancer cell death. But the NCI's in vitro testing procedure is set at 48 hours because the NCI assumes that it will always be dealing with a toxic material. For toxic materials, it makes sense to limit the duration of the test because the human body can only tolerate a toxic substance for a limited period of time. However, Cancell®, being non-toxic, could be taken *indefinitely* without harming the body. At the time of this testing, people who had used Cancell® to fully recover from their cancer had used it for much longer periods than 48 hours.

The benefits to using a non-toxic treatment approach for cancer cannot be overstated. Besides the fact that toxic treatments can have extremely serious side effects (such as liver, kidney, and heart damage) to the point that the side effects themselves can be life-threatening, there is also another issue. This is the issue that toxic conventional approaches such as chemotherapy and radiation do not allow for *continual use*. They are so toxic that continual use would kill the patient before the cancer could. So, toxic treatments are always administered with treatments spaced out in some way. But cancer's best attribute is its ability to grow new cells fast. This means that, in-between the toxic treatments, the cancer cells grow back. And those cells that grow back the fastest are those cells that have some amount of resistance to the treatment.

In other words, when a cancer patient needs a few days or weeks for their body to recover from the toxic cancer treatment being given them, the cancer cells may also recover during this time. They may even start to grow faster than before due to the body's immune system having also been weakened by the toxic treatment. Eventually, a person's body may not be able to recover anymore because it has been too weakened by the treatment.

With *non-toxic* treatments, however, this vicious cycle is avoided. For instance, Protocel® can be safely taken four or five times a day *every single day* for many months. This allows a therapeutic level to be kept in the body continually which *never* gives the cancer cells a chance to grow back because it keeps attacking them 24 hours a day, seven days a week. Because it is non-toxic, Protocel® can even be taken for many years if a person chooses to in order to ensure that the body stays free of cancer.

What was obvious from the 1990 NCI tests on Cancell® was that, as a cancer treatment in the initial stages of testing, it passed with flying colors. The only logical conclusions as to why it was never pursued further would have to be that either: (1) the institutionalized procedural bias was too strong, or (2) the NCI just didn't want to pursue it even though they could see that it worked.

The final blow to Cancell® occurred on Friday, November 13, 1992, when a federal judge enforced an FDA injunction to stop all distribution of Cancell® for the purpose of treating any disease. This injunction legally blocked Ed Sopcak from being able to ship Cancell® across state lines to people with cancer. Sopcak and Sheridan had never sold the product to anyone anyway, since they had always just given it away to people who needed it. But by prohibiting its distribution, the injunction also effectively prohibited them from giving the formula away.

What was the official injunction based on? It was based primarily on the fact that Jim had never had an LD-50 toxicity test run on the latest version of his formula!

Although Jim Sheridan never gave up trying to get Cancell® officially evaluated and accepted, his successful non-toxic formula for treating cancer was effectively kept from widespread availability to the public through a variety of "official" actions over a span of many years. As with other successful non-toxic alternative cancer treatments, his formula *should* have been fairly evaluated by official organizations and, if found effective, incorporated into mainstream medicine.

The *American Spirit Newspaper* published an interview with Ed Sopcak in their January/February issue of 1994. In the article, written by Nancy Burnett, Sopcak stated:

> It's outrageous that we have in our files probably 10,000 people that we have helped and who are living today because of Cancell. And this was all done freely with no exchange of money involved. Now I am considered a criminal. That's how panicky these people are. You become a criminal to help your fellow man.

When asked *who* brought the lawsuit and injunction against him, Sopcak answered:

> Actually they didn't have a plaintiff. The FDA represented it but the FDA cannot be a plaintiff. It really was the American Medical Association who uses the FDA as an enforcement arm. Furthermore, the National Cancer Institute lied and said they never ran the test.
>
> . . . When investigators for the FDA went out and interviewed people trying to find a harmed party they got all positive responses. They got the names illegally by going to the United Parcel Service and getting the names of the people I had sent it to. Then when they couldn't get a harmed party that way they solicited oncologists to try to get one to sign a complaint against me. But none of them would sign a complaint.
>
> So they went to trial without a plaintiff. And because they didn't have a plaintiff, there was never a hearing. I never saw the judge. They just did this all in paperwork and the judge illegally issued a permanent injunction. The law says I have a constitutional right to face my accuser. I didn't have that because there was no accuser. Furthermore, the law says the judge has to issue a temporary injunction to determine if the product does irreparable harm. He didn't do that. He issued a permanent injunction.

Referring to the 1990 tests that the National Cancer Institute performed in vitro on Cancell® (graphs presented earlier), Sopcak commented:

> According to the law, if they find one positive result out of the testing done, one case where a tumor was reduced in size or eliminated, they have to continue testing. What they did in this case is they said there was no reason to do any further testing. And they dropped all tests. It was completely unlawful.
>
> . . . We erroneously think that all we have to do is just modify the

law. But they're not following the law anyhow. What difference does it make if you modify it?

Because of the FDA injunction to stop all distribution of Cancell®, the exact version of Jim Sheridan's formula was not available for about seven years (between 1992 and 1999). But in April 1999, the Sheridan family was able to get the formula produced once again—this time for sale to the public. It was re-named "Protocel®" and was brought onto the market as a general health supplement to rid the body of non-productive anaerobic cells. It is now being legally sold in the United States by two distributors; one located in South Carolina, and one located in Ohio. (See last page of Chapter 12 for contact information.) Though neither company makes any claim that the product cures cancer or any other disease, they make available to the public Protocel® Formula 23, which is the reproduction of Jim Sheridan's original Entelev®, and Protocel® Formula 50, which is the reproduction of Jim Sheridan's and Ed Sopcak's original Cancell®.

As to the official toxicity test, another LD-50 test was requested and run on the formula before Protocel® went into production. This time, the test was achieved without any difficulty. (Possibly, the test wasn't blocked this time because the FDA-approved laboratory that performed it did *not* recognize the "Protocel®" name and did not know it was connected to the earlier Cancell® formula. Or possibly the test was allowed because the Protocel® product was not going to be sold as a cancer treatment.)

At any rate, Protocel® passed the toxicity test superbly! In fact, the LD-50 test results indicated that a quarter teaspoonful of Protocel® taken four or five times a day is *less* toxic to the body than taking one aspirin a day. The non-toxic aspect of Protocel® has also been verified by many people who have used it for years with no toxic side effects. There is even a report of one woman who did not understand the instructions and drank one-quarter bottle of the formula all at once (about a two-week supply), instead of one-quarter teaspoonful. She merely ended up with two hours of diarrhea, and then she was fine.

The important thing to remember is that, although Jim Sheridan's formula was officially suppressed and successfully kept out of mainstream medicine, it did *not* die. Over the years, thousands of people have found one way or another to use the formula (either under the name of Entelev®, Cancell®, or Protocel®) and treat their cancers with amazing success.

12

Protocel®
How to Use It For Best Results

Chapters 9, 10 and 11 make it clear that Protocel® is a unique product that was developed specifically for treating cancer and that it has brought about countless cancer recoveries over the past two decades. However, the National Cancer Institute and FDA were *not* interested in pursuing it as a cancer treatment. So, the only way this remarkable approach could be made available to the public was to sell it as a dietary supplement. As in other similar cases, this created the unfortunate conundrum that any company selling Protocel® cannot legally advise people on how to *use* it effectively for cancer or any other disease.

Thus, because distributors are limited in what they can say about using Protocel®, this chapter has been a much-needed comprehensive source of information since 2004. And, in keeping with the fact that *Outsmart Your Cancer* is still the definitive source of information on Protocel®, when the updated second edition was produced this chapter was significantly *expanded* to include even more information.

Since this chapter is very detailed and only about how to use Protocel® for best results, those readers who are NOT planning to use Protocel® at the moment may want to skip over this chapter and move on to Chapter 13.

On the other hand, for those who are currently using or planning to use Protocel® to treat their cancer, this chapter has *critical* information in it and may even make the difference between achieving a full recovery or not. In fact, Protocel® users may benefit from *re-reading* this chapter at various intervals after they have started treatment to remind themselves of important usage information.

In general, using Protocel® for cancer is quite easy. (Especially when compared to conventional cancer treatment or even many other alternative methods that involve mountains of pills, frequent juicing, or detoxifying enemas.) For best results, the basic rules are:

1. Space the doses out over each 24-hour period as evenly as possible and try to *never* go more than six hours between any two doses.

2. Shake the bottle vigorously immediately before each dose.

3. Make sure you are *not* taking any vitamin, mineral, herbal remedy, or other type of cancer treatment that might interfere with Protocel®'s action.

4. Be sure to drink plenty of good water each day, *besides* other liquids. (Preferably, at least a half gallon of water a day.)

5. Try to promote at least one bowel movement every day to support your body's ability to process out lysed material. (Use extra fiber or a mild laxative if needed.)

But, even though using Protocel® is a very easy and simple approach, there are still many details to understand for optimum usage.

Dosing Instructions

First of all, it is important to vigorously shake your Protocel® bottle before measuring out each dose. This is because a small amount of sediment-like substance settles at the bottom and you want that substance to be as evenly mixed into the formula as possible.

Once the Protocel® dose (generally between ¼ and ½ teaspoonful) is measured out, it can then be squirted into the bottom of a cup or glass and water added to help drink it down. Distilled water is best to use whenever possible. If that is not available, any form of non-chlorinated water can be used to dilute your dose. (This would include filtered water or spring water.) The amount of water to add is often suggested as 5 oz., but this does not have to be exact.

Most people do not mind the taste of Protocel® too much, but for those who do, a very small amount of juice can be mixed with the Protocel® instead of water. (Just enough to cover the taste and gulp it down quickly. Protocel® should *not* be allowed to sit in juice for any length of time). Or, a person can add just enough water to their dose to gulp it all down at once and then follow that with a glass of pure water to wash it down.

The following instructions apply to *basic* starting doses. For certain situations, or after being on Protocel® for a while, people may want to increase their dose size or frequency for better results. To read about variations on dosing, see the upcoming section entitled "Variations on Dosing."

Protocel® Formula 50 (Jim Sheridan's original Cancell®) is generally taken *four* times around the clock with each dose being a quarter teaspoonful. These doses should be spaced out as equally as possible over each 24-hour period. For one person, taking their doses at 6 A.M., 12 noon, 6:00 P.M., and midnight might be convenient. For another, taking their doses at 8 A.M., 2 P.M., 8 P.M. and 2 A.M. might be easiest. It doesn't matter what time of day you take your doses so much as it matters that you space them out as equally as possible around the clock.

For optimum results, it is best *not* to let more than six hours lapse between any two doses. The goal with Protocel® is to try to keep a steady therapeutic level in the body at all times. Most people find that taking a dose in the middle of the night is not so difficult as it seems, especially when they realize that their chances for becoming cancer-free are better that way. Those who know they will be getting up during the night to use the bathroom anyway may not need to set their alarm, but simply place their dose of Protocel® in a cup or bottle of distilled water and leave this in the bathroom when they go to bed. Others may decide to set their alarm to be sure they get up and take their middle-of-the-night dose at a set time. Some make this dose easy to take by placing it in distilled water by their bedside so they don't have to get out of bed to take it and can just roll over and go back to sleep quickly. Remember, pre-mixing your middle-of-the-night dose must always be in distilled water.

Protocel® Formula 23 (Jim Sheridan's original Entelev®) on the other hand, is generally taken *five* times around the clock for cancer with the daytime doses being ¼ teaspoonful, and the middle-of-the-night dose being ½ teaspoonful. These doses should also be spaced out as equally as possible over each 24-hour period. Again, never going more than six hours between any two doses is going to facilitate the fastest recovery. Thus, a sample schedule for Formula 23 for cancer might be 7 A.M., 11:30 A.M., 4:00 P.M., 8:30 P.M., and 2 A.M.

With either the Formula 50 or the Formula 23, some people like to double their bedtime or middle-of-the-night dose to give their cancer an extra punch, and that's okay. But if cancer breakdown starts happening too fast, all the doses can be kept at the same amount. Doubling the dose at bedtime was originally recommended to people who could not get back to sleep if they took a dose in the middle of the night, and it was thought that a double dose before bed would help the Protocel® remain active for 8 hours until their next morning dose. Many people *have* been able to achieve full recoveries this way, however going 8 hours between doses overnight tends to work better for the slower-growing cancers or cancers caught very early. For aggressive cancers, late-stage cases, or for anyone who wants to give themselves the very *best* chance for a full recovery, never going more than 6 hours between any two doses—even overnight—is the optimum way to use the Protocel® formula.

Some people find it difficult to accurately measure their dose with the medicine dropper that comes with the formula. If this applies to you, one tip is to go to a drug store and look at the baby supplies section. Usually, you can find a plastic baby medicine syringe that sucks up medicine and has markers for ¼ and ½ teaspoonful, etc. This works quite well for Protocel® dosing and may help in keeping your dose size accurate and consistent, whether you are sticking to the recommended ¼ teaspoonful or are increasing your dose to ⅓ teaspoonful or more. (See later section called "Variations on Dosing.") Some people find that simply using a measuring spoon works best for them, which is also fine. The important thing is to pay attention to detail and maintain a consistent accurate dosing *without* missing doses for as many months as are needed to get rid of your cancer.

Don't Give Your Cancer Cells a Bowl of Soup!

Ed Sopcak, who had the best track record of recoveries from cancer patients he helped to use Cancell®, used to stress the importance of taking doses with rigorous regularity around the clock every day. Sopcak would tell people that the formula metabolizes and dissipates from the body fairly quickly. He urged people to understand that, even though Protocel® may remain to some extent in the body for more than 8 hours, after about six hours the amount of the formula in the body may drop below the therapeutic level. Thus, going longer than six hours between doses could be counterproductive to healing.

An explanation for this is the following. Protocel® works by significantly interfering with the ATP production of anaerobic cells. The small effect Protocel® has on our healthy cells does not bother them because they have plenty of ATP energy to spare and they have more pathways by which they can produce energy. But cancer cells cannot tolerate the affect Protocel® has on them since they rely on the much less efficient method of energy production called "glycolysis." By taking Protocel® in regular, evenly spaced out doses, without missing doses, a person can systematically *starve their cancer cells to death*.

However, *beyond* six hours after any dose, the level of Protocel® remaining in your body may not be able to perform its job 100 percent. With the goal being to starve your cancer cells to death, going *more* than six hours between any two doses is like giving your cancer cells a little bowl of soup, so-to-speak, on the seventh or eighth or ninth hour between doses. Your cancer cells are not going to starve to death if you keep feeding them every night (or any other time you go more than 6 hours between doses). Thus, for optimum results, never go more than 6 hours between doses so that you *don't give your cancer cells a bowl of soup!*

For adults and children, Protocel® is best taken on an empty stomach whenever possible (about 30 minutes before a meal). But it will still work if there is food in the stomach, and sticking to an evenly spaced schedule is preferable to postponing or missing doses. One of the reasons we know that Protocel® works even when food is in the stomach is because it has generally been administered to pets by mixing the formula directly into their food and this has consistently shown great results. (See upcoming section called "Protocel® Works for Pets, Too!")

Although mixing Protocel® into juice and drinking it immediately is okay if a person does not want to take it in distilled water, leaving Protocel® in juice for any length of time is not recommended. If a person wishes to carry one or two premixed doses of Protocel® in a small plastic bottle for a day trip, for example, it is important that the Protocel® be mixed into distilled water only. As long as distilled water is used, these premixed doses can then be carried in one's pocket, purse, or glove compartment and kept for hours at a time. Alternatively, a small plastic bottle of pure Protocel® can be carried while traveling and mixed on the spot with juice to drink immediately. But never use more juice than is needed to simply cover the taste and gulp the Protocel® down in one gulp. More juice than that might give your body too much vitamin C when used multiple times each day.

Protocel® does not need to be refrigerated, but it should not be left in direct sunlight or high temperatures for long. It can easily be kept on a shelf, in a cupboard, or carried around under normal conditions.

Some people find it easiest to premix their four or five doses every morning, even if they are not travelling that day. They use small empty bottles and fill them with distilled water each morning, then measure out one dose into each bottle. As long as distilled water *only* is used to dilute the Protocel®, this can be a very convenient method, as you can see all your doses on the counter and simply take one at each dosing time throughout the day and night.

Protocel® has a shelf life of many years. It does not spoil after the bottle has been opened, therefore it requires no refrigeration. The best way to store it is simply on a shelf or counter where it is not in direct sunlight. Pre-prepared doses can be carried around during the day for hours in small containers if that helps a person stick to their schedule, or set out in a small closed container overnight—but only if mixed in distilled water. Protocel® can also go through airport scanners without detriment to the formula, so it is easy to travel with.

Once again, when measuring out the formula, be sure to shake the Protocel® bottle vigorously each time, then quickly measure out your dose. If you do not shake the bottle vigorously right before each dose, then by the time you are into the latter half of the bottle, there will be a higher ratio of sediment to liquid than there was in the first half of the bottle. Jim Sheridan and Ed Sopcak used to always tell people to shake the bottle vigorously to get an even amount of liquid to sediment, and virtually all the people who have used this formula successfully have done so.

Protocel® Formula 50 and Protocel® Formula 23 are *virtually* the same thing. They have the same ingredients and are made only slightly differently with slightly different ratios of those ingredients. Formula 50 used to be considered a little faster-acting, but over the years most Protocel® experts have agreed that this is not the best way to look at it. What appears to be more accurate is that either formulation will usually work for any anaerobic condition or type of cancer, however the Formula 50 seems to work a little better for some types of cancer and the Formula 23 seems to work a little better for others. Any possibility that the Formula 50 is stronger in some cases is made up for by the fact that people generally take the 23 *five* times around the clock, while people using the 50 generally take it four times around the clock. Thus, when a person takes the 23 for a type of cancer known to respond well to the 23, such as prostate cancer or breast cancer, people will usually have a faster recovery with that formulation, rather than with the 50.

The following guide may be used for ascertaining which formulation to start with for various health conditions. It is important for people to remember, though, that this guide is NOT set in stone. It is based on customer usage (anecdotal information) and individuals should feel free to try one particular formulation for a while, then switch to the other formulation if they need to according to how their progress is going. (If your particular health condition is *not* listed below, start with Protocel® Formula 50.)

Anecdotal Guide for Which Formulation to Start With

Formula 50	*Formula 23*
Adenocarcinoma	Bladder cancer
Cervical cancer	Brain cancers (other than GBM)*
Colon cancer	Breast cancer
Esophageal cancer	Kidney cancer (renal cell)
Glioblastoma	Leukemia—acute
Leukemia—chronic	Multiple Myeloma
Liver cancer (primary)	Neuroblastoma
Lung cancer	Prostate cancer
Lupus	Wilmes tumor
Melanoma	Viral infections***
Non-Hodgkin's lymphoma	Auto-immune disorders
Ovarian cancer	Crohn's disease
Pancreatic cancer	Endometriosis
Sarcomas	IBS or UC
Stomach cancer	Multiple Sclerosis**
Squamous cell cancer	Parkinson's
Throat cancer	Pets with any condition****
Uterine cancer	Psoriasis
Viral infections***	
Mononucleosis	

*   For people with primary brain cancer, Formula 23 has been the preferred version except for use against glioblastomas. The 23 has had an excellent track record with all types of astrocytomas and oligodendroglioma. However, if one is dealing with Glioblastoma Multiforme, they may want to use Formula 50, which appears to have had the best track record with that particular type of brain cancer. For all other types of cancer in the brain that are NOT primary (in other words it is metastasized cancer from some other part of the body), then users should pick the formulation that applies to the "primary" site. In other words, for a person with lung cancer mets to the brain, the Formula 50 is indicated for lung cancer and should be used. If they have breast cancer mets to the brain, then Formula 23 is indicated for breast cancer and should be used. Whenever dealing with cancer in the brain of any type, one needs to be cautious of not promoting too much edema too quickly, and the prescribed use of steroids or anti-seizure medications may be necessary until Protocel® has had time to reduce enough of the cancer load so that pressure in the brain is not an issue. Steroids and seizure meds will not interfere with Protocel®'s action.

** Many people with multiple sclerosis have experienced wonderful improvements in their condition through the use of Protocel®. Multiple sclerosis is so named because it is a condition where multiple areas of scar tissue (sclerosis) build up around neurons and this then interferes with proper functioning of the nervous system. One way it is thought that Protocel® helps people with MS is by breaking down the anaerobic scar tissue that has built up around their neurons. As Protocel® causes this scar tissue to break down, the nerves gradually regenerate and people find their normal functioning returning. To help support this process of nerve regeneration, people using Protocel® for MS may also want to supplement daily with: 1,000 mg borage oil, 3 tablespoons granular lecithin, and 2 tablespoons extra virgin cold pressed olive oil. These extra supplements are thought to help the body rebuild new myelin sheath. Another way it is thought that Protocel® helps MS is through its anti-viral activity. (Some theories regarding MS include a viral component.) Cortisone medications and the "ABC&R" drugs often prescribed for MS are suspected to interfere with Protocel® and should probably be avoided when using this formula.

*** Many people with various viral conditions have also experienced remarkable recoveries, and both the Formula 23 and the Formula 50 have been successfully used against viruses. The reason that Protocel® can help the body overcome viral challenges is the following: When viral infections occur, the virus must invade our normal healthy cells to replicate. While viruses circulate throughout our bloodstream, they have a special protein coating that protects them from attack by our immune system. But when they invade healthy cells to replicate, they have to shed their protective protein coating. These previously healthy host cells then become damaged anaerobic cells after becoming viral-infected. Protocel® causes these types of anaerobic cells to lyse and fall apart just as it does with cancer cells. When the viral-infected anaerobic cells fall apart, the viruses are then released back into the body, but *without their protective protein coatings.* When this happens, the body's natural defenses can attack and destroy the unprotected viruses. Numerous people have experienced amazing improvements with their herpes, hepatitis, mononucleosis or other viral conditions—even including HIV. Cats given Protocel® for FIV have experienced complete recoveries and some cases of dogs recovering from viral conditions have been reported as well.

**** Pets often require fewer or smaller doses of Protocel® for their recovery process, depending on their size, but still require rigorous, consistent dosing. (See upcoming section called "Protocel® Works for Pets, Too!" for more details.)

Because both formulations are so similar and both work for any condition involving anaerobic cells, the particular formulation one starts with is not as important as making sure to use Protocel® correctly in general. Keeping to your daily schedule and not missing doses unless absolutely necessary is critical. Watching your progress and increasing the dosage over time if needed can also be very important.

Only take Formula 23 or Formula 50 at any given time. In people's efforts to fine-tune their own lysing process and recovery, they may end up with part of a bottle of Formula 23 and part of a bottle of Formula 50. If this happens, do *not* mix the two formulations together. Formula 50 and Formula 23 should always be kept in separate bottles, and people should only use one or the other for any given period of time.

Avoid Taking Any Supplement or Treatment That Might Interfere With Protocel®

Finally, it is important to understand that certain supplements can interfere with Protocel®'s action and should therefore be avoided. Since Protocel® works by depleting ATP energy production, the most common way that supplements or herbs can interfere are those that *promote* the ATP energy production of cells. These supplements can be counter-productive to what Protocel® is trying to do to on a cellular level and can seriously interfere with a person's recovery.

The main supplements or treatments you should definitely avoid are listed below. (Keep in mind, this is not a *complete* list since not every supplement or treatment has been studied in terms of its compatibility with Protocel®. In other words, you should *not* assume that anything NOT on this list is okay just because it is not on this list.)

Definitely AVOID While Using Protocel®

Supplements or Therapies To Avoid
Because They Promote ATP Production:

Vitamin C	Vitamin E	CoQ_{10}
Selenium	Essiac Tea	Hoxsey Therapy
Poly-MVA	Acetyl-Cysteine	L-Cysteine
Alpha lipoic acid	Ginsengs of all types	LifeOne
L-Lipoic Acid	L-Carnitine	Burdock Root
Creatine	Taurine	Iodine
Glutamine	Resveratrol	Rhodiola Rosea
Fish Oil	Flax Oil	D-Ribose
Homeopathics	MSM	

Supplements or Therapies To Avoid
Because They May Interfere with Protocel® for Other Reasons:

Ozone	Cesium	Zeolite
Rife Treatments	714X	Modified Citrus Pectin
Cat's Claw	Flaxseed Oil with Cottage Cheese	

Most chemotherapy drugs (except for 5FU and Xeloda)
Hormone-blocking drugs for men or women (see pages 180–1)

All of the above items are certainly very beneficial and health-promoting when people are using a different approach than Protocel®. But, when using the Protocel® formula, they should be avoided because they may seriously interfere with what Protocel® is trying to do to the cancer cells on the cellular level. Both Jim Sheridan and Ed Sopcak used to discourage the use of a lot of supplements in general while using this formula and urged people to get balanced nutrients from their food instead. Though Sheridan used to say a one-a-day multiple vitamin was okay, the multi-vitamins in his day (twenty years ago) were not nearly as strong nor effective as they are today. Thus, it is most likely best to avoid even a once daily multi-vitamin.

As indicated on the "Avoid list," most of the items to avoid are those supplements or treatments known to promote ATP production in cells. However, there are also supplements or therapies to avoid even though they do *not* promote ATP production. Those are explained here:

Ozone. Although ozone treatments administered to people *not* using

Protocel® can be very beneficial for many types of health recovery, they should be completely avoided when using this particular treatment. Ozone can chemically interact with the Protocel® formula in an undesirable way. Most supplements that help oxygenate the body, such as germanium-132, work fine with Protocel® because they help to bring "O_2" to the cells. But because ozone is "O_3," it chemically interacts with the formula and this interaction produces toxic aldehydes as a byproduct. These toxic aldehydes are not good for the body and can make a person sick. Worse yet, when ozone and Protocel® are combined and they interact with each other, you no longer have ozone or Protocel® left. Thus, you get neither the benefit from the Protocel®, nor the benefit from the ozone.

While it is important to avoid ozone treatments when taking Protocel®, drinking water that has been disinfected with a small amount of ozone is fine. This is because, when ozone is used on municipal or bottled water for disinfectant purposes, the ozone has virtually always dissipated completely or converted back to O_2 by the time you drink it.

Cesium. Many people who read how powerful both Cesium High pH Therapy and Protocel® are want to do the two at the same time. Though more study needs to be done to be absolutely sure, it is has been theorized that cesium chloride may chelate to the Protocel® (or bind to it) and render it less effective. Anecdotal cases of people who tried the two together have shown mixed results. Thus, it appears to be safest to only do one approach or the other—not the two together.

Zeolite. For a similar reason, though not because of chelation, it appears that Zeolite may be best to avoid as well. This is because Zeolite may "trap" the Protocel® (as it traps toxins in the body) and render the formula less effective that way.

Rife Treatments. Jim Sheridan was alive when Royal Rife was also alive and promoting his Rife Technology for cancer treatment. Jim Sheridan looked into the Rife technology and reportedly stated that he thought Rife treatments and Protocel® should not be done at the same time. It is unclear as to what his specific reasons were, but given that he knew his formula very well, it has been suggested that people not do Rife treatments along with Protocel®.

714X. The compatibility of 714X and Protocel® are unknown, so it would be best to avoid doing the two together.

Modified Citrus Pectin. It is thought that modified citrus pectin products should be avoided because MCP might bind to the Protocel® and chelate it out of the body.

Cat's Claw. The compatibility of Cat's Claw and Protocel® is unclear, however according to anecdotal cases, it appears that people don't seem to respond as well to Protocel® when they use Cat's Claw at the same time. So it would be best to avoid doing the two together.

Flaxseed Oil and Cottage Cheese. It is still not certain whether the flaxseed oil and cottage cheese approach will interfere with Protocel® or not, but there is some suspicion that it might. Therefore it would be best to avoid. The suspicion is based on the fact that Dr. Johanna Budwig, developer of the flaxseed oil and cottage cheese approach, stated that her method of treatment helped to "normalize" cancer cells. Since Protocel® is trying to make cancer cells more "primitive" (which goes in the opposite direction), the two approaches may counteract each other.

Most Chemotherapy Drugs. Jim Sheridan stated that chemotherapy may interfere with this formula by changing the level on the oxidation-reduction ladder at which Protocel® works. Thus, it is best to avoid doing chemo along with this formula if possible. The only two exceptions are the chemo drugs 5FU and Xeloda. (See upcoming section called "What About Doing Radiation or Chemotherapy Along With Protocel®?")

MAY Be Taken While Using Protocel®

Any Type of Enzymes	Coral Calcium *(without vitamin C)*
AHCC	Larch
Shark Liver oil	Collostrum
B Vitamins	Reishi Mushrooms
Milk Thistle	Willard's Water *(clear)*
Ellagic Acid *(or Ellagitannins)*	Vitamin D_3
Hydrazine Sulfate	Potassium
Paw Paw	Graviola
Primrose Oil	Calcium
Borage Seed Oil	Magnesium *(not in mega-doses)*
DIM	Indole-3-Carbinol (I3C)
Laetrile	Saw Palmetto
B_{17}	Natural Progesterone
Germanium-132	Ambrotose *(without vitamin C)*
Low Dose Naltrexone	Turmeric
Probiotics *(friendly bacteria)*	Curcumin

Keep It Simple

Even though the previous list shows a large number of supplements that are considered compatible with Protocel®, that does *not* mean it is a good idea to take as many of them as you can. Truly, the safest thing to do when using the Protocel® approach is to "keep it simple." For best results, take as few other supplements, herbs, or remedies as possible and make sure anything you do take is known to be compatible with Protocel®. This is difficult to do sometimes in our age of supplementation, especially when everyone you know may be telling you to take this or that supplement for your cancer. But many of the best recovery cases have been those that took either *nothing* but Protocel®, or took no more than two or three of the supplements on the "May Be Taken" list along with their Protocel®.

Keep in mind that many alternative non-toxic approaches to cancer follow the philosophy that one must flood the body with nutrients, detoxify the body, and follow a very strict diet. That is because those approaches tend to rely primarily on making the body as strong as possible so that one's own immune system can get rid of the cancer. Protocel® follows a different philosophy. Protocel® does *not* rely on the immune system to get rid of one's cancer. Instead, it kills the cancer directly by starving it to death. The more supplements, herbs, juices, green drinks, etc., that people take, the more likely they will be working against Protocel®'s ability to starve the cancer cells.

Another thing to remember is that when Ed Sopcak was giving out Cancell® in the early 1990s and cancer patients were achieving phenomenal recoveries, people did not have the Internet in their homes. They did not have easy access to tons of alternative cancer treatment information and they did not even know about alkalizing the body. As a result, the vast majority of those people who had great recoveries took nothing but Cancell® and possibly some Bromelain (an enzyme) along with it. That was it! They didn't alkalize, they didn't juice, they didn't drink green drinks, they just ate what was considered to be a normal healthy diet.

Those people who do want to use other supplements while taking Protocel® can consult the previous list for items that are believed to be compatible. However, restricting one's use of these supplements to as few as possible is still advisable.

When in Doubt, Do Without

Since it is so important *not* to interfere with the way the formula works, it is best to avoid any supplement, herb or treatment while using Protocel® unless you *know* from the literature sent with the product, or from anecdotal reports, that the item you wish to take will *not* interfere with what Protocel® is trying to do on a cellular level. In other words, "When in doubt, do without." Remember, if you are considering a particular supplement, and it is not on the "Avoid" list, that does not mean it is compatible with Protocel®. Many supplements are still in question as to whether they are compatible or not.

Check Ingredients

Always look at the ingredients list for any item you are considering using at the same time as Protocel®, even if the item is listed on the "okay" list. For example, DIM is listed as compatible with Protocel® but many DIM supplements have vitamin E added. You may do best finding a DIM supplement to use that is a brand with no vitamin E added. Another type of situation is the following: A woman might wish to use Haelen, which is a powerful cancer-fighting beverage made from fermented soy beans known to help fight breast cancer. Because soy isoflavones are listed as compatible with Protocel®, and soy isoflavones are the key cancer-fighting ingredient in Haelen, the woman might think that Haelen is compatible with Protocel®. But a quick online search of Haelen to find out the wide array of nutrients in it reveals that the drink is *also* "rich" in proteins, selenium, zinc, and vitamins A, B_1, B_2, B_{12}, C, D, E, and K. Thus, at first glance, Haelen may sound good, but anything rich in selenium, vitamin C and vitamin E should be avoided when using Protocel®.

Prescription Medications and Hormone-Blocking Drugs

Many people have successfully used Protocel® for their cancer while they were also taking blood pressure medication, insulin, steroids, anti-seizure medications, antibiotics, or pain medication. This has given most experts the idea that, in general, prescription medications do not interfere with Protocel®. Thus, if you *need* to take a prescription medication for reasons other than treating your cancer, by all means take it.

However, since there have been no studies done to assess the compatibility of *all* medications with Protocel®, there *could* be some that are not compatible. For instance, at least two experts have had suspicions that using the drug Tamoxifen may be counter-productive to Protocel®. Tamoxifen is a hormone-blocking drug given mainly to women with breast cancer and it changes the metabolism of the cancer cells to some extent. (Refer to Chapter 19 to read about how Tamoxifen is a "cytostatic" drug that blocks estrogen and puts cancer cells into a sort of sleep state.) This alteration of the cancer cell metabolism may interfere with how Protocel® was designed to work on the cell respiration of cancer cells. Unfortunately, some women who have used Protocel® and Tamoxifen together have not done as well as expected. It is unclear whether *other* forms of estrogen-blocking drugs for women, such as Raloxifene, might interfere or not, but the risk is probably not worth taking.

Similarly, there is some suspicion that testosterone-blocking drugs, such as Lupron and Casodex, that are given to men with prostate cancer may also be less compatible with the Protocel® formula than previously thought. Though they don't *directly* interfere with Protocel®, testosterone-blocking drugs make a man more estrogen-dominant and estrogen fuels prostate cancer growth. Thus, taking a testosterone-blocking drug may make it harder for Protocel® to stop the cancer growth. (For more information, refer to Chapter 20.)

Since not all prescriptions drugs have been evaluated for compatibility with Protocel®, the fewer taken the better. If you are taking a life-saving prescription medication, definitely continue with it as prescribed. However, if you don't really need to be on a medication while you are using Protocel® to fight your cancer, you may want to consider discontinuing it.

Whenever possible, take prescription medications *separate* from your Protocel® dose. In other words, try not to put the medication in your stomach at the same time as Protocel® just to be on the safe side. Rarely will there be a chemical interaction, but caution is best in order to give Protocel® its very best chance of working. For instance, many people take a medication such as Nexium® for their heartburn or acid-reflux. Nexium® changes the pH of the fluids in the stomach. If one were taking their Protocel® into the stomach at the same time, this might alter the pH of Protocel® also in an undesirable way.

Anecdotal observation has shown that the use of Protocel® can often *improve* other health conditions a person may have, such as high blood pressure, arthritis, chronic fatigue, some forms of diabetes, Crohn's disease, multiple sclerosis, viral infections, endometriosis, hemorrhoids, and psoriasis. So it sometimes happens that while a person is using Protocel®

for cancer, he or she may see an improvement in these conditions and require *less* prescription medication over time. It is important, therefore, for people to be aware of this and carefully monitor the dosage of any prescription medications they are taking—*especially* in cases where a person is taking blood pressure medication or insulin. People who require insulin should monitor their blood-sugar levels more than once a day while on Protocel® and people on blood pressure medication should monitor their blood pressure closely in case they end up needing less of the prescription medication. Protocel® will not cause blood sugar or blood pressure to rise abnormally, so if a person notices either of these going too high, they should look to other reasons as the cause.

Diet

No rigid dietary restrictions are required while using Protocel®. The simple most common recommendations are to:

1. **Eat a healthy, well-balanced and varied diet.** This includes fresh organic vegetables and fruits, good sources of protein (eggs, yogurt, cottage cheese, meat, fish, poultry, legumes), and plenty of good water. (But NOT specialized high-alkaline waters.) It is not necessary to be vegetarian or vegan. However, vegetarian or vegan cancer patients should be conscientious about making sure their non-animal source protein intake is balanced and sufficient so that their body has enough good quality protein to rebuild tissues during their recovery. Junk food should be kept to a minimum for general health (especially soft drinks), but caffeinated coffee or tea is fine.

2. **Avoid refined sugar.** This is by far the most important restriction because cancer cells thrive on sugar. Table sugar, pastries, cookies, candies, ice cream, and all other sweets made with sugar should be avoided. Stevia or Xylitol do not raise blood glucose levels and are good sugar substitutes. Refined wheat (white flour) turns readily into glucose in the body and should also be avoided or greatly reduced, but whole grain breads are fine. Fructose ingested by eating whole fruits (not juiced fruits) is okay as long as the amount of fruit in one's diet is not excessive. Protocel® works against cancer by interfering with the cancer cells' ability to have enough glucose for their energy needs. So, eating refined sugar while taking Protocel® is like trying to put out a fire while dousing that fire with gasoline at the same time! The less sugar you eat, the better you will do.

NOTE: If a cancer patient using Protocel® is in the hospital, they should make sure they are NOT given an I.V. solution full of glucose unless absolutely necessary. Glucose in I.V.s feeds cancer growth.

3. **Restrict alcoholic beverages.** Though some people have done fine with a small glass of wine once in a while or some other minimal drink of alcohol on occasion, just remember that alcohol intake can raise blood sugar levels in some people and lower blood sugar levels in other people, depending on a variety of factors. One factor is that alcohol can interfere with insulin metabolism, making blood sugar levels fluctuate in unpredictable ways. Since you don't want your blood sugar unduly high at any time because that could feed your cancer cells, the wisest choice is to avoid alcohol altogether.

4. **Avoid concentrated foods, such as juices.** The daily intake of juices or other concentrated foods may be too high in fructose, vitamin C or other nutrients such as selenium. Common fruit juice, concentrated green drinks and exotic juices like Goji, Mangosteen, or Noni should probably all be avoided the way many supplements must be avoided. However, foods in their whole natural form that may be high in vitamin C, such as citrus fruits, broccoli and strawberries, are fine in reasonable (not excessive) amounts.

Lysing Symptoms

The Protocel® formula produces no *direct* negative side effects in people. Any symptoms associated with taking Protocel® are *indirect*, and are a result of the anaerobic cells of the body lysing, or breaking down, and being processed out of one's system. Therefore, any symptoms that occur during one's recovery process while using Protocel® are referred to as "lysing symptoms." In other words, a perfectly healthy person could take Protocel® everyday and not experience any symptoms at all, because they won't be having a lot of lysing occurring. Protocel® is non-toxic and *very* safe to use. However, when a person has a significant amount of cancer and it is responding well to the Protocel®, they will very likely experience lysing symptoms. Sometimes, these symptoms are quite remarkable in themselves and can involve a lot of mucousy or white material coming out of the body in various ways.

Lysing of anaerobic cells most likely begins internally within the first 24 hours of starting Protocel®, but may not be noticed through outward signs or symptoms for a while. The onset of noticeable lysing symptoms will vary from person to person, with some people experiencing signs of lysing within a few days of starting Protocel®, yet others not noticing any for weeks or months. Visible, outward indications of lysing are not always apparent, even when cancer cells are actively lysing inside. Some people have even fully recovered from their cancer with no outward signs of lysing at all. People with only a small amount of cancer or slow-growing cancer are less likely to notice signs of lysing, whereas people with a lot of cancer or fast-growing cancer will often see signs of lysing on an almost daily basis.

The one type of lysing symptom that appears to be unique to Protocel® is a mucousy excretion of egg white-like material that may be noticed draining out of the nose, being coughed up from the lungs, or coming out in the feces. This is because, as the cancer cells lyse, they break down into their basic protein parts and the body has to process this "dead cancer cell debris," or protein material, out through any orifice it can. A runny nose is quite common, and as long as the mucous is not a greenish color and there is reason to believe it is not from a cold or allergies, it is usually an indication of lysing. For anyone using Protocel® for cancer and having a clear, whitish, or slightly yellowish mucous draining from the nose, it is best *not* to use a cold medicine to dry this up. Just keep lots of tissues handy and let it come out.

Some people may also experience some crust around their eyes in the morning. When mucous material comes out through the urine or feces, it may be clear or a little yellowish, or even sometimes very white. White mucousy material or chunks of white stuff are very good signs. When bowel movements are sluggish, some people have done enemas and found that a copious amount of white mucousy material then comes out after being on Protocel® for a while. This is lysed material and a good sign that the Protocel® is working well. All these types of excretion are visible forms of evidence that lysing is occurring inside the body and can be encouraging when noticed. When this material comes out, it is simply the body's way of housecleaning the unwanted broken down cancer cell parts.

Tiredness within the first few weeks is also a common symptom for people who have a lot of lysing going on, but may not be experienced at all for people with less cancer. Tiredness does *not* mean that Protocel® is draining energy from one's normal cells. It just means that the body is working hard to process out the lysed material (or broken down cancer.) Thus, extra tiredness is simply a detoxing symptom. If a person has very little cancer in their body to begin with, such as right after having a tumor removed surgically, then they will most likely *not* experience any tiredness at all because there won't be that much cancer lysing at any given time and their body should be able to deal with it without feeling tired.

Some other lysing symptoms that may be noticed are similar to common "detoxing" or flu-like symptoms. These may be short periods of mild nausea, elevated temperature, upset stomach, or headache while the body is working on processing out lysed material. It could also involve a temporary increase in normal body waste functions, such as an increased frequency or volume in urine or bowel output or sweating. Usually these symptoms will not last long, or they may occur sporadically for a while. This is also why increasing the amount of water one drinks while using Protocel® can be really important. (To help flush everything out.)

Other possible experiences due to lysing are: "bubbly" or "foamy" urine or pimply bumps on the skin or a temporary rash. Less common symptoms are excess earwax, excess hair oil and vomiting. (Vomiting is *not* common, but if it does happen because of lysing, it will often contain unusual-looking material that does not look like normal food vomit.) It seems our bodies have many ways to rid themselves of unwanted material.

Another lysing symptom can be sharp needle-like pains. These are not a common occurrence, but can sometimes happen. When they do, they appear to be related to broken-down cancer debris moving through very narrow lymph vessels. These types of pains are most commonly experienced by women using Protocel® for breast cancer and may occur in the chest area, abdomen, or under the arms. Some find relief by increasing their intake of water and doing movements to assist the flow of the lymph fluid through the body. One excellent way to improve lymph flow is to very gently bounce on a mini-trampoline for about 10 minutes twice a day. But not all women with breast cancer experience this and everyone's experience is different.

To review, 5 common types of lysing symptoms that may occur are:

1. Initial tiredness in the first few weeks (this could last longer in some cases, especially for those people who are dealing with a *lot* of cancer.)

2. Possible flu-like symptoms (fever, sweating, weakness, loose stools.)

3. An increase in normal body waste output (increased frequency of bowel movements and urination.)

4. Possible excretion of mucousy material through the nose, bowels, and

urinary tract (bubbles or foam in the urine in the toilet bowl), which could be either clear, slightly yellowish, or white in color.

5. Possible needle-like pains in or near the cancer area. These are usually so fleeting when they do occur that they are not a problem. However, if difficult, try getting the lymph fluid to flow better by increasing your water intake and doing gentle physical movement.

Also, Protocel® appears to work faster on fast-growing cancers and slower on slow-growing cancers. This may be because fast-growing (aggressive) cancers have a higher rate or percentage of anaerobic activity going on and this is what Protocel® targets. Thus, people with aggressive cancer may observe more lysing and have their tumors regress more rapidly than people with slow-growing cancer. This does not mean that Protocel® won't work on slow-growing malignant cancers, it just means that those people with a slow-growing cancer may need to be more patient.

For people using Protocel® for brain cancer, lysing symptoms may involve a return of the person's initial brain tumor symptoms for a short period around the fourth to sixth week after starting Protocel®. This may involve dizziness, foggy thinking, or motor problems if those were the initial symptoms when diagnosed. The reason for this is that when a tumor or tumors are starting to lyse in the brain, the resulting effect may be a mild edema. Most people will get through this period just fine if they know what to expect. If any of the lysing symptoms get to be *too* much, adults can reduce their Protocel® dosage down to ⅛ teaspoonful four times a day until the lysing becomes more manageable (preferably no more than a few days), then work back up to the normal dose. Do *not* stay on a lower than recommended dose for any longer than you have to.

It has also been shown that many brain cancer patients using Protocel® need to be on a prescription steroid for edema or a prescription anti-seizure medication. These types of meds are often necessary to control pressure and fluid build-up in the brain long enough to allow Protocel® to work. Over time, these meds can be reduced gradually under the supervision of a doctor as the cancer goes away.

What if You Start Getting Headaches While Using Protocel®?

Daily headaches are *not* a normal lysing symptom except when there is cancer in the brain. If a person starts getting regular headaches while taking Protocel®, or headaches that are getting worse and worse, they may want to consider getting an MRI or PET scan of the brain to see whether or not they have cancer in the brain. Sometimes people dealing with cancer in other areas of the body don't know that it has already metastasized to the brain and it can be very important to know. This is because headaches can occur as a result of pressure in the brain due to either the cancer itself or the breakdown of the cancer. If a person *does* have cancer lysing in the brain, this does not always, but may in some cases cause headaches due to increased pressure. (The brain processes out lysed material more slowly than other areas of the body, so sometimes the lysed material builds up in the brain faster than the body can eliminate it.) These situations will often require that a steroid be prescribed by a doctor to control the pressure and give Protocel® time to work.

Unfortunately, some people are unaware that their cancer has already gone to their brain when they start taking Protocel®. This type of situation has come up a number of times with women dealing with breast cancer, for instance. Because breast cancer does *not* readily go to the brain within the first few years, oncologists don't tend to give these cancer patients brain scans. However, through the use of surgery, they can often slow the progression of the disease by a number of years. As a result, many women dealing with breast cancer have been fighting it for six, seven, eight, or more years. Over these years, since the cancer was never completely gone, it may have had time, in some cases, to metastasize to the brain. In these cases, stopping the Protocel® for a few days might cause a lessening of the headaches because the lysing activity stops temporarily, but that is just a confirmation that anaerobic cells in the brain are breaking down, and one will need to get back up to the regular dosing with the help of steroids in order to get the cancer to go away.

Thus, anyone experiencing regular or progressively worse headaches after starting Protocel® should consider getting a brain scan to find out if they have cancer in the brain so that they can get onto a steroid medication for the pressure, if needed to allow Protocel® time to work. This has the added benefit of giving the patient one more area of the body that can be seen through scans for assessing their progress.

Cancer Marker Tests May Elevate

Another possible outcome of lysing that is extremely important to know about® is that, as one's cancer is stabilizing and then starting to dissipate, one's cancer blood marker tests may dramatically elevate. Not all types of cancer can be tested for through blood cancer markers. But for those types of cancer that can, such as breast cancer, ovarian cancer, intestinal cancer, and prostate cancer, many doctors will want to run cancer marker blood tests at various intervals. However, any person using Protocel® should be aware that cancer markers often rise quickly within the first 3 to 6 months of being on Protocel® as their cancer is lysing. Eventually (depending on how much cancer you have and how fast your cancer is lysing), those markers will come back down, but in the initial stages, seeing the markers rise can often be scary and cause doctors as well as patients to become discouraged.

When using Protocel®, you can get cancer marker blood tests if you want to, but you should not rely on them until the numbers have peaked and already started coming back down. Thus, in the first 6 months or so of using Protocel®, it is often a better idea to rely on scans and lysing symptoms to assess one's progress.

Unfortunately, doctors interpret higher cancer marker results as "more cancer." However, when using Protocel®, this is not necessarily the correct interpretation. Most cancer marker tests are *general* indicators of how much cancer is in a person's body because they measure certain substances that go along with, or are released by particular types of cancer cells. For some types of cancer, the marker tests will be measuring a type of enzyme that is released by that particular type of cancer into the bloodstream. For other types of cancer, the marker tests will be measuring a type of protein released by the cancer cells, and so forth.

But when Protocel® is doing its job, the breakdown of the cancer cells causes them to *release* their enzyme or protein markers into the bloodstream even more quickly than they would if alive. Remember, Protocel® operates in a fundamentally different way than doctors are used to. This means that lysing symptoms, such as temporarily elevated cancer markers, will not necessarily be understood correctly by oncologists or other doctors. Some people may choose to *not* get cancer marker blood tests at all in the first six months or so in order to not have to deal with doctors being alarmed. Others just explain to their doctor that the alternative approach they are using *causes* marker levels to rise as the cancer breaks down and that other types of diagnostic tests may be best to use for a while.

Assessing Your Progress and Using Scans

Some people using Protocel® will be able to fairly quickly see that their cancer is going away. This often happens when a person is able to feel or see their tumor, such as a breast tumor close to the surface or a lymph node tumor on the neck. But most people are dealing with internal tumors or various areas of metastases that are not readily observable. In these cases, how do people know they are making progress?

Often, the use of diagnostic scans can be helpful. X-rays, ultrasounds, thermograms, CT scans, MRIs, and PET scans are all possible choices. The particular type used is often determined by where the cancer is and what type of scan is most effective for that part of the body (which people should consult their doctor about.) Most people will find that within the first two to four months on Protocel®, their cancer diagnostic tests will show a stabilization of their cancer, and their scans often show that previously aggressive tumors have stopped growing or spreading. This halting of the progression of the disease is a very good sign and means that the Protocel® is working. At the same time, other types of lysing symptoms will often be noticed to confirm that the cancer is indeed breaking down. By the third month, or sometimes not until the fourth month, most people will start to see a decrease in tumor size.

However, just as tumor marker tests may be affected by lysing, scan results may also be affected by lysing in ways that doctors don't understand. So, interpreting scans when using Protocel® can be tricky. Thus, it is important for people using Protocel® to be discerning when they assess their progress, and to take into account the "whole picture" of their situation, rather than rely on the results of just one diagnostic tool. This whole picture may include the results of other diagnostic tests, the amount and frequency of lysing symptoms the person is experiencing, and the whole history of how they have been feeling.

One consideration is that, in some cases, tumors will actually show up just a little bigger on scans in the first few months of being on Protocel®, even though they are breaking down. This is because tumors may sort of liquefy and spread a little as the cancer cells lyse (like an ice cube melting and forming a puddle). And very large tumors may take so much time decreasing in density that they don't actually show reduction in size until the fourth month or so. However, smaller tumors do often show a decrease in size on scans within the first few months, sometimes even as quickly as after just a few weeks on Protocel®. The rate of tumor reduction may also depend on how fast-growing or slow-growing the cancer is because, as mentioned before, it appears that fast-growing cancers lyse faster and slow-growing cancers lyse slower.

Another important thing to be aware of is that sometimes a scan may be taken at a time when lysed material has not yet been processed out of the tumor area. CT scans and MRIs don't always differentiate between active cancer and lysed material. So, if scan results do not appear consistent with other signs of progress (such as how the person feels or lysing symptoms), then the person may want to request a PET scan.

PET scans are more expensive and sometimes doctors won't order them or insurance companies won't pay for them. But, at least in some cases, they may be able to help differentiate between active cancer and broken down cancer cell debris (lysed material). The reason is that PET scans are the only type of scan that uses the administration of a slightly radioactive sugar solution with a short half-life just before the scan is given. The fact that sugar is used to transport the slightly radioactive material (which is what highlights on the scan) is the important thing. Because cancer cells gobble up sugar about 17 to 20 times faster than normal cells, they tend to be the cells that highlight the most on the scan. However, they will only gobble up the sugar if they are alive and metabolically active. Lysed cancer is merely broken down cell parts and therefore will not gobble up sugar.

A good example of this type of confusion is the story of a man who was treating his oligodendroglioma brain cancer with Protocel®. Before starting Protocel®, his MRI scans were showing that he had advanced cancer in two places in his brain: the frontal lobe and the brain stem. After being on Protocel® 23 for six months, he got another MRI. The doctor was horrified at the results and proclaimed that the MRI showed the cancer had spread throughout his entire brain. This man and his wife were confused about this result since the man was feeling great and had been working full-time and exercising three days a week for many months. How could he feel so good with that much cancer in his brain? So the man requested a PET scan, which was done just two weeks later, and the results presented a completely different picture from the MRI. According to the PET scan, there was no more active cancer in the frontal lobe at all and only a tiny spot of active cancer left in the brain stem. Thus, the MRI had most likely highlighted lysed cancer that had not yet been processed out of the brain. (This type of phenomenon may be more common in the brain than other areas of the body since the brain is notoriously slow at processing out large amounts of lysed material.) If this man had only relied on the MRI, he would have thought the Protocel® wasn't working and would probably have stopped taking it.

However, PET scans have their problems, too, and are not always perfect diagnostic tools even without the factor of lysing. For instance, highly inflamed or rapidly healing tissues will also uptake sugar faster than normal tissue. Thus, a recent surgical area or broken bone may highlight on a PET scan in a way that looks like cancer. Even radiation treatments may cause tissue to highlight on a PET scan. Once again, it cannot be overstressed that the whole picture of what is happening with a person must be considered when evaluating any diagnostic results. Blood marker tests, ultrasounds and other forms of scans can be used, and often should be used at regular intervals. But using common sense and considering all possible sources of information is also critical in order to determine one's progress accurately.

Will Protocel® Work on Benign Tumors or DCIS?

It is possible that tumors must be malignant for Protocel® to work on them. This has not yet been proven and some people seem to experience some effect on benign tumors. But there have also been cases where Protocel® has not appeared to affect truly benign tumors, probably because there is not enough anaerobic activity going on. (The more malignant a tumor is, the more anaerobic metabolism is used.) This may also be the case with DCIS (ductal carcinoma in situ). Though classified as "Breast Cancer" by conventional medicine, many medical researchers believe the "in situ" breast cancers such as ductal carcinoma in situ and lobular carcinoma in situ are really *pre-cancerous* conditions that have not fully turned malignant. Some anecdotal cases appear to indicate that DCIS or LCIS may not respond to Protocel®. Thus, for benign tumor cases, Protocel® can be tried, but if it doesn't work the person may want to switch to another approach that has had success with benign tumors.

Will Protocel® Work on Skin Cancer?

Yes, Protocel® works well on life-threatening skin cancer, such as malignant melanoma, as well as non-life-threatening skin cancer, such as basal cell cancer. Most people use the Formula 50 for skin cancers and it should be taken orally the same as for any internal cancer. For extra benefit, some people choose to *also* put some Protocel® on topically wherever lesions are accessible on the surface, but this should only be done in *addition* to taking Protocel® orally, not instead of it.

Variations on Dosing

Taking ¼ tsp. of Formula 50 every 6 hours (*four* times around the clock) and ¼ tsp. of Formula 23 every 4 to 5 hours (*five* times around the clock) are the basic starting doses for the Protocel® formulations. And, for many people, that is the exact dosing that they stay on throughout their entire cancer recovery. However, sometimes varying the dosing can be a good idea and may even in a few cases make the difference between full recovery or not.

Higher Doses. To give themselves the best possible chance, some people may wish to start out at ⅓ teaspoonful each dose instead of ¼ for either formulation. This may not sound like a big difference, but with Protocel® it can be significant. Increasing the dose usually causes more lysing to happen more quickly. Since Protocel® is non-toxic, higher doses won't be harmful to the body and it is not uncommon for some people to take ⅓ teaspoonful each dose or even ½ teaspoonful in some cases. However, one does need to be concerned about whether increased lysing is something the body can handle or not. In most cases, increased lysing is not going to cause any real difficulty, and if a person experiences too much lysing they can go back down to the ¼ teaspoonful dose. But, as already mentioned, people with very little cancer in their bodies will often not even notice lysing symptoms at all.

Thus, starting out at ⅓ teaspoonful is particularly safe for people who have very little cancer in their body. (They are in remission or their cancer has been caught early.) Increasing to ⅓ teaspoonful is also a good idea if a person has been taking Protocel® for a month or two at ¼ teaspoonful and they don't feel their cancer is responding as well as they'd like it to. If one's cancer appears to be still progressing after a month, for instance, it is always possible to increase the dose to ⅓ teaspoonful.

The most common individual dose size is either ¼ or ⅓ teaspoonful, with some people needing as much as ½ teaspoonful every dose. More than that may be used, but is not common. Also, sometimes people will "power dose" (see next page) at regular intervals to push the limit on their dosing and ensure optimum results.

But there are some situations where people should NOT go higher than ¼ teaspoonful until they see how their body processes out the lysed broken down cancer. The two main situations where one should be *not* go higher than ¼ teaspoonful are:

1. When there is any cancer in the brain. This is because cancer break-down occurs just as fast in the brain as anywhere else, but the brain does not process out lysed material very efficiently and

2. When there is a tumor in a restricted passageway. (Such as in the esophagus, urethra, or other narrow area.)

Power Dosing. "Power Dosing" is the term used for any increase in one's Protocel® dose size or frequency for a short period of time. (Usually not more than 5 to 7 days at a time.) This is one added way that people can take charge of their recovery and push their Protocel® use to the limit. For instance, if a person has been using Protocel® for a number of weeks, is feeling fine and not seeing much in the way of lysing signs, they may choose to power dose for a short period to increase their rate of lysing. If they have been using Protocel® 50, for instance, at ¼ teaspoonful every 6 hours, they might want to power dose with ⅓ teaspoonful every 4 hours for 5 days to see what happens, then go back to their normal dose. If they don't experience any increase in lysing symptoms, then they may want to slightly increase their normal dose. (For instance, to ⅓ teaspoonful every 6 hours.)

Pushing the limit on one's dosing can be helpful in many cases when you don't know whether you are progressing or not, or when you just want to give your cancer an extra "kick" for a short period. A good example of this can be found in the book, *The Breast Stays Put*, by Pamela Hoeppner. Hoeppner gives a personal account of how she used power dosing to make sure Protocel® was able to completely get rid of her very aggressive breast cancer. And she explains some of the intense lysing symptoms she experienced as a result. Though power dosing can be a very effective way to improve one's chances for full recovery, it is important to remember that it should probably *not* be done by people who have cancer in the brain, because it could make the lysing go too fast for the brain to handle.

Middle-of-the-Night Dose

The middle-of-the-night dose was instigated by Ed Sopcak. Sopcak was the man who manufactured Cancell® (the original name for Protocel® 50) at his own expense and *gave* away more than twenty-thousand bottles of it to cancer patients. He always told people to spread their doses out evenly around the 24-hour clock and never go more than 6 hours between any two doses.

Ed Sopcak had the best track record of cancer recovery for those people he helped to use this formula. Years later, some people found that a lot of people could still get well if they doubled their bedtime dose and took their next dose in the morning 8 hours later. This certainly has worked in many cases, particularly for those cancers that are either slow-growing or have been caught very early. (Such as prostate cancer caught early.) However, this author believes that taking a dose in the middle of the night and never going more than 6 hours between any two doses is still the most optimum way to use Protocel® for cancer. And, in cases where there is a lot of cancer or the cancer is particularly fast-growing, there have been cases where the middle-of-the-night dose has appeared to be *necessary* in order for Protocel® to be able to get on top of the cancer growth effectively.

Sopcak used to say that the "life" of the formula in the body was 6 hours. (It is unclear as to what Ed meant exactly, but he may have meant that after 6 hours whatever Protocel® was still in the body would have dropped below the therapeutic level—in other words, *below* the level where it can effectively cause cancer cells to lyse.) That is why he always told people to never go more than 6 hours between doses. Thus, it really appears that most people will have their best chance for recovery if they get up sometime during the night to take a dose and space all their doses out as evenly as possible around the 24-hour clock.

How Long Does Protocel® Take?

It is impossible to give a time-scale for recovery that would apply to every cancer patient. Keep in mind that Protocel® does not work as quickly as cytotoxic agents like chemotherapy. This is because it is not a fast-acting dangerous poison. Instead, it is designed to break down cancer in a steady methodical way that is safe and effective and not too much for the body to handle at any given time.

The more cancer one has, the longer it will generally take for it to go away. Also, as already stated, slow-growing cancers appear to lyse slower and fast-growing cancers appear to lyse faster. It is best to think of each person's recovery time as unique. There have been people who have seen tumors start getting smaller within the first month and became cancer-free in about six months time, while others have not seen obvious tumor reduction until the third or fourth month and have needed to use the formula for a year or several years to become totally cancer-free.

As a general rule, most people using Protocel® for cancer will notice some lysing symptoms within the first few weeks of starting the formula, and many will also experience a reduction of pain or an increase in well-being within the first month. (Though people experiencing a particularly good response to Protocel® and who have a lot of lysing going on may also feel tired until the cancer load is reduced.) But as already mentioned, the first two months or so may simply involve the Protocel® formula stopping the progression of the cancer and stabilizing tumor growth. This, in itself, is a wonderful thing. It generally takes *longer* than two months for most people to experience a noticeable reduction in the size of their tumors, but some cases do see tumors go down within the first couple of months.

It helps to keep in mind that the speed at which Protocel® can totally rid someone of their cancer is still remarkably fast when compared to conventional treatments like chemotherapy and radiation. These conventional treatments may cause fast tumor regression, but because they so often do not completely get rid of the cancer, tumors will many times grow back and must be treated a second or even a third time over a several-year period. The initial reduction of tumors under these circumstances (called "remission") may be fast at first, but short-lived—and rarely results in a fully cancer-free state. Whereas, with Protocel®, the reduction in tumor size may be slower at first in some cases, but *permanent* when one continues to use the formula correctly over a period of time.

What About Doing Radiation or Chemotherapy Along With Protocel®?

This is a *very* important question. Radiation will not interfere with the action of Protocel®. In fact, it appears that radiation treatments work synergistically with Protocel®. This is mainly because radiation also reduces cell voltage. But it is important to make an *informed* decision whenever considering the use of radiation treatments. Ask your doctor about all the side effects that are possible from radiation treatments and try to make sure that you will not be risking damage to vital nerves, tissues, or organs by doing it. Radiation to the brain can be effective against cancer for short-term results, however long-term tissue damage can occur that may cause other problems down the line. If a tumor is so big or life-threatening that it needs to be dealt with through radiation to help ensure the survival of the patient or to give Protocel® enough time to work, then it is probably a good idea to do radiation and Protocel® together until the tumor is reduced to a safer size, then continue with the Protocel® alone.

If this is not the case, however, then it might be best to either decline the radiation or at least make sure that the radiation treatments are considered low-dose or short-term. People doing Protocel® and radiation at the same time generally do not need to complete the full course of radiation that would normally be prescribed for the same situation without Protocel®. In other words, if one does choose to use radiation at the same time as Protocel®, one can usually get by with less radiation than would normally be prescribed.

Chemotherapy, on the other hand, often works *against* Protocel® and should be avoided in most cases to give Protocel® the best possible chance of working. Years ago, Jim Sheridan wrote,

> Chemotherapy can bring the percentage of success down, because chemotherapy changes the level on the oxidation-reduction ladder where Entelev/Cancell works.[1]

Therefore, if at all possible, it is best to *not* combine chemotherapy with Protocel®.

The only exception to this rule is when the chemotherapy agent is an "anti-metabolite" type of chemo drug. The anti-metabolite chemo agents push the energy level of cells down and therefore tend to work well with Protocel®. However, there are very few of these types of chemo. Basically, there are just two that are known at this time to be compatible anti-metabolite chemo drugs that won't interfere with Protocel®. They are:

1. 5FU (Fluorouracil)

2. Xeloda (Capecitabine)

But people also need to be well informed whenever they make a choice to use chemo. Even anti-metabolite chemotherapies can damage normal, healthy cells. Any chemo is toxic and can potentially cause serious side effects and possible long-term damage to the heart, liver, kidneys, brain, and nervous system. Thus, the risks versus the benefits must be weighed.

When it comes to any other type of chemotherapy besides the two listed above, one should consider that there is a risk that the chemo will make the Protocel® less effective or even possibly *completely ineffective*. This is no small matter since chemo can rarely cure a person and Protocel® can if it isn't interfered with. Thus, in most cases, people should seriously consider *declining* the use of chemo if they are using Protocel®.

Too many people hear of someone that did fine while using chemo-therapy and Protocel® at the same time, and think they will do fine as well. They may not realize that the type of chemo the other person used was one of the two above and that any other type of chemo could inhibit Protocel®'s action.

One eye-opening case I personally followed was of a woman with metastasized ovarian cancer who had been on chemo for a long time. While she was in-between chemo treatments, she started using Protocel® and began experiencing signs of lysing and saw positive changes in a lymph node tumor on her neck. She also began feeling better. But her oncologist soon convinced her to go back on the chemo and she didn't feel she could say no to her doctor. Though she stayed on Protocel®, all her signs of lysing stopped as soon as she resumed the chemo and she had no more indications that the Protocel® was working for her. Since the chemo itself was ineffective against her disease, she died 5 months later full of cancer. In her case, it was very clear that the chemo drugs kept the Protocel® from being able to work effectively. This unfortunate woman felt she could not say "no" to her oncologist, but by doing so she took away Protocel®'s ability to save her life.

Some people advise that Protocel® can be taken with any type of chemo and it will help reduce the side effects of the chemo. This may be true. Protocel® is a powerful anti-oxidant and it may help reduce some of the serious side effects of chemo because of that. However, Protocel® does not get rid of people's active cancer by being a powerful anti-oxidant. The anti-oxidant capacity of Protocel® is simply a nice "side-benefit." By using a chemo drug other than the ones known to be anti-metabolite chemos, cancer patients may be negating Protocel®'s ability to work effectively on their cancer cells—and that is not a good trade-off.

When to Stop Using Protocel®

Most people using Protocel® for cancer continue to take it for at least one year *after* their doctor has given them the "all-clear" according to all diagnostic tests that can be done. (Some people prefer to use it for up to two years or more after the all-clear point, just to be on the safe side.) The reason for this is to make sure that all the cancer cells have completely lysed before stopping the treatment. Keep in mind that current diagnostic techniques may not always detect cancer unless there are about 10 million cancer cells or more all in one place. This means that if you have as many as 9 million cancer cells, *diagnostic techniques available today may not reliably detect them.* Therefore, if a person stops using Protocel® as soon as their scans or other tests show no more signs of cancer, there may still be a significant number of cancer cells in their body that are still alive and ready to begin proliferating again. There have been some people who stopped using Protocel® 4 to 6 months after their "all-clear" diagnostic point, and later found they hadn't gotten all the cancer.

Continuing to use the formula rigorously for at least one year after the "all-clear" point is the best safeguard.

In some cases of treating primary brain cancer, a person may have been able to reduce and stabilize a large brain tumor that, instead of completely disappearing, has simply shrunk somewhat and stopped highlighting on scans. In these cases, it appears the tumor has turned into a benign or dead mass. For some cases, surgery at this point might be an option for removing the dead mass. But if that is too risky and some amount of the original mass continues to remain in the brain, the person may want to stay on Protocel® indefinitely to avoid the possibility that the mass might start highlighting and growing again. As shown in Case Story #10, stopping Protocel® simply because the mass is no longer highlighting can risk the tumor becoming active again months or even years later.

The length of time each person continues to take Protocel® after their cancer is no longer detectable is up to each person. Since Protocel® is not toxic to the body like chemotherapy or radiation, people can continue taking it indefinitely if they choose to. At least one woman has taken it for over 15 years with the only effects being that she feels great and never seems to come down with a cold or flu (since Protocel® helps the body fight viral infections, too.)

Do Not Reduce Your Dose for Maintenance Purposes

One of the biggest mistakes people make when using Protocel® to treat their cancer is stopping too soon. Another mistake people often make is reducing their dosing after the all-clear point. One woman used Protocel® 23 to get her bladder cancer to completely disappear from all scans and to no longer show up through a scoping procedure up the urethra. She was at the diagnostic all-clear point. But she made the mistake of thinking that she could then reduce her dosing of the Protocel® to only one dose three times a day. Within a few months, scans and scoping showed the cancer growing again. Keep in mind that *there is no scientific evidence that anything less than 4 doses a day of Protocel® will work effectively on cancer in humans.* Having less cancer does not mean you can take less Protocel®.

Some people do choose to use Protocel® just once or twice a day for health purposes, but in those cases they are receiving the anti-oxidant benefits of the formula only—*not* its ability to get rid of active cancer. By all observations, Protocel® must be taken at least 4 times every day in order to work effectively on cancer in people, even if they are dealing with only a small amount of cancer. If you use less than that you are risking the cancer growing and spreading again.

Protocel® Works for Pets, Too!

Many people have helped their beloved pets with Protocel®, and it is exciting that some veterinarians have even started using or recommending the formula for their canine and feline cancer patients. It also works remarkably well for any viral condition, so giving your dog or cat Protocel® for either cancer or a viral disease is well worth trying. Most animals appear to respond *faster* than humans and, though dosing 4 times a day is still often optimal, 3 times a day usually works for pets. (For some exciting dog recovery testimonials, visit the home page of www.OutsmartYour Cancer.com.)

Although there is a lack of information about using Protocel® for birds or reptiles, excellent reports have come in about giving Protocel® to a dog, cat, or horse. Most likely any *other* mammal, such as a ferret, goat, or pot-bellied pig, would also respond quite well. Usually, pet owners will mix the formula into any type of pet food or other treat the animal likes. One colorful story comes from a family that treated their female dog "Dink" for cancer by putting a few drops of Protocel® onto a piece of bread and throwing the bread up into the air. Dink would then happily leap up, grab the bread in her mouth, and gulp her cancer treatment down. Other pet owners choose to mix the Protocel® into canned pet food, meat baby food, or meat broth to get their animals to eat it. Just be sure the animal eats the entire amount over a short period of time to make sure they are getting their full dose.

Another way to administer Protocel® to a dog or cat is to first mix the dose in a small amount of distilled water or broth and then suck that up into an eye-dropper or plastic syringe and squirt the entire amount into the animal's mouth. Sometimes just holding the lip aside and squirting into the area between the lip and gums works well. One woman said her dog didn't like the taste and would shake it out of his mouth if she squirted the Protocel®/water mixture into its mouth directly. Luckily, she found that mixing the Protocel® dose into a small serving of cat food was enough to cover the taste and the dog would eat that up readily. She also found that mixing it in a very small amount of broth and putting the bowl down where the dog could lick it up worked well, too. This woman was then easily able to give the dog ¼ teaspoonful of Protocel® every 8 hours (three times a day).

A great horse story was related by one woman who treated her 20-year-old horse named "Ladd" for melanoma with Protocel®. Ladd was a white Arabian-Bay mix and was suffering from a type of melanoma that light-skinned horses often get. Ladd had melanoma spots on various parts of his body and one bulging tumor that had originated inside his right ear that was growing outward as well as inward. A biopsy was done on the tumor mass and the resulting diagnosis was "dermal sarcoid with acanthosis and hyperkeratosis." This type of melanoma is not necessarily fatal, but Ladd's veterinarian said that if nothing was done, the mass would eventually cut off the horse's hearing in that ear. Also, it could become quite painful if allowed to keep growing. As the mass grew steadily larger and larger, Ladd became more and more uncomfortable and could not tolerate anyone or anything touching that side of his face.

The woman who owned Ladd had, herself, recovered from life-threatening cancer using Cancell® and decided to try Protocel® on her horse. Every morning and evening, she would core an apple, put 1 teaspoonful of Protocel® into the inner part of the apple, and give the apple to her horse. (Thus, the horse received 1 teaspoonful of Protocel® twice each day). Ladd loved the taste of the formula so much that if any accidentally spilled on the ground, he would eagerly lick it up. After about three to four months of doing this regularly, all of Ladd's melanoma was gone, and he was a completely normal horse again with no spots and no bulging mass in his ear.

To confirm the stories I heard about using Protocel® for pets, I contacted a veterinarian in Illinois who had been using Protocel® on a few of his dogs and cats. An example of a success story he had was with an adult boxer dog that had been diagnosed in early January 2002 with adenocarcinoma of the stomach. The dog was extremely sick and was experiencing frequent vomiting. Within a month of starting Protocel® Formula 23, the dog was feeling a lot better and, in the second month, stopped vomiting altogether. The dog continued to feel better and better throughout the year, and by October of 2002 all of his tests and blood work were completely normal. In about nine months, this extremely sick dog showed no more signs of cancer.

The most remarkably fast recovery that this veterinarian observed, however, was when he used Protocel® to try and help a small male cat that was so sick from FIV (Feline Immunodeficiency Virus), that he was almost dead. This cat was not expected to live through the night, so the vet assumed it wouldn't hurt to try one last thing. He began administering Protocel® Formula 23 to the cat. By the next morning, the vet was astounded to see the cat sitting up and drinking water. This alone was amazing. By the third day on Protocel®, the cat was energetic and eating normally. After only one more day in the hospital, this almost dead cat seemed to have made a full recovery and was sent home to its family. He remained completely healthy after that.

According to one veterinarian, the *most* effective way to give Protocel® to a pet would be four times a day, spaced evenly around the clock. (Every 6 hours.) If this schedule is possible, it is worth trying. But, due to work schedules and other commitments, many people have difficulty giving their pet a dose that frequently, and the pet may not respond well to be awakened in the middle of the night for a dose. Luckily, most dogs and cats do quite well with just 3 doses a day, spaced out every 8 hours. (Two examples are: 7 A.M., 3 P.M., and 11 P.M.; or 6 A.M., 2 P.M., and 10 P.M.)

Some general dosing guidelines for pets are the following:

- For cats and *very* small dogs (toy variety): 1/8 teaspoonful of Protocel® 23 every eight hours. (Three times, spaced out as evenly as possible, over every 24-hour period.)

- For medium sized dogs: ¼ teaspoonful of Protocel® 23 every eight hours. (Three times, spaced out as evenly as possible, over every 24-hour period.)

- For large dogs: 1/3 teaspoonful of Protocel® 23 every eight hours. (Three times, spaced out as evenly as possible, over every 24-hour period.)

- For horses: 1 whole teaspoonful of Protocel® 23 every 8 if possible; every 12 hours otherwise. (Can be placed on the inner part of a cored apple or other treat.)

Administering the 3 daily doses as evenly spaced out as possible, every 8 hours, keeps a level amount of Protocel® in the animal's body, and this is important for optimum effectiveness. For people who can logistically do 4 times a day, that might be even more effective. *The one thing pet owners should not do is give their pet the Protocel® just twice a day.* This would most likely *not* be enough to effectively get rid of cancer. I have seen at least one case where a dog owner was told that simply giving her dog a double dose of Protocel® every 12 hours would be sufficient. Unfortunately, that turned out to be bad advice and her dog did not have a recovery. So, if a pet cannot be given the Protocel® every 8 hours because of the owner's work schedule or for any other reason, then a different alternative approach for that pet's cancer should probably be chosen.

Pet owners will want to watch their pets closely when giving them Protocel® for cancer. It is a good idea to make sure the pet's cancer is responding by watching for signs of lysing and by observing the tumor or tumors if possible. Try to see if the tumor or tumors are getting softer at first, then smaller. (If the cancer is not visible, then at least look for signs of lysing.) If, after a month or 6 weeks, the cancer does not appear to be responding effectively enough, then the owner may need to increase the dose size a little to meet their animal's specific needs. Or if the Formula 23 is being used and it doesn't seem to be stopping the cancer growth effectively, Formula 50 can be tried instead. But usually the Formula 23 is a good choice for pets in general.

IMPORTANT NOTE FOR TREATING PETS: Just as with humans, an animal taking Protocel® for cancer will often exhibit signs of lysing. For instance, the pet may become more tired in the first few weeks on Protocel®. Look for a possible runny nose or mucousy egg-white like material in their bowel movements. Chunks of white material may even come out in their feces. Dogs or cats whose cancer is responding well to the Protocel® may vomit up lysed material, too. If this happens, there is typically little or no food stuff in the vomit, and it may look like whipped egg whites.

As with humans, more frequent bowel movements or mild diarrhea may occur as a detox symptom while the body is trying to process out lysed material. Thus, it is important for a dog or cat getting Protocel®

for cancer to be able to go to the bathroom as frequently as they need to. A dog that is closed up inside the house with no access to a yard may have an accident on the rug due to cancer breakdown. And a dog that is crated during the day may be particularly at risk for having to sit in its own vomit or excrement until its owner comes home from work. So, if your dog does *not* have outdoor access or someone to let it out when it needs to go to the bathroom, Protocel® might not be the best choice and a different alternative treatment approach might need to be looked into. Usually, cats that are kept indoors have cat boxes they can access any time, so they should not have the same problem.

How Effective Is Protocel® for Cancer?

This is a question that cannot be answered with specific numbers because no formal clinical trials or even informal human case studies have ever been done on Entelev®, Cancell®, or Protocel®. What we do know is that countless cancer patients have achieved full recoveries through the use of this formula alone and that their stories along with the NCI in-vitro studies done in 1990 (see pages 159–163) show that this formula kills cancer very well.

However, whether or not a person achieves a full recovery depends on many factors and these factors greatly impact its success rate. Obviously, it is extremely important that Protocel® be used correctly for it to be effective. It is also important that people don't wait until they are too far along in their disease process to use Protocel®. In other words, some may use the formula correctly and see evidence that it is killing their cancer, but they still may not recover because their body has already been too damaged by either their cancer or previous toxic conventional treatments they used. One's body must be strong enough to process out the lysed (broken-down) cancer cells and able to build new healthy cells in order to achieve a full recovery.

It is also a good idea to avoid doing anything that could weaken the body while working on one's recovery. For instance, it is recommended that people consider avoiding flu shots while using Protocel® since they usually contain mercury, formaldehyde and other toxic substances. These can weaken the immune system and put a toxic load on the body.

And too many cancer patients have successfully reached the "all-clear" point according to diagnostics only to stop too soon and then suffer a cancer recurrence. Friends or family of these people may think that the

Protocel® "didn't work" because the person eventually died of their cancer, when in reality the Protocel® worked perfectly but the person simply stopped treatment before they got rid of every last cancer cell.

Last but not least, Jim Sheridan thought that people were at their most vulnerable around age 7, during the teen years, and in the menopausal years (for both men and women.) He felt this was because there was so much going on in the body in terms of growth spurts and hormonal changes. He was very concerned that certain cancers at these junctures were harder to treat with any kind of therapy, including his own formula, and that the success rate would be lower than otherwise for people undergoing growth spurts or hormonal changes. This is not to say that Protocel® will not work during those periods, but simply means it may be a more difficult situation and progress should be carefully monitored to gauge the response to the formula. Again, in these situations, larger or more frequent doses may be needed. (Some people even increase their dosing of Protocel® to every four hours, which is six times around the clock, and do well on that schedule.)

Unfortunately, because the Protocel® formula has been opposed by the ACS, FDA, and NCI in the past, no formal studies have been done on it to provide us with reliable official statistics. Of the thousands of people who have used this formula for cancer, many have had great recoveries while others have not. For some of those who did not, it was evident they did not use the Protocel® in an effective way, by either taking too many other supplements with it or chemo at the same time, or by going too long between doses overnight. A few have used it correctly but did not have the best response for reasons that are not understood. Thus, even though Protocel® has been curative for many, many cancer cases, people should be advised to not just take it and *assume* it is working. As with any approach to cancer, people should be diligent in assessing whether their treatment is working or not and should follow their progress through the use of scans whenever possible, increasing their dosing if needed, and switching to a different approach if all else fails.

But even without a cancer cure rate that can be quoted, more and more people are choosing to assess Protocel®'s success by the numerous real-life stories from people who have used it. As can be seen from the small sampling of true cases listed in this text, there have been amazing recoveries of all types—some that even involved cancer patients who were not expected to live more than a few weeks.

There are even *more* real-life recovery testimonials on the audio CD at the back of this book, on the various pages of www.OutsmartYour Cancer.com and at ElainesMiracle.com. Many of these people faced the grim reality that there was nothing in conventional medicine that could save them and were told by their doctors that they should go home and get their affairs in order. In my search into alternative cancer treatments available today, I could not find any other approach that appeared to be *more* successful than Protocel® for all types of cancer, including late-stage cancer.

As far as anyone knows, there is no known type of malignant cancer that Protocel® will not work on at all. And, as with most types of cancer treatments, there are some types of cancer that respond particularly quickly. Just from my own personal observation of cases, some of the *best* responders may be cervical cancer, bladder cancer, kidney cancer, prostate cancer, colon cancer, astrocytoma brain cancer, and acute leukemia. On the other end of the spectrum, the types of cancer that Protocel® can work on, but are not the best responders, so they may require more rigorous attention and monitoring of progress are squamous cell cancer, rhabdosarcoma, ovarian cancer, and glioblastoma multiforme brain cancer.

Resources:

Protocel® is available for purchase by phone or online from the following distributors:

Vitamin Depot (Ohio, U.S.A.)
(330) 634-0008
Mon.–Thurs. 10:00-8:00 / Fri. 10:00-6:00
www.YourVitaminDepot.com
For questions about using Protocel®, ask for
Dr. Kimberly Cassidy (Doctor of Naturopathy)

WebND (South Carolina, U.S.A.)
(888) 581-4442, or (864) 962-8880
Mon.–Thurs. 9:00-5:00 / Fri. 9:00-4:00 EST
www.WebND.com
www.RenewalandWellness.com

To find out about Protocel® distributors *outside* the U.S., go to www. OutsmartYourCancer.com, click on "What is Protocel," then "How to Order Protocel."

Cost of Treatment: Protocel® is relatively inexpensive. The average cost in the U.S. is approximately $100–$120 per month. (Dosage amount and frequency may vary from case to case.) Please note that international pricing will vary based on shipping costs, import fees and exchange rates.

Books

Elaine Hulliberger. *Winning the Battle Against Cancer, 2nd Ed.* Lightning Source, 2010. (See Amazon.com and www.ElainesMiracle.com.)

Websites

www.EntelevHome.net

www.ElonnaMcKibben.com

www.ElainesMiracle.com

www.BradMatznickStory.com

www.BeatingCancerWithoutBreakingASweat.com

Private Protocel® Support Forum

www.elonnascorner.com

13

Flaxseed Oil and Cottage Cheese

A truly remarkable all-natural cancer recovery approach is the "Flaxseed Oil and Cottage Cheese" diet developed by German biochemist Dr. Johanna Budwig. Dr. Budwig held a Ph.D. in natural science, went through medical training to become a physician, and was schooled in pharmaceutical science, physics, botany, and biology. Because of her important contributions to science and medicine, she was nominated by her peers to receive a Nobel Prize seven different times!

Dr. Budwig's most important contribution to the world involved her pioneering research into the roles of essential fatty acids. Her discoveries began in the 1950s, and over time, she illuminated a common causative factor behind many of our modern degenerative diseases, including cancer. In a nutshell, Dr. Budwig found that the widespread dietary habits of our modern world tend to promote a dangerous deficiency in the essential fatty acids so important to good health. She discovered that, as a result of modern food industry practices, we no longer eat enough good oils in their natural states, and instead, eat too many chemically altered oils that are damaging to our health. This tends to create a situation where we become deficient in two of the most important categories of essential fatty acids: the omega-3 and omega-6 fatty acids.

Dr. Budwig found that in order to mass produce and distribute food products high in oils (e.g., salad dressings, cooking oils, margarine, etc.), modern food manufacturers put these products through chemical processes to deliberately alter the makeup of the oils. These alterations are done because most healthful oils easily go rancid once they are processed out of the natural foods they are found in, such as vegetables, fish, seeds, and nuts. Once these oils are exposed to heat and sunlight for periods of time, as they would necessarily be through shipping and storage, they can easily degrade into a spoiled state. Thus, manufacturers of common food products such as margarines and bottled oils used in cooking or salad dressings, must put the oils they market through chemical processes so they can be packaged, shipped, and left to sit on store shelves for long periods of time.

The process of chemically altering natural oils is good for the manufacturers' profits, but bad for the consumer's health because these processes turn good, healthful, natural oils into harmful oils, or "pseudo" fats, as Dr. Budwig called them. Some of the most health-damaging pseudo fats are the hydrogenated and partially hydrogenated fats and oils, but many of the processed poly-unsaturated fats can be harmful as well.

It might surprise many people that *all margarines* and *virtually all fried foods* include these extremely harmful fats. Many other common foods contain harmful fats as well. For instance, any solidified peanut butter that does *not* show a layer of oil at the top of the jar when sold is made up of altered, harmful oils.

History and Theory

It wasn't until the late 1920s that essential fatty acids were beginning to be understood and categorized by researchers. Although food industries were producing substances such as margarine since the 1930s, they did not understand all the effects these altered oils would have on people. When Dr. Budwig began studying them in the 1950s, she was able to discover much more about the metabolism of oils in the body than had previously been known to the scientific world. She began her research by first studying and categorizing thousands of blood samples from people who were seriously ill, then comparing those samples to the blood of people who were healthy. One of the things Dr. Budwig discovered was a strange greenish-yellow substance in the blood of people with debilitating chronic illnesses. This was *not* found in the blood of people who were healthy. What was alarming was that this greenish-yellow substance appeared in place of healthy, red oxygen-carrying hemoglobin!

Dr. Budwig saw this greenish-yellow substance over and over in the blood of people with cancer, in particular. She also discovered a marked *lack* of phosphatides (an important fatty compound) and lipoproteins (fats bound to proteins) in the blood of cancer patients. After more research, Dr. Budwig discovered that these anomalies were linked to a severe deficiency of omega-3 and omega-6 essential fatty acids (EFAs). They are called "essential" because they are critical to good health and are substances our bodies can't make and therefore must be supplied through diet.

There are a variety of omega-3 and omega-6 essential fatty acids which are found in many different natural foods that we eat. In general, certain ocean fish—particularly the oily, cold-water fish such as tuna, salmon, and mackerel—are the foods highest in the omega-3 essential fatty acids, and certain seeds and nuts are the foods highest in the omega-6 essential fatty acids. (I like to remember this general rule by saying to myself, "Omega-3 from the sea; omega-6 from the sticks.")

Some food sources have both types of EFAs, however. When Dr. Budwig discovered a link between the deficiency of these essential fatty acids and many degenerative diseases, she looked for a natural way to replenish them. She settled on flaxseed oil because it is an extremely rich source of both omega-6 and omega-3 fatty acids—and because it is *particularly* high in the very important omega-3's, which tend to be the most deficient. Unrefined, cold-pressed flaxseed oil contains a whopping 15 to 25 percent linoleic acid (omega-6), and an incredible 50 to 60 percent alpha-linolenic acid (omega-3). (**NOTE:** Flax seeds are called "linseeds" in many places, so the term "flaxseed oil" refers to the same thing as the term "linseed oil.")

Dr. Budwig discovered that omega-3 and omega-6 essential fatty acids play a critical role in protecting us from cancer, especially in the following three ways:

1. They help maintain the health and integrity of cell membranes

2. They help promote oxygen transport into cells

3. They are required in the body's production of prostaglandins

She also found that people tend to be more deficient in the omega-3's than the omega-6's. This may be because people in the modern world tend to have more sources of omega-6 EFAs from other seed oils in their diets, such as safflower oil, sunflower oil, corn oil, sesame oil, and soybean oil.

Lipids and Cell Wall Integrity

Every cell in our body is covered with a protective membrane, or cell wall, that is made up of lipids (fats). In his book, *How to Fight Cancer and Win*, William L. Fischer states:

> Each cell in this miracle we call the body is protectively covered with a sheath of fats. The cell body (plasma) is interlaced with little lipid veins, often called the "nerves of the cell." These lipid veins are the connection between the nucleus and the outer membrane. They influence the care and feeding of the cell and the process of normal cell division by the use of tiny electrical impulses.[1]

Dr. Budwig came to believe that cancer was a result, not of "too much" cell growth, but of "faulty" cell growth, or cell division. She proposed that this faulty cell division was caused by not enough essential fatty acids in the cell membrane along with an accumulation of harmful manmade fats in the cell membrane. In her book, *Flax Oil as a True Aid Against Arthritis, Heart Infarction, Cancer and Other Diseases*, Dr. Budwig explains the important role of the "lipoid" membrane in the process of cell division:

> In growing cells, we find a dipolarity between the electrically positive nucleus and the electrically negative cell membrane with its highly unsaturated fatty acids. When the cell divides, it is the cell nucleus which begins this. The cell body and the daughter cell are then separated and tied off by the lipoid membrane. When a cell divides, its surface area is larger and must, of necessity, contain enough material in this surface with its fatty acids, to be able to divide the new cell completely from the original. Normal growth is always distinguished by a clearly defined course of action. In all our skin and membranes, in that of adults too, there are continual growth processes. The old cells have to be shed with new ones being formed underneath. When this process is interrupted, it means the body is beginning to die.[2]

Dr. Budwig reasoned that the common deficiency of essential fatty acids in cancer patients—evidenced by a marked lack of phospholipids in their blood—was why cancer cells often have multiple sets of chromosomes. The normal cell would attempt to divide but wouldn't have enough lipids necessary to complete the formation of the new cell membrane. Rather than one mother cell becoming two daughter cells, the mother cell would become one daughter cell—but the mother cell's chromosomes would have already divided and replicated themselves. Thus, according to Dr. Budwig, the daughter cell becomes an abomination with too many chromosomes due to lack of material for building new cell walls.

Lipids and Oxygenation

The oxygen utilization of every cell in our body depends on essential fatty acids. For instance, without natural, unaltered linoleic acid (omega-6), the body cannot produce hemoglobin. And without hemoglobin, the blood cannot carry oxygen to all the body's cells. Another way that EFAs oxygenate cells is by *attracting* oxygen to the cell via the cell membrane. When a cell has a normal and healthy cell membrane, this membrane is full of highly unsaturated essential fatty acids. The "unsaturated" aspect of the lipids means that they have lots of unbound electrons looking for something to bind to. One thing they love to bind to is oxygen. This then brings oxygen to the cell, which supports and stimulates the respiratory process of the cell itself and promotes better transport of oxygen into the cell.

Taking a closer look at the mechanics of cells, every cell wall (or cell membrane) is made up of lipids (or fats). The most common lipids in the membrane are the omega-3 essential fatty acids and cholesterol. The polyunsaturated EFAs found in virgin, cold-pressed, unrefined flaxseed oil are electron-rich. These natural polyunsaturated fats greedily bind to oxygen and proteins. When absorbed into cell walls, they attract oxygen to the cell. When bound to sulfur-based proteins, they are water-soluble and free-flowing and their electron-rich characteristic is reserved as a form of energy that the body can use when it needs to.

The problem with "pseudo" fats and oils that have been chemically refined and altered for marketing is that, in order to extend the shelf life of these oils, the vital electron cloud of the essential fatty acids has been destroyed. The resultant effect is that these essential fatty acids can no longer bind to proteins to make them more assimilable by the body, and they can no longer attract and bind to oxygen. William L. Fischer explains this in *How to Fight Cancer and Win*:

> The chemical processing of fats destroys the vital electron cloud, demonstrated in the foregoing material to be of immense importance to the functioning of every cell in the body. Once the electrons have been removed, these fats can no longer bind with oxygen and actually become an obstacle to the process of breathing. The heart, for instance, rejects these fats, and they end up as inorganic fatty deposits on the heart

muscle itself. As we pointed out earlier, a diseased heart and its aortas clearly show deposits of these worthless, electrically dead lipids.

Chemically processed fats are not water-soluble when bound to protein. They end up blocking circulation, and they damage heart action, inhibit cell renewal, and impede the free flow of blood and lymph fluids. The bioelectrical action in these areas slows down and may become completely paralyzed. The entire organism shows a measurable loss of electrical energy that is replenished only by adding active lipids to the diet.[3]

Unfortunately, the amount of manmade, partially hydrogenated oils known as "trans-fatty acids" is extremely high in modern Western diets. These trans-fats are so similar to cholesterol that our bodies cannot tell the difference. They are mistakenly used by the body in place of good cholesterol to build cell membranes. This then causes these cell membranes to lack a vital electrical charge that would normally attract oxygen. Without sufficient oxygen, the cellular environment becomes more and more anaerobic. The damaging trans-fats also impede the cellular exchange of nutrition and waste products through the membrane, or cell wall. They may even contribute to adult-onset diabetes because insulin is a large molecule that cannot easily pass through cell walls made up of manmade "pseudo"-fats.[4]

As mentioned in previous chapters, Dr. Otto Warburg believed that insufficient oxygen is the *key* reason that normal cells turn into cancer cells. He also reportedly proved that, by reducing the oxygen levels in tissues by about 35 percent, he could consistently induce the development of cancer. Dr. Budwig stated that Dr. Warburg believed the insufficient uptake of oxygen by cancer cells was somehow linked to fat metabolism and that Warburg tried to prove this theory by working with oils. But according to Dr. Budwig, Warburg was not successful because he did not use the *right type* of oils in his studies.[5]

When Dr. Budwig discovered the role that omega-3 and omega-6 fatty acids play in oxygenating cells, she believed that she had found the missing link Dr. Warburg had been looking for. In other words, she had found the *reason* cells sometimes resorted to anaerobic functioning!

Lipids and Prostaglandins

Another important function of the omega-3 and omega-6 essential fatty acids is that they can be converted by the body into "prostaglandins." Prostaglandins are hormone-like substances that have far-reaching effects on many different systems of the body. There are more than a dozen different prostaglandins that our bodies manufacture, none of which can be biosynthesized without sufficient essential fatty acids from our diet. EFA-derived prostaglandins regulate kidney function, inflammation response, and immune functioning in our bodies. They also help to keep blood vessels elastic, regulate blood pressure, influence platelet stickiness, and are necessary for proper metabolization of cholesterol. (These last functions of prostaglandins are largely why sufficient EFAs in the diet are important to cardiovascular health.) Thus, the prostaglandins play many roles in a healthy, well-functioning immune system and help the body to resist the development of cancer. And natural, unaltered EFAs are critical to the production of prostaglandins.

So, What Does Cottage Cheese Have to Do With It?

By now, you are probably wondering what cottage cheese has to do with anything. Obviously, what Dr. Budwig discovered was how important essential fatty acids are. The way that cottage cheese comes into play is the following. In researching how to most efficiently get the depleted essential fatty acids back into our bodies, *Dr. Budwig found that the body's assimilation and use of essential fatty acids was greatly enhanced when the fatty acids were combined with sulfur-based proteins.* In fact, nature has provided this combination already for us since most of the natural sources of essential fatty acids, such as milk, nuts, and seeds, also contain sulfur-based proteins.

Sulfur-based proteins are also found in many other foods, such as onions, leeks, chives, garlic, and yogurt. In her attempt to reverse advanced degenerative diseases, Dr. Budwig believed she needed to quickly replenish her patients' bodies with sufficient EFAs, and flaxseed oil was the highest source around. Then, she searched for the richest dietary source of sulfur-based proteins to go with the flaxseed oil. She finally settled on a food called "Quark." Quark is common in Germany and is similar to cottage cheese and yogurt. However, Quark is difficult to obtain outside of Germany. Next to Quark, cottage cheese is the richest source of sulfur-based proteins and is the most commonly used option around the world for the Budwig cancer approach. By combining flaxseed oil with the sulfur-based proteins in Quark or cottage cheese, the essential fatty acids bind to the sulfur-based proteins, and this makes them water-soluble and much more bio-available to the body.

Dr. Budwig also discovered that there were certain vitamin and mineral "co-factors" that aided the body in its use of the essential fatty acids. The primary co-factors are vitamins B_3, B_6, and C, and the minerals magnesium and zinc. These nutrients are all required by the body to make prostaglandins.

Thus, though the essential fatty acids are the main dietary factor needed for recovery from degenerative diseases such as cancer, simply ingesting flaxseed oil alone will not work as well as combining the flaxseed oil with foods rich in sulfur-based proteins. In fact, there is some evidence that taking flaxseed oil daily *without* sufficient sulfur-based proteins in the diet may even be harmful. (This is why some recent scientific studies that test the use of flaxseed oil alone for cancer do not show results anywhere near what Dr. Budwig was able to achieve.)

In case after case, Dr. Budwig found that thoroughly mixed flaxseed oil with cottage cheese was an efficient and successful way of replenishing the body's levels of essential fatty acids. She proved that, through the use of her special dietary approach, the anomalous greenish-yellow elements in her patients' blood would disappear over about three months and would be replaced by healthy red blood cells. Normal levels of phosphatides and lipoproteins would reappear in the blood as well, and tumors would disappear. Dr. Budwig reportedly accumulated over 1,000 documented cases of cancer recoveries with her special dietary approach!

As a result of her in-depth research and clinical practice, Dr. Budwig claimed the following:

- Lipoproteins can be found in all biochemically active tissues and always contain highly unsaturated fatty acids and sulfur-rich proteins.

- Anesthetics and certain drugs, such as barbiturates, sleeping pills, and painkillers, can separate highly unsaturated fatty acids from sulfur-containing proteins.

- Hard carcinoma tumors can be dissolved with serums high in essential fatty acids and organically bound sulfur.

- Polymerized pseudo-fats of marine origin (such as fish and whale oils) that have been radically altered by being subjected to high temperatures for use in margarines, have been isolated from soft tumors.

Opposition and Suppression

History tells us that the many health benefits of flax have been appreciated for thousands of years. Flax was cultivated in Babylon as early as 5,000 B.C. Hippocrates wrote about the healing benefits of flax. And ancient scripts from India claim that a yogi must eat flax daily in order to achieve the highest state of contentment and joy possible.[6]

Unfortunately, in the modern world, big businesses have gotten in the way of some of our most ancient healing traditions. Dr. Budwig met with ferocious opposition from various powers in the food industry, particularly from the margarine producers. She was the first scientist to oppose the modern practice of altering of oils for commercial distribution purposes. Her conflicts started with Professor H.P. Kaufmann, who was the head of the German Institute she was doing her research at. Kaufmann also happened to be a very famous lipid expert who had been nicknamed "The Pope of Fats and Oils." He held patents for some of the hydrogenation processes that produced the very polymers Dr. Budwig claimed were harmful to our bodies and which she had isolated from soft tumors. Thus, even though her research was sound, he had a strong financial interest in the use of these polymers, or pseudo-fats, particularly by the margarine industry.[7]

According to Johanna Budwig, Dr. Kaufmann tried to bribe her with money to keep her from publicizing her discoveries about oils. She refused his bribe, whereupon he supposedly denied her any further access to the research institute facilities he headed. When Dr. Budwig tried to move to another institute where she could continue her research, she found her access blocked by what she felt was an industry-wide conspiracy against her. Apparently, the "Pope of Fats" and margarine industry moguls had mobilized in some way to keep her from continuing her work in modern scientific laboratories. She also found herself blocked from publishing her research in scientific journals. Her only recourse then was to write books and share her information with the public that way.

The one good that came from Dr. Budwig's banishment from further laboratory research was that she spent more time working with patients in a clinical setting. It is unfortunate, however, that she was not able to continue her formal research, which might have given us an even better understanding of fat metabolism and its connection with serious illnesses such as cancer.

Dr. Budwig's Dietary Protocol

Anyone wishing to use Dr. Budwig's approach should be aware of the protocol she recommended. The *basic* rules of her approach are listed below, but I do not recommend that readers rely solely on what is written here. If you are interested in using the flaxseed oil and cottage cheese diet to recover from an illness, please refer to the books and Internet sites listed at the end of this chapter for more detailed information about what other dietary restrictions or supplements may be helpful.

Primary ingredient: Thoroughly mixed low-fat cottage cheese (preferably 1 percent organic) with unrefined, virgin, cold-pressed flaxseed oil. The ratio of these two items may vary depending on the severity of disease, but the minimum ratio is 1 tablespoon flaxseed oil to ¼ cup cottage cheese. For patients with serious illnesses such as cancer, Dr. Budwig suggested anywhere from 3 to 6 tablespoons of flaxseed oil per ½ cup of cottage cheese per day. Using a blender or other sort of electrical mixer is important to optimally mix the oil and cottage cheese and thus bind the essential fatty acids with the sulfur-based proteins. Various fresh or frozen fruits, honey, and/or stevia can be added to the mix to make it tasty. Lowfat or skim milk or unsweetened fruit juice can also be added. Keep the blended mix refrigerated and eat it throughout the day.

If preferred, low-fat plain yogurt may be substituted for cottage cheese. However, since yogurt is not quite as high in sulfur-based proteins as cottage cheese is, one should triple the amount of yogurt used.

People who are allergic to dairy products have varied responses to this mixture. Some find that, even though they are generally lactose-intolerant, they tolerate the FSO/CC mixture just fine. Others may want to look into different sources of sulfur-based proteins that may be used instead of cottage cheese or yogurt (though it may be difficult to achieve the optimum effect with other substitutions.) One possible non-dairy substitution is a special supplement in capsule form that contains dried sulfurated proteins. "Nature's Distributors," based in Arizona, sells this type of supplement. Their phone number is (800) 624-7114, and their non-dairy substitute for cottage cheese sulfurated proteins is called "Companion Nutrients." Nature's Distributors claims that one capsule of Companion Nutrients can activate the essential fatty acids in one tablespoon of flax oil.

Along with eating one of the above mixtures every day, Dr. Budwig included some dietary restrictions in her healing approach to help promote recovery. These restrictions are the following:

Foods to Completely Avoid

- Refined sugar (Unsweetened grape juice and honey okay)

- All animal fats

- All salad oils, including commercial mayonnaise

- All meats containing chemicals, hormones, or preservatives

- Butter

- Anything "hydrogenated" (such as margarine or fried foods)

Fresh vegetable juices, such as carrot, celery, apple, and red beet, are fine. Dr. Budwig also thought it essential to drink a warm tea, such as peppermint, rose hips, or grape tea, three times a day. (Black tea before noon is okay.) For those who would sorely miss butter and mayonnaise, there is a special flaxseed oil "spread" that can be prepared and used as well as a special flaxseed oil "mayonnaise." (For more details on how to prepare these, refer to Chapter 7 of Fischer's book, *How to Fight Cancer and Win*. Chapters 6 and 7 of Fischer's book present an excellent in-depth description of Dr. Budwig's protocol for cancer.)

Remember to use only unrefined, cold-pressed flaxseed oil that is sold in a dark (light-blocking) bottle and kept refrigerated at all times. Barleans is an excellent brand and is very high-quality oil. For best results, use the bottled liquid oil rather than capsules and keep the bottle refrigerated. It takes about 14 capsules of flaxseed oil to equal just 1 tablespoon of the bottled oil, and many times the bottles of capsules are allowed to sit on store shelves or warehouses in the heat which can cause the oil to become rancid.

Flax seeds freshly ground at home in a coffee grinder *and used immediately* can be added to the daily mixture. But do not grind your flax seeds at a health food store, then drive home and expect them to still be good. Dr. Budwig claimed that the oils in freshly ground flax seeds can go bad in just 10 to 15 minutes! There are more details to this diet that can be obtained from the resources listed in the back of this chapter. These should be studied and followed carefully if you have life-threatening cancer and choose to use this approach.

Although some people have a remarkably fast disappearance of tumors using this approach—sometimes in just a few months—others may take longer. Dr. Budwig recommended that people using this dietary treatment for serious illnesses stay on it for three to five years to achieve complete healing. According to Dr. Budwig, people who break the rules of the diet (for example by eating preserved meats, candy, etc.) may grow rapidly worse to the point where they cannot be saved. However, some people have just used flaxseed oil thoroughly mixed into cottage cheese on a daily basis, without adhering to the other aspects of Budwig's dietary protocol, and have still done quite well. To be on the safe side, however, it is probably best to stick as closely to her original protocol as possible.

Here are two simple recipes that can be tried. The first creates a soft-yogurt consistency and can be poured into a bowl to eat with a spoon. The second creates a milkshake consistency and can be poured into a glass to drink.

1. Mix in a blender these five ingredients:

   1 cup low-fat, organic cottage cheese
   4 tablespoons unrefined, cold-pressed flaxseed oil
   2 fresh peaches (sliced), or other fresh fruit
   1 tablespoon honey
   Juice from ½ lemon

2. Mix in a blender these nine ingredients:

   1 cup unsweetened grape or pineapple juice
   1 banana, cut up
   1 ½ cups frozen, dark cherries
   ½ cup low-fat cottage cheese
   1 cup plain, nonfat yogurt
   ¼ cup freshly ground flaxseeds
   2 tablespoons raw wheat germ
   2 to 3 tablespoons flaxseed oil
   1 to 2 tablespoons honey

You can create your own unique recipes for combining flaxseed oil and cottage cheese. Pineapple is another tasty fruit to mix with it, for example. Just be sure to also supplement with co-factors that help the activation of the essential fatty acids. A daily multiple B vitamin (or wheat germ) and a daily multiple mineral supplement of some sort are a good idea. There are some excellent cancer recovery stories to be found in Fischer's book,

How to Fight Cancer and Win, and there are many others that can also be found on the Internet. (www.healingcancernaturally.com has an excellent compilation of recoveries using this diet for both humans and pets with cancer.) The following case stories were recorded from interviews with people I contacted and spoke with myself.

Case Stories

Case Story #1—Metastasized Prostate Cancer

Cliff Beckwith is an American man who has done a great deal to spread the word about the use of flaxseed oil and cottage cheese for cancer. (I use his full name here because he publicly posts his story on his website: www.beckwithfamily.com.)

In January of 1991, Cliff was diagnosed with prostate cancer. Initial bone scans and other tests indicated that the cancer had not spread, so surgery was recommended. During the operation, however, Cliff's surgeon discovered that his cancer had in fact metastasized to his lymph glands. Because of this, Cliff was diagnosed as stage IV, and the operation was *not* completed. His doctor said that, since the cancer was in his lymph system, it would not do any good to cut it out locally at the prostate gland.

At that point, it was decided to use the drugs Lupron and Eulexin to block his production of testosterone. Cliff went on the drugs, but in the meantime, he also found out about Dr. Budwig's flaxseed oil and cottage cheese approach. He read that most people are about 80 percent deficient in omega-3 and that Dr. Budwig had worked with cancer patients who sometimes had only a few hours to live and restored them to health.

So Cliff gave it a try. For two and a half years he put about half a cup of cottage cheese and some fruit, such as crushed pineapple or frozen strawberries, mixed with just 2 tablespoons of flaxseed oil and a little honey, in the refrigerator. He ate that throughout the day. When he was first diagnosed, Cliff's PSA count was 75. After just six months of eating the flaxseed oil and cottage cheese on a daily basis, Cliff had another PSA test done. He got a call from his doctor's office the following Monday and the office girl exclaimed, "Mr. Beckwith! Your count is completely normal!" Cliff's PSA was down to 0.1.

For the first four years, Cliff continued to get PSA readings at six-month intervals, and every time, his count was between 0.0 and 0.16. He had continued on the hormone blockade throughout these years, so the flaxseed oil and cottage cheese mixture was not the only thing he was doing. Cliff knew that the hormone-blocking drugs could also effectively lower PSA counts for a while. But when he asked his doctor if he had expected the counts to go down that much, the doctor said, "No way!"

After 1995, Cliff was no longer on the Eulexin and Lupron and was just using flaxseed oil and cottage cheese. In the years since stopping the hormone-blocking drugs, his PSA level has varied just a little more. As of this writing, in August 2003, Cliff is still doing great and has no clinical signs of metastasis to other organs. He is 82 years old, and his PSA count has remained in a normal range for a man of his age. Best of all, Cliff has already lived about 12 years longer than his doctor thought he would.

Over the years, Cliff has helped many people with his Internet site and also with an audiotape about flaxseed oil and cottage cheese that he created to give out to people who needed information. He has known of over 100 people who have successfully used this method of treatment to help them recover from all types of cancer. He has even known some stories of flaxseed oil and cottage cheese working to help dogs recover from cancer.

Unfortunately, Cliff has *also* known people who were getting well using the FSO/CC combination (their cancer markers were going down, symptoms were going away, etc.), but were convinced by their doctors to do more chemotherapy or radiation. Many of these people who had been beating their cancer by replenishing their essential omega fatty acids then died after doing conventional treatment. Apparently, many of these people's doctors could see that their patient was recovering from cancer but couldn't accept that they were doing it without the help of conventional medicine.

Case Story #2—Metastasized Pancreatic Cancer

William is a 72-year-old man whom friends and family have always called "Huck." About 10 years ago, at the end of 1993, Huck suddenly became very ill. He was overcome with extreme pain and nausea, and was rushed to a nearby hospital emergency room. Doctors there were unable to find the problem, so they sent him home. However, the symptoms kept returning, with Huck suffering from about a half-dozen painful attacks by the end of January. He was finally admitted to the hospital in late January of 1994 to undergo more tests. The doctors suspected a problem with his pancreas but hospital tests still showed nothing. A CT scan also showed nothing unusual.

Because of his severe pain, Huck requested that his gallbladder be removed in case that was the problem. This surgery was done on February 7th and went smoothly. For a few days, Huck seemed to feel better, but then the pain returned in the same place it had been before. He saw some other specialists, but they couldn't find anything, either. Toward the end of April, Huck had lost 50 pounds and suffered his worst attack of pain ever.

Finally, in May of 1994, another CT scan was done, and this time it showed some serious changes in his pancreas. The doctors could now see that Huck's pancreas had tripled in size since his first scan in January. He was referred to a pancreatic surgeon, who tried an endoscopic procedure to learn more details of what was going on. Unfortunately, that did not reveal anything either. So the next day, Huck went into surgery. After opening him up, the surgeon found malignant pancreatic cancer that had metastasized (stage IV). Huck's primary tumor in the pancreas was about the size of two slightly flattened lemons. It was also obvious now that the tumor had reached out and grown around the blood vessel running between the pancreas and liver, as well as around another primary blood vessel.

The surgeon knew there was no way he could surgically remove all of the cancer and didn't even try to cut it out. The only thing the surgeon did before sewing Huck back up was to take a few fine needle biopsy samples. (The needle biopsies came back from the lab indicating that the type of pancreatic cancer was "adenocarcinoma.") After surgery, Huck was told he would probably not live more than three months. Huck and his wife, Nan, were told that neither chemotherapy nor radiation would help, so no treatment was recommended.

Huck and Nan left the hospital with a terrible diagnosis, but they didn't give up. They looked into alternative approaches. First, Huck started drinking six 12-ounce glasses of fresh vegetable juices each day and improved his diet. By the end of June, he also started getting Laetrile treatments at an alternative clinic. Every day (except Sundays) for three weeks, he received intravenous Laetrile along with DMSO and massive amounts of vitamin C. After that, Huck switched to oral Laetrile tablets. Huck added other supplements to his daily regimen, too, as well as Essiac tea. Then, around mid-August, Huck and Nan found out about flaxseed oil and cottage cheese, so he started taking 1 tablespoon of flaxseed oil with 1 tablespoon of cottage cheese after every meal. His total intake of oil was 3 tablespoons a day.

Huck never did any conventional treatment for his cancer but gradually began to feel better and better. In December 1994, he was feeling very well and had put back on 25 pounds. Another CT scan was performed, and unbelievably, just seven months after being diagnosed with metastasized pancreatic cancer, his doctor could not find anything abnormal on the scan at all! The doctor was stunned. He called in the radiologist to look at the scan with him, but the radiologist could not find any cancer or anything else out of the ordinary, either.

On December 28, 1994, a blood test was taken to measure levels of a pancreatic cancer marker. This test is called the CA-19-9. For this test, the normal range is between 0 and 37. Huck's test came back at 17. Over the years, Huck continued to get regular CT scans. Every time, the results showed him to be clear of cancer. In April 1997, he had another CA-19-9 test done. His count this time was 14.

Huck gradually stopped using the flaxseed oil and cottage cheese as well as the Laetrile tablets. He went back to eating a normal, healthy diet, and he continues to take some supplements. He has had no recurrence of cancer since, and his doctor has had a hard time believing it. At first, Huck would receive a phone call from his doctor's office about every three months, just to see how he was doing. After a while, his doctor's office only called him every six months, then once a year. Finally, the doctor's office stopped calling him.

Huck's story is truly an amazing one. People who are diagnosed with stage IV pancreatic cancer are given virtually no chance for long-term recovery by standard medical practices. Probably everything Huck did worked together to help him get well. Laetrile treatment can be a very powerful approach but does not appear to have high success rates for metastasized cancer when the intravenous part of the treatment is only done for three weeks. Usually, patients must keep coming back for intravenous Laetrile treatments in order to fully recovery. Although it is hard to be sure, Huck and Nan believe the flaxseed oil and cottage cheese combination had the biggest impact.

Case Story #3—Breast Cancer

Huck's wife, Nan, now has her own cancer story. In October 2002, Nan's breast started hurting and she noticed a big lump that had not been there before. She had undergone a mammogram just a couple of months before, and, strangely, it had showed her to be fine. But with the lump clearly observable now, she was given an ultrasound. The ultrasound showed that Nan most definitely had a tumor, and a needle biopsy came up with the diagnosis of "lobular infiltrating carcinoma."

Nan's doctor immediately recommended a mastectomy followed by chemotherapy. Nan had seen too many other people die after going through chemo for cancer, and she had also seen her own husband recover without it. So, she refused all surgery and chemotherapy. She started eating flaxseed oil and cottage cheese every day instead. Her conventional doctor refused to monitor her progress if she didn't do the standard treatments, so she had to look around for another doctor who would. Luckily, she found one with whom she could work.

Nan did not do any Laetrile treatments as her husband had done because the doctor who administered them to Huck had since moved. She started with 6 tablespoons of flaxseed oil mixed with cottage cheese every day. She also cleaned up her diet, avoided all junk food, and took lots of vitamin and mineral supplements. After a few months, Nan reduced her intake of flaxseed oil to 3 tablespoons a day.

When Nan had been diagnosed with breast cancer in October 2002, her tumor was almost as big as a golf ball. Another ultrasound in January 2003 showed that the tumor was stable in size (showed no increase). A full-body CT scan was done, and there was no indication that the cancer had spread to any other areas. In July 2003, the breast tumor was down to the size of a marble. The pain in Nan's breast has been gone since mid-November, and she feels great otherwise. Nan continues to diligently eat her flaxseed oil and cottage cheese on a daily basis.

Case Story #4—Prostate Cancer

Because of Cliff Beckwith's influence, many other men with prostate cancer have found out about using flaxseed oil and cottage cheese and have their own great success stories. Seventy-eight-year-old Chester is one of them. Seven years ago, Chester was diagnosed with prostate cancer. At diagnosis, his PSA count was 24. Chester's doctors administered radiation five days a week for a total of 39 treatments. Chester also started taking flaxseed oil and cottage cheese on a daily basis.

For the first five months or so, Chester took 6 tablespoons of flaxseed oil a day. After that, he went down to 2 tablespoons a day and has stayed on that ever since. Chester just puts the oil in a bowl, stirs in about half a cup of cottage cheese, and eats it. From 24, his PSA count went down to 12, which is the level it stayed at for over three years. Then, his count went down even more, and for the last few years has remained at 5.

Chester feels great and still works in his own barbershop, where he tells anyone who is interested about the healing wonder of flaxseed oil and cottage cheese.

Case Story #5—Brain Cancer

Tom Rolland was only 37 years old when, on February 10, 2002, he was rushed to the hospital with a splitting headache and projectile vomiting. He thought he just had a very bad migraine, but was to find out instead that he had a malignant brain tumor. Two days later, he was rushed into surgery, and the resultant biopsy on his tumor came back with a diagnosis of "glioblastoma multiforme," stage IV.

Although Tom's surgeon said he had removed all of the cancer he could see, Tom was told he would probably only live about six months if he did *not* undergo post-operative radiation treatments, and only about a year if he *did* do the radiation. This prognosis was due to the reality that glioblastomas virtually always grow back quickly, even if all of the "visible" tumor has been removed. And radiation is only a palliative treatment in these cases, not a curative one. Tom gave the radiation a try, but stopped it after only five days of treatments because it made him feel so awful.

Being Christians, Tom and his wife, Kelly, decided it was time to seek guidance, and they went to their church. They had Tom anointed with oil and hands laid on him in prayer by the elders of the church (according to James 5:14). They also began to look into holistic methods of fighting cancer. After all, there was nothing conventional medicine could do that would offer him a chance of long-term cure.

Through other members of the church, Tom and Kelly then found out about Dr. Budwig's flaxseed oil and cottage cheese treatment and they started Tom on this in March 2002. For the first three months, Tom mixed ¼ cup of low fat (2 percent) cottage cheese with 1 tablespoon of flaxseed oil twice a day. Thus, every day he took a total of just 2 tablespoons of flaxseed oil with cottage cheese. He also took three 750 milligram capsules of shark cartilage three times every day. On top of that, Kelly frequently rubbed frankincense oil on Tom's head because they had heard that this oil has anti-cancer properties.

Three months after his diagnosis and surgery, Tom's MRI looked very good. His brain was clean and the hole where they had removed the tumor was empty except for a tiny line around a portion of the inside. Tom's doctor thought this line could be either (1) scar tissue, (2) a benign bit of tumor, or (3) re-growth of the glioblastoma. After the three-month mark, Tom and Kelly added Graviola tincture to his daily regimen. (Tom took the Graviola for about nine months.) They also had Tom take daily supplements of borage seed oil, CoQ_{10}, and a barley/mineral supplement called "AIM Garden Trio." And he cut back on his intake of meat and sugar.

At the six-month mark, Tom had another MRI, and this time his brain was completely clean! There was no cancer visible anywhere. Tom's doctor said it was a miracle, and that in 14 years of practice, he had never seen anything like it. All of Tom's MRI's since then have been clean, and he just had his 18-month MRI. *Still no sign of cancer!*

Tom has been given his life back, and he and Kelly have posted his story on the Internet to help others. Their website address is: www.flaxoflife. com. They don't know what caused his brain tumor, but they suspect that it may have been caused by artificial sweeteners. Before he was diagnosed, Tom had been regularly drinking at least 2 liters of diet soda every day. Now, of course, he no longer ingests artificial sweeteners, and he, Kelly, and their two children are *very* happy he found out about flaxseed oil and cottage cheese. Tom and Kelly feel very strongly that their prayers were answered and say, "We believe that the Lord provided all of the information to get Tom well and we have to give Him the Glory."

Cliff Beckwith reports that most of the people he has seen recover from cancer by using flaxseed oil and cottage cheese did *not* know about Dr. Budwig's other rigid dietary requirements. Thus, it appears that it is possible to get well without following her full strict protocol. But according to Cliff, some of those who did *not* keep up the flaxseed oil and cottage cheese after their cancer went away found themselves facing a recurrence of cancer in a few years. It is possible that if one does not follow Dr. Budwig's full dietary protocol for three to five years to fully heal the body, then one may have to stay on the daily flaxseed oil and cottage cheese indefinitely to avoid having their cancer come back.

Some experts believe that although flaxseed oil is effective in treating degenerative diseases, it might be too rich in omega-3 fatty acids to be used on a daily basis for more than five years. In other words, at some point, a person should go back to consuming a two-to-one ratio of omega-6's to omega-3's. Udo Erasmus, author of *Fats That Heal, Fats That Kill*, states that a person using flaxseed oil as their sole source of essential fatty acids will develop an omega-6 deficiency over time. He claims to have remedied this problem by creating his own mixed oil blend with added sunflower and sesame oils. This product is called "Udo's Choice Blend." It also contains the omega-9 essential fatty acids, and may be something to consider using once normal health has been regained.

However, it is rare that a person will be using the flaxseed oil as his or her sole source of EFAs. This is because most people do get some significant amounts of the omega-6 fatty acids from other dietary sources. For anyone wishing to check the levels of omega-3 and omega-6 fatty acids in their bodies, there is a laboratory in Asheville, North Carolina, that can tell you what your levels are from a simple blood test. (For contact information, see Resources at the end of this chapter.)

It is still somewhat unclear as to why Dr. Budwig chose flaxseed oil as the best way to replenish EFA deficiency when much of her research seemed to indicate that the omega-6 EFAs were the *more* important deficiency involved in cancer. It is speculated that, though the omega-6's are extremely important, we tend to be more deficient in omega-3's. This may be because there are numerous other vegetable oil sources of omega-6's in our diets. Thus, we tend to be much more deficient in omega-3 than omega-6. Regaining a balance between these two EFAs is very important in the process of regaining health. Dr. Budwig's clinical results from working with very ill people certainly proved that the flaxseed oil combination of essential fatty acids is extremely effective.

Treatment and Guidance

Unfortunately, Dr. Budwig died in 2003 at the age of 94. She had suffered a fall from which she was unable to recover. Specific doctors or clinics that specialize in the use of Johanna Budwig's approach to healing are not easy to find, so the flaxseed oil and cottage cheese diet is almost always a self-administered cancer therapy at this point. The exception to this rule is the Budwig Center in Spain. It uses an omega-3 approach, along with other supportive non-toxic techniques, and I have heard they have a very high cure rate for cancer.

For those people who are not able to attend the Budwig Center, there are some very helpful Internet support groups dealing with the use of flaxseed oil and cottage cheese for cancer. These can be searched for online using the common abbreviations "FSO/CC," or "FO/CC." In addition, there is a cancer coach named Bill Henderson whose contact information and book are listed below. Bill is an expert on many different alternative cancer treatment methods and is particularly experienced in helping people to use Dr. Budwig's approach for optimum results. I have heard great reports from people who have worked with him and I highly recommend his book and coaching service.

Resources:

The Budwig Center   Phone: +34 952 577 369
Malaga, Spain   www.budwigcenter.com

Coaching Service

Bill Henderson, author of *Cancer-Free: Your Guide to Gentle, Non-toxic Healing, 3rd Ed.*, provides coaching for those who wish to use the flaxseed oil and cottage cheese approach along with other supportive supplements or treatments. To find out about his service, go to www.beating-cancer-gently.com.

Books

William L. Fischer. *How to Fight Cancer and Win*. Baltimore: Agora Health Books, 2000.

Bill Henderson. *Cancer-Free: Your Guide to Gentle, Non-toxic Healing*, 3rd Edition. Booklocker.com, Inc., 2008.

Bill Henderson and Andrew Scholberg. *How to Cure Almost Any Cancer At Home for $5.15 a Day*. Online Publishing and Marketing, LLC, 2009. (plastic comb binding)

Udo Erasmus. *Fats That Heal, Fats That Kill*. British Columbia, Canada: Alive Books, 1993.

Dr. Johanna Budwig. *Flax Oil As a True Aid Against Arthritis, Heart Infarction, Cancer, and Other Diseases*. Vancouver, Canada: Apple Publishing, 1994.

Websites

www.budwigcenter.com

www.whale.to/cancer/budwig.html

www.healingcancernaturally.com

www.beating-cancer-gently.com

www.aspartame.ca/page_c1.htm

www.beckwithfamily.com

www.mnwelldir.org/docs/cancer1/budwig.htm

www.road-to-health.com/news/36/budwig.htm

www.fatsthatheal.com

14

The Rife Machine

In this chapter, we'll look at another of the early non-toxic cancer treatments. This approach from the early 1900s may have been the *most* effective method of treating cancer ever developed, but it is a difficult approach to acquire in its original form these days. Still, since it is an option many people will hear about, and since it will hopefully be resurrected in its original form someday, it is an approach worth knowing about.

In the 1920s and 1930s, an American named Royal R. Rife developed an audio frequency-emitting device that, when directed at a person with cancer, was able to send frequencies into the person's body that would destroy micro-organisms he found to be causally associated with cancer. Over a number of months of treatments, cancer patients of all types got well. This approach involved a theory of cancer that we have not yet discussed. This theory has to do with the concept that certain types of micro-organisms are involved in the development of cancer. It may sound hard to believe, but the fact is that research by numerous highly respected scientists has supported this theory repeatedly.

To the misfortune of the entire world, Rife's approach was never fully accepted into mainstream medicine and was never used in a widespread way. However, there are still some forms of Rife Machines in existence today and some people claim to have achieved complete cancer recovery through their use. The current difficulty for cancer patients is determining *which* of the machines available today are similar enough to the original

Rife Machine to be effective. It appears that *none* of the Rife machines sold today are exactly the same as the one Royal Rife developed and used. Although some modern Rife Machines may be close to the original and be effective for some people, others may be quite far from authentic with little effectiveness.

Therefore, if you are considering using a Rife Machine for cancer, it is important to understand the history and issues to look into. Hopefully, someday, the original Rife method will be reproduced in all of its authentic aspects and will once again be available to the world.

History and Theory

Royal Raymond Rife was born in the late 1800s and was undoubtedly one of the great scientific geniuses of the 20th century. At a young age, he became interested in becoming a medical doctor and attended Johns Hopkins University to pursue this dream. During his studies, he realized he was really more interested in the field of bacteriology, and decided to specialize in that. Rife began photographing specimens for Heidelberg University, and because of his great contribution to that institution, he was awarded an "honorary" doctorate of parasitology in 1914.[1] Realizing the restrictions of microscope technology, Dr. Rife became very involved in the field of microscope development, and studied for a while with some of the world's top German microscope specialists.

Jobs in bacteriology were scarce, however, so when Dr. Rife returned to the United States he took a position as a chauffeur for a wealthy businessman in San Diego, California. This businessman was Henry Timkin, a leader in the ball-bearing industry. Timkin discussed with Rife some of the production problems he was having, and Dr. Rife was able to develop a new type of motor for Timkin's business. The motor and other innovative improvements to Timkin's ball-bearing business ended up saving Timkin millions of dollars and, in appreciation, Timkin set up a life-time stipend for Dr. Rife.[2] The stipend's monthly payments allowed Rife to focus his efforts on his work in bacteriology. A number of other wealthy people also believed in Rife's abilities and helped finance a privately owned and fully equipped laboratory for his work.

Finally free to do his work in microbiology without restriction, Rife began to experiment with a bold new idea he had been toying with—that of electrically stimulating micro-organisms as a method of affecting them. Rife then made a discovery that should have been heralded later in all the history books. He discovered that, by using audio frequencies, he could actually *kill* micro-organisms. Finding that different frequencies were required to kill different organisms, he named each specific frequency the "M.O.R.," or "Mortal Oscillatory Rate," for each particular organism.

Rife soon faced a big problem, however. He wanted to include viruses in his study and realized that, in order to see such small organisms, he would have to somehow get around a limiting problem. This was the problem that standard microscopes could only magnify up to 2,500 times diameter. It was a mechanical problem that resulted from how microscopes were made, and was due to the limiting factor that no micro-organism could be seen if it was smaller than half a wavelength of light in size.[3]

By 1920, Rife had solved this problem by single-handedly developing a new type of microscope. Rife's innovative microscope could magnify up to 9,000 diameters with clarity! This was far more powerful than any other microscope yet developed in his time. He then began seeing and categorizing forms of micro-organisms that had never been clearly observed by anyone before.

But Rife soon encountered another problem. There were even *more* micro-organisms that he and other researchers could not see because the organisms themselves were smaller than the molecules in the dyes or acids used to stain specimens for observation. To get around this problem, Rife devised and patented a totally new way to observe specimens under a microscope *without staining* by focusing on the spectrographic light properties which coordinated with the chemical makeup of the micro-organisms he was trying to study.[4] In order to do this, he employed numerous quartz lenses immersed in glycerin. What Rife did is difficult to explain in simple terms, but basically he figured out a way to "stain" his specimens with light instead of dye. Rife's new microscope was eight times more powerful than the best microscopes used by physicists of his day.

Throughout the 1920s, Dr. Rife kept searching in his laboratory for the cause of cancer. He believed it would be a virus-like organism. In 1932, he found two forms of just such an organism. One form, which he called "BX," was the organism that caused carcinomas, and the other form, called "BY," was the organism that caused sarcomas. He also found that this virus-like organism was pleomorphic. In other words, the cause of cancer was an organism that could take more than one form. In one form, it was benign and *not* cancer-causing—in another form it *was* cancer-causing.

"Pleomorphism" was an idea supported by the 19th-century French scientist, Antoine Bechamp. In those early days of microbiology, Antoine Bechamp and Louis Pasteur were the leaders in a huge battle of ideas regarding the forms microbes could take. Pasteur believed that microbes were distinct organisms with distinct, or unchanging, characteristics. In other words, every microbe is either a particular form of bacteria, or a particular form of virus, yeast, or fungi throughout its life cycle, and there is *no* crossover between forms. Pasteur's theory of microbes is referred to as "monomorphism."

Bechamp, on the other hand, argued that micro-organisms may not necessarily be limited to one distinct form. In his view, micro-organisms were capable of being pleomorphic, or capable of having *more than one form* in a given life cycle. This meant that the *shape* of a microbe could drastically change (i.e., a rod-shaped bacteria could turn into a spheroid-shaped bacteria) and the *size* of a microbe could drastically change during the life-cycle of a single organism. Bechamp argued that micro-organisms could undergo these changes in response to the state of health of the host organism in which the microbe lived.[5] Bechamp believed, for instance, that bacteria could actually "devolve" into a much smaller form which he called "microzymia."[6] His theory of pleomorphism included the possibility that bacteria could turn into *virus*-sized organisms in some situations as a response to their environment.

A key turning point in history occurred when Pasteur's ideas won out, which caused monomorphism to become the basis of today's modern views in microbiology. But many reputable scientists of the 20th century have since proven Bechamp's ideas of pleomorphism to be correct and have continued to debate the issue.

One important aspect of Rife's work to understand is that, in the early 1930s, viruses were just beginning to be defined. Scientists knew quite a bit about bacteria already and had devised special filters that could filter out certain bacteria from the media or environment they were in. The size of an average bacterium is about 1 micron (or 1/25,000 of an inch in length). But the largest virus is only about ¼ to ⅓ this size.[7] This means that most viruses are too small to be seen by any normal light microscope. (Although they *can* be seen now under an electron microscope, the electron microscope kills the specimen, so they can not be seen in their *living* state.)

Because viruses could not be seen in the early 1900s, scientists had to rely on the process of *filtering out* viruses from cultures and then detecting them by other means. The filtering process was done using filters with pores too small for bacteria to pass through. Scientists decided that any-thing that passed through these special filters *must* be something different from bacteria, and they referred to the organisms that passed through as "filterable viruses." (Eventually, the word "filterable" was dropped and they were just called "viruses.") In the early days, this filtering process was the *only* way to designate the difference between bacteria and viruses. Although more ways of defining viruses have since become accepted, there is still debate as to whether certain organisms are actually viruses or bacteria, and some organisms previously categorized as viruses have since been proven to be "filterable" bacteria instead.

Given the many shortcomings in microbiology in the 1930s, Dr. Rife's discoveries were phenomenal. He was not only able to *find* a micro-organ-ism involved in the development of cancer for the first time in history, but he was also able to *prove* the organism was pleomorphic, with the smaller life-cycle forms having the characteristics of a virus! Eventually, Dr. Rife identified four distinct forms that this cancer-causing organism could take within its life cycle:[8]

1. The BX virus (cause of carcinoma)

2. The BY virus (cause of sarcoma and larger than BX)

3. Monococcoid form (can be seen through standard microscopes in the blood monocytes of more than 90 percent of cancer patients)

4. Crytomyces pleomorphia fungi

Amazingly, Dr. Rife was able to culture the BX cancer virus from a fungoid organism. He then used this virus to directly produce cancer in hundreds of laboratory animals. He also proved that any of the above four forms of one organism could change back into the BX cancer virus within 36 hours. In fact, he was able to complete the cycle of virus to cancer and back to virus 104 times. He could observe and document all of this with his powerful microscope, something other scientists could not do. There is no doubt that Rife found a micro-organism involved in the development of cancer. And his discovery was verified and documented by other prominent microbiologists who visited his laboratory.

Even now, with the electron microscope, the back and forth culturing of a micro-organism from bacterial form to viral form *cannot* be observed because the electron microscope virtually destroys any virus that is put under it. What Dr. Rife discovered was—and still is—ground-breaking news. However, although he proved a micro-organism connection to cancer, he also discovered that *this did not mean cancer is an "infectious" disease.* The key is that the organism is pleomorphic and only takes a cancer-causing form when a person's inner environment, or state of health, is poor or unbalanced. So, this micro-organism was not something people could "catch" from one another. In fact, it was something we all have in us in its healthy form. It is only when our inner environment becomes unhealthy that this organism turns into its unhealthy form.

Royal Rife was not some unknown "kook." Over the years, he was given 14 government awards for scientific discoveries, was visited and acclaimed by world experts in medicine and microbiology, and had his accomplishments written up in many newspapers and magazines. A prominent professor, Arthur I. Kendall, Ph.D., and a prominent physician, Milbank Johnson, M.D., soon began collaborating with Dr. Rife. Drs. Kendall and Rife both observed normal tuberculosis bacteria convert to a filterable type of bacteria the size of a virus, something not previously observed. Dr. Kendall, Dr. Johnson, and many other medical specialists were *extremely* impressed with Dr. Rife's accomplishments and whole-heartedly supported his work.

But Dr. Rife did not stop at simply *finding* the pleomorphic micro-organism responsible for cancer—he also found a way to destroy it. To do this, Rife experimented with a wide variety of audio and light frequencies to find just the right frequency, or M.O.R., that would kill what he called the "cancer virus." He only used "sine waves," which are pure tones or frequencies. (Most sound is made up of a jumble of frequencies, as is most light. However, a sine wave is a single frequency.) X-ray tubes were the prominent medical technology of the day, so Rife worked with that mode of delivery. Once he found the cancer virsus's M.O.R., he could then deliver that devastating frequency to the organism. Rife could liter-ally *see* cancer viruses moving around alive under his microscope, then briefly zap them with the correct frequency from his "ray tube," and immediately observe that all the viruses on the same slide, which had been moving around only seconds before, were now dead! This way, with the help of his microscope, he could determine which sine waves would kill the organism in a particular human.

Since audio waves do not broadcast efficiently, more research and experimentation was required for Rife to be able to successfully deliver the mortal oscillatory rate of frequency to cancer organisms *deep* inside tissues of living animals. Rife solved this problem of delivery by using a "carrier wave." In other words, the audio frequency which turned out to be the specific M.O.R. for the cancer virus would not penetrate tissue deeply enough for many internal cancers, so Rife ingeniously modulated (or "piggy-backed") the desired audio frequency to another frequency that *could* penetrate deep tissue. If he hadn't done this, he would have only been able to treat cancers on or near the surface of the body. The two frequencies travel together but remain separate and distinct. Rife's records later showed that he used frequencies ranging from the audio range to 17 MHz, and that he also experimented with many different carrier frequencies.

Rife's theory that the BX virus caused cancer was proved to be sound when he injected 411 laboratory mice with the BX virus and produced 411 corresponding tumors.[9] Then, he was able to use his ray tube to completely eliminate the cancers in many of these animals. Rife's method was *not* directed at killing the cancer cell itself. Rather, he found the BX or BY virus to be *inside* each malignant cancer cell and that killing this micro-organism would cause the malignant cell to also die off.

In 1987, after doing a great deal of research, author Barry Lynes wrote the definitive book on Royal Rife and his cancer cure. This excellent book, *The Cancer Cure That Worked: Fifty Years of Suppression*, is packed with fascinating information and is available today and well worth reading. According to Barry Lynes, "By the end of 1932, Rife could destroy the typhus bacteria, the polio virus, the herpes virus, the cancer virus and other viruses in a culture and in experimental animals."[10]

In 1934, Dr. Milbank Johnson set up a committee of leading medical experts to oversee human trials in a southern California clinic where Rife could start treating terminally ill patients who had no other hope for cure. The initial results were astounding. In just 70 days of treatment, this committee of physicians pronounced 14 out of 16 patients with terminal cancer "cured." Thus, this first human trial showed a success of 87.5 percent. Moreover, after 60 more days of treatment, the remaining two patients from the original trial were also pronounced cured. This meant that within 130 days, or just a little over four months, all 16 terminally ill cancer patients were pronounced cured by the committee of medical experts.[11] After this amazing success, other doctors obtained ray tubes and operated them in their own clinics with a general success rate of about 90 percent.

The cancer treatment itself was totally non-toxic. It caused no tissue damage whatsoever, and a person receiving Rife's frequency treatment could not feel or hear anything. They merely saw a tube light up for three to five minutes, and the treatment was done. The only slightly toxic aspect of the treatment resulted from the die-off of the cancer micro-organisms. In fact, Rife discovered with his human cancer patients that the treatment was *most* effective when given at the rate of only three to five minutes exposure to frequency *every other day*. This was because he found that if he treated his patients every day, the toxins released by the dead micro-organisms accumulated too fast in the patients' bodies and caused toxic overload.[12] When he limited treatment to every other day, however, patients responded with incredible recoveries.

During the 1930s, Rife collaborated with many cancer researchers and doctors. Several reputable physicians began using Rife's frequency instrument on their patients with great success. They began seeing cancers of all sorts disappear. They also observed other conditions unexpectedly resolving after treatments with the ray tube. These other conditions included syphilis and gonorrhea.[13]

But the original ray tube Dr. Rife built was too cumbersome and expensive to market to doctors and clinics worldwide. It filled almost a whole room. So he signed an agreement with business colleagues to form a company called Beam Ray Corporation that would begin building Dr. Rife's frequency instruments for the purpose of selling them to medical practitioners. Unfortunately, however, not all of the businessmen involved were conscientious enough to make sure the machines were built correctly and according to Rife's specifications. His first business partner, Philip Hoyland, built the machines to emit *harmonics* of frequencies in order to save money, rather than building them to just emit specific, clean frequencies. Beam Ray Corporation's machines understandably performed poorly and Dr. Rife was not happy with what the corporation was doing.

Then, events took place that ended up bringing about the final downfall of the Rife frequency technology. These events began when Morris Fishbein, the head of the American Medical Association (AMA), tried to buy into Beam Ray Corporation. Basically, Fishbein was attempting to take control for his own financial gain, but he only wanted to give Royal Rife a small royalty on the machines. (This was the same man who had tried to gain ownership of the Hoxsey therapy for his own profit.)

After all of Dr. Rife's work, the business deal Fishbein offered was scandalous. Dr. Rife refused Fishbein's unfair business deal, and as a result, Fishbein went all out to destroy Beam Ray Corporation. The AMA filed expensive lawsuits and Beam Ray went bankrupt as a result of legal battles. To complicate matters, Philip Hoyland reportedly turned against Rife and also tried to take over total control of Beam Ray Corporation. Court transcripts from a 1938 trial show that Hoyland even tried to claim *he* was the originator of some of the technology, instead of Rife.

Later, in the 1950s and early 1960s, Dr. Rife worked with another man, John Crane, with whom he formed a company called "Life Labs." They modified the technology again to produce a slightly different version of his instrument. This one was also portable but used round disks that came in contact with the body. However, once again, Crane disregarded some of Rife's suggestions when he built the product. Then, Crane started making changes he did not tell anyone about. For instance, he lowered Rife's frequencies *by a factor of 10* so that the machines would fall below the 10,000 hertz level. It is believed that Crane did this to avoid FCC regulations that were just coming into place at the time. This drastic lowering of frequencies meant that the 1950s Rife machines could no longer achieve the impressive results of Rife's earlier 1930s machines.

Thus, Life Labs Rife Machines were not working as well as they could have. At the same time, Morris Fishbein was continuing to do everything he could to stifle Dr. Rife's technology. Doctors were put under pressure from the AMA to *not* use Rife's machines anymore. As with Harry Hoxsey's herbal remedy, Morris Fishbein used his power as head of the AMA to stop any progress on treating cancer that he himself could not profit from. Then, with just the right timing to put the final blow on Dr. Rife's technology, penicillin and other marketable antibiotics began to take the limelight in medicine. Since Rife had refused to sell Beam Ray Corporation to Fishbein, Fishbein made sure that the AMA pushed the concept of fighting diseases with antibiotics rather than with Rife's technology. Tragically, fighting microbes with frequencies soon fell out of medical favor.

Nevertheless, Dr. Rife did not give up. He continued to improve his machine, and in the 1950s, he tried again to get the medical community interested in his methods. Dr. Rife had developed a smaller and less expensive form of equipment to try to entice doctors to buy them. Unfortunately, doctors were still being influenced to use antibiotics, and the medical community never showed significant interest in Dr. Rife's technology again. In 1971, Rife died without ever seeing a widespread use of his incredibly successful method of treating cancer.

In *The Cancer Cure That Worked*, Barry Lynes sums up Morris Fish-bein's influence as follows:

> ... within the few, short years from 1934 to 1939, the cure for cancer was clinically demonstrated and expanded into curing other diseases on a daily basis by other doctors, and then terminated when Morris Fish-bein of the AMA was not allowed to "buy in." It was a practice he had developed into a cold art, but never again would such a single mercenary deed doom millions of Americans to premature, ugly deaths.[14]

Partly as a result of Barry Lynes's book, an "underground" interest in the Rife Machine sprang up once more in the 1980s and 1990s. Many different engineers started building Rife Machines according to blueprints and records from Rife's original papers. Pros and cons about current-day Rife Machines abound—some seeming to work well and others seeming to not work at all.

One problem is that many of the modern frequency machines claim-ing to be Rife Machines do *not* use any carrier wave. Yet, the carrier wave was an important aspect of Rife's technology and the only way to get the mortal oscillation sine wave to deep tissue cancers. Another problem is that some current-day machines do not transfer the frequencies prop-erly for various reasons. Even though the specific frequencies that Rife discovered to be M.O.R.s for many different organisms and diseases are actually presented on the Internet, the method of delivery is critical for these frequencies to be effective. And this appears to be the main reason why many modern day Rife devices are not as effective as the original technology was.

It is worth mentioning again that, although Rife found a micro-organism to be a causal factor to cancer, this did *not* mean he was proving cancer to be an infectious disease. In fact, it is most likely that the cancer-causing micro-organism Dr. Rife identified is within each and every one of us. Rife agreed with and confirmed Bechamp's earlier theory that it is a body's *inner* environment which ultimately influenced the form the pleomorphic cancer organism would take. If a person's inner environment was healthy, then it would remain in its harmless form. If, on the other hand, a person's inner environment was *not* healthy, it could devolve into one of the forms that might cause cancer. (See the next chapter on 714X for a similar conclusion made by the French hematologist, Gaston Naessens.)

Thus, to some extent, both Rife and Antoine Bechamp looked at various pleomorphic forms of bacteria as the *symptom* of disease, not the *cause* of disease. Royal Rife, himself, said:

> In reality, it is not the bacteria themselves that produce the disease, but the chemical constituents of these micro-organisms enacting upon the unbalanced cell metabolism of the human body that in actuality produce the disease. We also believe if the metabolism of the human body is perfectly balanced or poised, it is susceptible to no disease.[15]

Thus, it is best to *not* conclude from this chapter that cancer is a disease that can be "caught" by being near someone who has cancer. Instead, we need to realize that our common ideas about how micro-organisms are linked to diseases have been molded by one narrow medical viewpoint—that of monomorphism. We must be open to the reality that ideas in science get molded by various ideas of the times. Barry Lynes makes the astute observation that Pasteur's monomorphic view of micro-organisms probably won out for two main reasons: (1) It was a simpler theory and much easier to understand. And (2) it applied more directly to *infectious* diseases which were the biggest problem of that era. (I would also add that monomorphism won out as the reigning viewpoint in part because no one had a microscope capable of "seeing" micro-organisms change from one form to another.)

It is time for medical science to rethink its reigning theories, especially since a huge problem of *our era* happens to be chronic degenerative diseases in their many forms—and some degenerative diseases, such as cancer, may be better explained by Bechamp's theory of pleomorphism. According to Barry Lynes, the powerful Memorial Sloan-Kettering Cancer Center in New York is currently a leading institutional opponent of the concept of pleomorphism—even though, in 1975, Sloan-Kettering's *own* studies reportedly showed pleomorphic bacteria-virus in *all* of their cancer blood tests. According to Barry Lynes, Sloan-Kettering buried these laboratory results.[16]

Last but not least, scientists still need to have the right type of microscope in order to view pleomorphism, and even today that type of microscope is not prevalent. Rife's "Universal Microscope" was virtually lost to medical science, and there is a rumor that there is only one original Rife microscope left in existence today. However, there don't appear to be any institutions trying to duplicate its technology. Although the average person probably believes that modern medical practices are always based on "true science," there is a great deal of evidence indicating otherwise. As can be seen with the history of Royal Rife's technology, a certain amount of medical practice is based on professional biases and profit margins of big business.

And, of course, unfortunate timing was a factor. Antibiotics were highly profitable for pharmaceutical companies to market. They also happened to work quite well for infectious diseases, so it was easy for doctors and the public to wholeheartedly support them. But the downsides to antibiotics are showing up more and more with virulent drug-resistant bacteria becoming more prevalent and side effects to antibiotics taking their toll. Medical frequency technology, such as Rife created, is much cleaner with no side effects, and does not create drug-resistant bacteria. Moreover it works on viruses, which modern medicine *still* has not been able to fully conquer.

It is very interesting to note that, in the May 2003 issue of *Reader's Digest*, there was an article about some new and promising treatments for breast cancer. On pages 64–67, the article talks about one of these "new" treatments, called "RFA" (radiofrequency ablation). RFA is a recently developed technique whereby a probe is inserted into or next to a tumor and a certain radio frequency is then emitted for about 23 minutes. With an ultrasound, the technician performing this procedure can then see the dark tumor mass become the same grainy gray as the rest of the breast tissue. Surgeons can then simply go in and remove the tumor, which has become dead tissue.

This *Reader's Digest* article stated that RFA has also been used on liver cancer since the early 1990s, and is currently being tried on breast, kidney, and lung cancer. One study at Houston's M.D. Anderson Cancer Center is referred to where 20 women with breast tumors were treated with RFA. This study was small but achieved great success. Out of the 20 subjects, 19 were shown to have had the cancer completely killed! The current success of RFA shows that Rife's frequency technology was based on sound principles, but I wonder if Rife's discoveries will ever be given credit. No mention of Rife is made in the *Reader's Digest* article and the modern RFA procedure is referred to as new and "experimental." Too bad the article does not mention that an even more powerful form of frequency treatment for cancer was administered totally noninvasively as far back as the 1930s.

Maybe one day, we will yet again have Rife's original technology available to us. Until then, anyone considering using a Rife Machine today or other similar type of device for cancer should thoroughly research the *specific* device being considered.

An interesting side note is that more and more people are finding modern Rife-type machines and other frequency devices extremely helpful for recovering from Lyme Disease. The main Lyme bacteria is a particularly difficult one to completely rid the body of because it pleomorphs into different forms as a defense mechanism against antibacterial agents and is also very good at hiding in low-blood flow tissues that antibiotics may not reach in full strength. Fortunately, the spirochete form of the Lyme bacteria is readily destroyed by a variety of modern Rife-type machines. Unfortunately, the process of recovery can be slow and challenging as one experiences die-off toxins and waits for all forms in one's body to pleomorph back into the spirochete form. Nevertheless, some severely affected chronic Lyme Disease patients have completely cured themselves with modern Rife-type machines.

For an excellent collection of in-depth books and DVDs about using frequency devices for Lyme Disease, go to www.biomedpublishers.com (also called www.lymebook.com).

Resources:

Book

Barry Lynes. *The Cancer Cure That Worked!* Ontario, Canada: Marcus Books, 1987.

DVDs

"Rise and Fall of a Scientific Genius: The Forgotten Story of Royal Raymond Rife." 2-DVD set, 125 minutes. To order, call (530) 541-7200, or go to www.lymebook.com.

Websites

www.rife.org

www.royalrife.com

www.scoon.co.uk/electrotherapy/rife/beamray/

www.rifevideos.com

www.biomedpublishers.com

15

714X

Another unique and fascinating approach that also addresses the relationship of micro-organisms to cancer is 714X. It was developed by Gaston Naessens, a French biologist and hematologist. While still in France, Naessens developed two anti-cancer products that created quite a stir. One was called "Ana-Blast" and the other was called "GN-24." In 1964, Naessens immigrated to Quebec and introduced his innovative cancer treatments to Canada. In the 1970s, Naessens replaced Ana-Blast and GN-24 by what he called 714X, which has now been used by thousands of people to help them recover from cancer and other degenerative conditions. Considered by many to be a genius, Naessens has become known in the world of alternative cancer treatments as "French Canada's Wizard."

Naessens's personal background illustrates his creative intellect. He was born in 1924 and, as young as five years old, built a small functional, automobile-like vehicle. Next, he built a homemade motorcycle. At age 12, Naessens built an airplane that flew![1] When Naessens was old enough to attend college, he studied physics, chemistry, and biology, and later went on to study hematology (the study of blood).

Early on, Naessens had a "premonition" of sorts that there were tiny particles moving around in blood. But with normal light microscopes of the 1940s, nothing like that could be clearly discerned. So, like Royal Rife, Naessens decided a more powerful microscope (in terms of resolving power) was needed and he enlisted the aid of some German optical specialists to manufacture aluminum mirrors for him. The optical specialists were not aware of what Naessens was going to do with the mirrors, but they were to go in the new microscope that Naessens was developing.

Naessens's new microscope, which he called the "Somatoscope," was much more powerful than any other light microscope commonly used at the time. It used an innovative combination of laser and ultraviolet light technology and produced a magnification of 30,000 times with a resolution of 150 angstroms! Any light microscope with a dark field condenser can observe live material, so that aspect of the Somatoscope was not unique. However, the conventional field of hematology has generally shown little interest in observing live material and the observation of living specimens has been a foreign concept to their staining methods. The Somatoscope did *not* require staining a sample before viewing it as other microscopes did, and this made a big difference in observing living organisms in blood.

The ability to observe behavior and life cycles of living microscopic organisms in blood made the Somatoscope in some ways superior to the electron microscope, which was developed later. As mentioned in the previous chapter, the electron microscope can achieve much higher magnification (enlargements into the millions of times), but can only observe dead or static specimens. Thus, it is of little value in observing actual behavior changes or life cycle changes that might occur in microscopic organisms.

Using his own special microscope, Naessens was able to study the tiny blood particles he had previously noticed. He could now observe them with detail and clarity in their living state. Eventually, he identified a number of different micro-organisms that he concluded were all stages of development for one sub-cellular organism commonly found in blood. Naessens called this organism a "somatid." He believed that somatids were distinct from bacteria and viruses and, because he could observe these organisms in their living state, he was able to discern two separate life cycles for them. One life cycle tended to occur in the blood of *healthy* people and the other life cycle tended to occur in the blood of *unhealthy* people. (This corresponds closely to what Royal Rife discovered and the work of each of these geniuses supports the work of the other.)

In healthy individuals, the somatids appeared to display what Naessens called a "microcycle" consisting of 3 different forms the somatids would take. In *unhealthy* individuals, however, the somatids appeared to display a much longer "macrocycle," consisting of 16 different forms that the somatids would take. This macrocycle was a more complex life cycle that Naessens observed in the blood of people with degenerative diseases. Naessens theorized that somatids play an important role in the body and that it is normal for them to be found in everyone's blood in their *microcycle* life stages. But he theorized that when somatids are exposed to trauma, such as pollution, radiation, and so forth, they can then enter into a wild and uncontrolled growth cycle (the macrocycle), which can lead to cancer.[2]

Just as interesting as Naessens's discovery that somatids have different life cycles in healthy versus unhealthy people was his discovery that somatids are *everywhere* in nature and seem to be an integral part of everything. In the human body, he found that somatids play a role in the cell division process of normal cells. According to one source,

> What Naessens discovered was that somatids were everywhere, in the sap of plants, in the blood of animals, and even in lifeless organic matter like ashes. When he cultured the somatid life cycle, he discovered that somatids are resistant to acids and bases as well as heat and that they cannot be cut with a diamond. Cell division cannot take place without the somatid. Somatids, according to Naessens's theory, release the growth hormone trephone, which enables cells to divide and multiply. Naessens believes that the electrically charged somatid is the original spark of life, the point in which energy condenses into matter.[3]

In other words, Naessens believed somatids to be "basic living particles indispensable to life,"[4] and by culturing the somatids and using his special microscope he could verify their "micro" and "macro" cycles. (Apparently, other scientists who observe these same particles with normal microscopes generally refer to them as "fibrin formations.") In terms of how they are involved in the division of normal healthy cells, Naessens's theory proposes that when somatids are in their healthy 3-stage microcycle, they produce just the right amount of a growth hormone-like substance. This substance keeps healthy body cells reproducing at their correct rate. Naessens called this hormone-like substance "trefons" (also spelled as trephones). However, when a person's body is seriously stressed or weakened, then the somatid shifts into its longer *unhealthy* 16-stage macrocycle that includes forms resembling bacteria, viruses and yeasts. In this extended cycle, the somatids produce excessive amounts of trefons and cause normal, healthy body cells to undergo abnormally fast cell growth, which can then develop into cancer.

Naessens theorized that a healthy body can hold somatids to their 3-phase cycle by having ample "blood inhibitors" to keep the somatids functioning normally. These blood inhibitors in a healthy person consist of certain enzymes, hormones, and minerals. Naessens believed that inadequate nutrition and stress could *reduce* the amounts of these inhibitors in the blood and thus allow somatids to shift into their longer 16-phase cycle.

Naessens's theory of reduced blood inhibitors being a contributing factor to cancer is consistent with many of the nutritional deficiency theories of cancer development. And his observation that, at different life cycle stages the somatids could resemble either bacteria, yeasts, or fungi, is also consistent with many findings over the last century that have indicated a connection between cancer and various yeasts or fungi.

Thus, there was no doubt in Naessens's mind that the somatid microbes were involved in the development of cancer, but it was not in the way that we normally think of microbial involvement. As Dr. Rife's research suggested, Naessens's research also suggested a type of pleomorphism whereby common microbes (somatids) in every person's body could, under certain conditions, *change into a different form of microbe that can cause cancer.* Some of these forms could be so different from the original microbe that to any observer it would appear that a common bacterium was actually "pleomorphing" into a virus or fungus.

An important aspect of Naessens's discovery was that when the somatids switched to their longer life cycles as a result of trauma and/or insufficient blood inhibitors to control them, they then started secreting excess amounts of their hormone-like substance, which would cause cells to replicate too fast. The resultant effect would be a conglomerate of cells multiplying at an accelerated rate in close proximity to each other and beginning to form a tumor.

Once Naessens had formulated his theory on how cancer gets started, he worked to find a solution for it, which he eventually did. To understand his solution, we have to understand another interesting fact Naessens observed. He realized that fast-replicating cancer cells required much more *nitrogen* to survive than normal cells do and that they would often "steal" the nitrogen away from healthy cells in order to subsist. Naessens also observed that, in a healthy body, the immune system usually attacks and destroys any out-of-control conglomerate of cancer cells before the conglomerate gets too big. But Naessens discovered that, if this group of renegade cells is able to reach a "critical mass," then the conglomerate of cells (or tumor) starts to act like its own *entity* and begins to emit a substance Naessens called "Co-carcinogenic K Factor" (CKF). Theoretically, CKF paralyzes the immune system by masking the cancer cells from recognition. CKF thus frees the young tumor from attack by the body and the cancer cells are able to steal as much nitrogen as they need from surrounding healthy cells.

Naessens felt that if he could *stop* cancer cells from producing this Co-carcinogenic K Factor, then a person's immune system would be able to recognize and attack the cancer cells. He was finally able to develop an aqueous solution he called "714X." 714X is an innovative mixture of camphor, nitrogen and mineral salts specifically created to supply the cancer cells of the body with the extra nitrogen they need so the tumor does not have to excrete CKF in an attempt to obtain more nitrogen. When it does not secrete CKF, it is *not* hidden from the immune system and the body's own defenses can then attack the cancer. Thus, the main way that 714X works against cancer is not by directly killing cancer cells, but by debilitating the cancer's ability to mask itself. The person's own immune system then kills the cancer cells.

Naessens found that camphor has a special affinity for cancer cells, so he used natural camphor as the base to carry the nitrogen to the cancer. Naessens also included ammonium salts in 714X because he believed that they could help to liquefy the lymph fluid and increase lymphatic flow. This could help the lymph system deal with toxins better and could activate certain "kinins" that inhibit abnormal cell growth.[5] Also found in 714X are 18 different minerals in trace element form.

Gaston Naessens designed 714X to improve the natural defenses of the body and to stimulate the immune system. It does *not* kill abnormal or cancerous cells, but rather helps the body defend against them and heal from degenerative diseases and immune-deficiency disorders. 714X is administered by injection directly into the lymph system. As a general agent for healing, it performs two distinct functions:

1. It removes toxins from circulation by liquefying the lymphatic fluid.

2. It helps the body to repair itself.

714X is not a cytotoxic product, such as chemotherapy, and can be used safely for any length of time with no negative side effects. Injections are self-administered just under the skin with a very small 3/8-inch needle and "perinodally" around a lymph node in the groin area. It is sold by Cerbe Distribution, Inc., located in Quebec, Canada. The product comes with very clear instructions on how to use it, and Cerbe also offers a phone service that answers inquiries.

714X is usually administered through perinodular injection once a day for 21 days straight. After two days of rest, the injections are repeated again for 21 days, and this cycle is repeated over and over until the person is disease-free. The perinodular injections are the *main* treatment and cover the main large lymphatic circulation. In some circumstances, where the disease is localized in the upper body and/or in the upper right areas, 714X may be given by inhalation as well to cover the small lymphatic circulation. This inhalation, or nebulizer method, is considered an "add-on" treatment to be used along with the injection, not instead of it. The nebulizer add-on is recommended when there is cancer in the right breast, the lungs, the esophagus, or anywhere in the head.

How long the treatment takes for each individual will vary. This is partly because each person metabolizes the product at his or her own pace, and also because the body tends to "clean" itself before repairing itself. Thus, the more a person has used toxic treatments such as chemotherapy or radiation prior to starting 714X, the more cleaning out needs to be done by the body before repair can begin. It is probably safe to say that the prognosis is best when 714X is started immediately after diagnosis. 714X can also be used safely while doing conventional cancer treatments, and in those cases, it can reduce the side effects of the toxic treatments. Cerbe Distribution recommends that 714X be used for a minimum of six to eight consecutive cycles when a confirmed cancer diagnosis has been received. Once a person is cancer-free, then a maintenance program of one or two cycles twice a year is recommended.

There is no doubt that 714X has brought about truly astounding recoveries for many people with late-stage cancer. Most of these people had reached the point where their disease was *not* responding to conventional treatments and their doctors had no other options to offer them. Many of these remarkable case stories have been documented by physicians or other reliable sources, and many others can be found throughout the Internet. Some examples that I found are the following:

> Jacques Viens was 39 years old when he had seven-eighths of his stomach removed, according to writer Stephanie Hiller. The cancer had already spread to the lymph. Since there seemed to be no hope of recovery,

his doctor offered him 714X. Four months after taking 714X he was healthy enough to go hunting and soon resumed his job.

Marcel Caron had intestinal cancer but refused to have his intestine removed. His wife's breast cancer had been successfully treated with 714X and so he tried it as well. Sixty-five days after he started treatment, no cancer was found in Caron's body. Eight years later he is still healthy.

Anne Vignal, wife of the former French Counsel General in Quebec, sought out medical opinions and was told she could not conceive children. She was also told that her infertility was due to a lethal form of leukemia and she had only three to five years to live. She took 714X. She is now cancer-free and the mother of a healthy son.[6]

The story of a 17-year-old boy named Luke Stevens is yet another remarkable story. In August 1995, Luke (the son of a South African chiropractor) developed a giant cell tumor on his knee. This grew so rapidly that it destroyed most of Luke's upper tibia. According to one source, "Surgeons removed the tumor and rebuilt the boy's tibia. Four months later, Mr. Stevens's body rejected his bone graft and the tumor returned with a vengeance, breaking through the skin and growing into a hideous, fist-sized mass. Stevens's father grew disillusioned with oncologists, ignoring their advice to amputate his son's leg and begin massive chemotherapy."[7]

Luke's father found out about 714X and his son began that treatment instead of undergoing amputation and chemotherapy. Luke's condition rapidly improved and, according to the same source as above, "the tumor disappeared. Subsequent X-rays documented 100 percent bone regeneration, considered medically impossible. Today, at 21, Mr. Stevens attends university and rows on his school's team. He gives all the credit to Dr. Naessens's therapy."[8] About two-and-one-half years after he was diagnosed with cancer, Luke's diagnostic tests showed him to be cancer-free and he has been cancer-free ever since.

Here are 714X testimonies from two different physicians:

Dr. Florianne Pier, a Belgian physician, reported that over a four-month period she had treated seven cancer patients with 714X. "The product prolonged the lives, and eased the deaths, of two terminally afflicted patients," she said, "and has allowed the other five who came to me with seriously advanced cancerous states, to see every one of their symptoms disappear and to take up their lives as if they had never incurred the disease."[9]

Dr. Raymond Brown of New York City, a former Sloan-Kettering cancer researcher, told a pretrial press conference how he had treated one of his own patients with 714X for a pancreatic cancer that had proven resistant to all other forms of treatment. Naessens's therapy had prolonged the patient's life well over expectancy and kept him free of side effects, he said. Dr. Brown declared that while 714X was not a panacea, it deserved a place in the arsenal of weapons available to official medicine.[10]

In Canada, 714X is still not a fully approved cancer treatment. It is only allowed for use against cancer "on an emergency basis" through the Canadian government's Special Access Program. This means that any Canadian physician wishing to *officially* use 714X for a cancer patient must request special authorization to do so on compassionate grounds. Since January 1990, when 714X was introduced as an emergency drug in Canada, to June 2003, 18,366 authorizations were given to 1,684 doctors to use 714X on behalf of 4,030 patients.

However, 714X can be obtained by individuals *outside* of Canada *without* a physician's authorization. Although 714X is not approved as a cancer treatment in the United States, people in the United States can order this non-toxic compound by simply phoning Cerbe Distribution in Quebec and having it mailed to them. The promise of cancer recovery through this form of treatment is somewhat difficult to ascertain for any particular person, and may have a lot to do with how soon one starts to use it after diagnosis. Unfortunately, since the law in Canada only allows 714X to be prescribed by doctors as an emergency drug, it is often given to patients who are so far along in their disease that they are beyond recovery through any means. Even in these cases, 714X has often been known to improve the patient's quality of life (less pain, more appetite, more energy, etc.). There is no risk associated with using 714X because there are no adverse side effects.

Many of the full recoveries involving 714X have been achieved without any other treatment used. But there have also been people who achieved remarkable recoveries when they combined 714X with other alternative, non-toxic treatments. For example, there is one well-known story of a teenage boy named Billy Best, who was cured of his Hodgkin's lymphoma in just two and one-half months by the combined use of 714X, Essiac tea, nutritional supplements, and a healthy diet. His story is presented at www.BillyBest.net.

As we have seen with many other effective alternative non-toxic cancer treatments, the general rule is that there will be attempts at suppression. Gaston Naessens, unfortunately, had to deal with this as well. In the mid-

1950s, Naessens started to have trouble with the medical authorities in France. When his unorthodox methods began having incredible success in the 1960s, his laboratory was closed by these authorities, his equipment was confiscated, and he was fined for practicing medicine without a license. This prompted Naessens to move to Canada in 1964 where he was able to continue his work for a number of years in a privately funded laboratory outside Montreal. However, in 1989, Naessens was brought to trial by the Quebec medical authorities. It was a long and difficult trial where testimony was heard from both patients and physicians who had used 714X for cancer, AIDS, and other degenerative conditions. Dozens of demonstrators rallied outside the courthouse throughout the proceedings and carried banners in support of Naessens.

Some impressive cancer recovery stories were brought to light throughout the court battle. For example, one man named Roland Caty testified that he had been diagnosed with adenosarcoma of the prostate. His conventional doctor recommended he have all of his sexual organs removed. When Roland refused, his doctor told him he'd be dead in three months. Instead, Roland began to inject himself with 714X and achieved a complete recovery. At the trial, Roland Caty told the press, "And here I am testifying to you, eleven years after I got well."[11]

Marcel Caron, another ex-cancer patient, testified with his story. Marcel had been diagnosed with cancerous intestinal polyps eight years earlier. As with Roland Caty, surgery was recommended to Marcel by his conventional doctors. However, Marcel refused because his brother had died after surgery years before for the very same condition. According to Marcel's court testimony, he used 714X instead, and after just 21 days of treatment he was cancer-free.[12]

Fortunately, this trial resulted in acquittal for Naessens in December of that same year (1989). In fact, the jury turned in "not-guilty" verdicts on all counts. In January 1990, the Canadian Federal Government then hurriedly introduced 714X for use as an emergency drug.

So, how has Canada's powerful neighbor, the United States, reacted to 714X? In 1974, Dr. Raymond Brown from New York's Memorial Sloan-Kettering Cancer Center visited Gaston Naessens and investigated 714X. He was *very* favorably impressed and wrote an extremely enthusiastic memorandum about Naessens's work. Below is an excerpted paragraph from what Dr. Brown wrote:

> What I have seen is a microscope that reveals with spectacular clarity the motion and multiplicity of pleomorphic organisms in the blood

which are intimately associated with disease states. The implications . . .
are staggering . . . It is imperative that what its inventor, a dedicated
biological scientist, is doing be totally reviewed. I am convinced that he
is an authentic genius and that his achievements cut across and illumine
some of the most pertinent areas of medical science.[13]

At first, Memorial Sloan-Kettering was reportedly very interested in
Dr. Brown's report. But then they supposedly lost interest in pursuing
714X. Some speculations are that Sloan-Kettering dropped their interest
in 714X like a hot potato when they found out that the American Cancer
Society had blacklisted Naessens. Apparently, the American Cancer Society
was Sloan-Kettering's biggest monetary contributor in the 1970s.

Then, in 2001, the U.S. National Cancer Institute suddenly put 714X
on a "fast-track" for review. This was supposedly in response to patients
in Massachusetts and media reporters making allegations that an investigation of 714X had been covered up the Dana-Farber Cancer Institute
in Boston. In August 2001, Cerbe, Inc. submitted 16 in-depth cases of
patients who had used 714X successfully for long-term recovery. Gaston
Naessens and his wife, Jacinte Naessens, attended a press conference in
Boston, and were accompanied by successfully treated 714X patients.

One of these patients, 14-year-old Katie Hartley, spoke at the press
conference. In April 1995, when Katie was seven years old, she was diagnosed with a malignant tumor (undifferentiated sarcoma) that was growing inside her head. It was first noticed when one of Katie's eyes started
to protrude from its socket. The sarcoma was the size of a tangerine, and
Katie's doctors from the Dana-Farber Cancer Institute prescribed chemotherapy. Katie went through nine of the thirteen weeks of chemo that
had been prescribed. She had to stop it early because of debilitating side
effects of the treatment.

Next, Katie went through six weeks of radiation, after which she was
too weak to continue any further conventional treatment. Her tumor began
to grow again and her doctors sent her home and told her family that she
only had a couple of weeks to live. Katie's mother frantically searched for
other options, and in January 1996, started her on 714X. They gave her
injections in the morning and nebulizer treatments at night. A year and
a half later, tests showed that Katie's cancer was completely gone.[14]

The NCI's Office of Cancer Complementary and Alternative Medicine
(OCCAM) was initially responsible for the review of 714X. After that,
it was supposed to go to the Cancer Advisory Panel for Complementary

Alternative Medicine (CAPCAM). At this point in time, it is unclear what the results of the NCI investigation have been or whether they did, indeed, investigate it.

714X is not expensive compared to conventional cancer approaches and costs about 300 U.S. dollars per 21-day cycle. The number of cycles required for recovery will vary from case to case, but is usually six to eight cycles, or until conventional tests show remission. No significant dietary changes are required, though it is recommended to reduce one's intake of red meat and dairy products. In terms of other supplements that may or may not be used in conjunction with this treatment, it is merely suggested that people using 714X stay away from supplementation of the following: vitamin E, vitamin B_{12}, and all anti-angiogenic herbs or drugs (e.g., bindweed, shark or bovine cartilage, or thalidomide). The amount of vitamin E or B_{12} ingested from a normal diet, however, is fine.

Gaston Naessens is considered by many to be a great contributor to the field of microbiology, and his work impacts the treatment of not only cancer, but other terrible diseases including HIV/AIDS as well. (These other applications of 714X are beyond the scope of this book.) Christopher Bird, co-author of the best-selling book *The Secret Life of Plants*, wrote a detailed book about Gaston Naessens and his struggles with organized medicine. His book is called *The Persecution and Trial of Gaston Naessens: The True Story of the Efforts to Suppress an Alternative Treatment for cancer, AIDS, and Other Immunologically Based Diseases.*

For those people who use 714X for cancer, the results can vary quite a bit and some people feel that the perinodal injections are too painful. However, sometimes recoveries are simply astounding. To read about and listen to more current recovery stories from people who have used 714X for cancer, go to www.714X.com and click on "Testimonials."

Resources:

CERBE Distribution, Inc.   (819) 564-7883
5270 Mills Street, Rock Forest   www.cerbe.com
Quebec, J1N 3B6
Canada

Book

Christopher Bird. *The Persecution and Trial of Gaston Naessens: The True Story of the Efforts to Suppress an Alternative Treatment for Cancer, AIDS, and other Immunologically Based Diseases.* Tiburon, California: H. J. Kramer, 1991.

Video

For around $10, you can purchase an information and instruction video about 714X by calling the above phone number.

Self-Treatment at Home: 714X is relatively inexpensive and costs only about $300 per month (and an extra $150 for those who also need to use the nebulizer). The number of months of treatment will vary for each individual.

Websites

www.cerbe.com

www.714X.com

www.luminet.net/~wenonah/new/naessens.htm

www.BillyBest.net

16

Cesium High pH Therapy

Cesium high pH therapy is yet another powerful and highly impressive approach for outsmarting cancer. It has brought about some remarkable recoveries for people with primary cancers as well as late-stage, metastasized cancers. Though temporary side effects from this therapy are often felt, such as diarrhea and tingling sensations in the skin, when used properly it is a non-toxic approach that targets cancer cells but leaves healthy cells unharmed.

A particularly positive aspect of cesium high pH therapy is that it can often quickly reduce the severe pain that accompanies advanced cancer. It is also sometimes able to reduce large tumors faster than many other approaches. Thus, for people whose disease is so far advanced that they may not have time for another alternative approach to work, or are in such severe pain that they are on heavy narcotics which may be shutting down their bodily functions, cesium high pH therapy may be their best treatment option. On the other hand, a downside to this approach is that it is difficult to find qualified experts who can give guidance for best results. Some are listed at the back of this chapter, but hopefully more practitioners will adopt this approach over time and become available for consultation.

Like Protocel®, this approach specifically targets anaerobic cells (i.e., malignant cancer cells as well as other damaged unhealthy cells of the body that have become primarily anaerobic to survive.) However, cesium kills cancer cells in a different way than Protocel® does. Whereas Protocel® biochemically interferes with the cell respiration of cancer cells by blocking their production of ATP, cesium raises the pH *within* the cancer cells to such a high alkalinity that the cancer cells can no longer function and they die off as a result. The premise for this approach is based on the fact that anaerobic cells are much more acidic than normal healthy cells and must maintain their acidic intracellular environment in order to survive. A more detailed explanation will follow in the next section but, in a nutshell, *cesium high pH therapy alkalizes cancer cells to death from the inside out*!

Cesium has been used to treat cancer in humans since the 1980s. But it has recently been made easier and more effective as a treatment with the development of "liquid ionic minerals." And as you will see, it is because of this liquid ionic form of cesium that this approach is now more available to the public for self-administration and bringing about some truly astounding recoveries for cancer patients.

History and Theory

The pioneer of cesium high pH therapy was physicist Aubrey Keith Brewer, Ph.D. Dr. Brewer lived from 1893 to 1986 and was a highly esteemed American physicist who focused his research on the study of cell membranes. For a period of time, he held the position of chief of the National Bureau of Standards Mass Spectrometer and Isotope section.

Dr. Brewer proved with spectrographic analysis that cancer cells have an *affinity* for cesium—meaning they readily absorb cesium through their cell walls. The fact that cancer cells have an affinity for cesium is also evidenced by the common current-day use of a radioactive isotope of cesium as a marker in conventional oncology for tracing how well chemotherapy agents get into tumors.

Dr. Brewer developed his theory of how cancer could be treated with cesium (the non-radioactive form) based on his understanding of the physics of cell membranes and the fact that cesium is the most alkaline mineral. He wrote a number of scientific articles on his theory, and in the late 1970s, initiated animal research studies at three U.S. universities— first using rubidium (the second most alkaline mineral), then using cesium chloride. (Cesium Chloride, or CsCl, is also referred to as cesium salts.) All three university studies proved that high pH therapy was, indeed, effective against malignant tumors in mice. In fact, these tests showed marked shrinkage of mouse tumors within just two weeks.

Being a Ph.D. physicist and not an M.D., Dr. Brewer could not legally conduct human clinical trials himself. However, he was able to follow and write about the clinical work done by several physicians who were administering cesium to some of their late-stage cancer patients—people who had been given up on by conventional medicine and had no other hope. Two of these physicians were Dr. Hans Nieper of Germany and Dr. H.E. Sartori of the United States. In 1981, Dr. Brewer was able to follow the treatment of 30 late-stage terminal cancer patients and the results were extremely positive—far better than any results conventional medicine could achieve.

In 1984, Dr. Brewer published his findings in *Pharmacology Biochemistry and Behavior*.[1] In the article, Dr. Brewer explained the cesium approach to cancer in great scientific detail, and also proposed his understanding of how normal cells can become cancer cells. Starting with the widely accepted knowledge that normal healthy cells have membranes which allow the free exchange of both oxygen and glucose and maintain stable intracellular environments at around 7.35 pH, Dr. Brewer proposed that there is a sequence of four main steps that occur as the healthy cell turns into a cancer cell. These steps are summarized below:

How a Healthy Cell Becomes a Cancer Cell

1. When carcinogenic materials, such as environmental toxins, attach themselves to the outer surface of the cell membrane, the membrane may become damaged. This process involves two factors: (a) the presence of carcinogenic-type molecules primarily of the polycyclic type, and (b) an energized state of the membrane, which may result from prolonged irritation. (Dr. Sartori also felt that X-rays, parasites, or other factors may damage the cell membrane as well.) At some point, the membrane of the normal cell may become so damaged and altered that it can no longer pass certain materials easily. In particular, the damaged cell membrane may no longer be able to readily pass magnesium, calcium, or sodium into the cell. Since oxygen transport depends on two of these elements, calcium and magnesium, the cell then becomes oxygen deficient. However, a damaged cell membrane *can* still pass potassium, cesium, and rubidium. Since glucose transport depends on potassium, glucose continues to be fully supplied to the damaged cell while oxygen is no longer being fully supplied. Without sufficient oxygen to maintain aerobic functioning for energy, the cell reverts to

the fermentation of glucose for energy in order to survive. Thus, it turns into an anaerobic cell.

2. Fermentation of glucose produces lactic acid as a byproduct, and this lowers the *intracellular* pH of the cell. The cell pH drops internally from the normal 7.35 to around 7, and then to the extremely acidic pH level of about 6.5. In very advanced stages of cancer, the cell pH may drop even further to 5.7. Thus, the damaged cell has not only become an anaerobic cell, but it has also turned into a cell with a highly acidic internal environment.

3. In the acid medium of the anaerobic cell, the genetic blueprint of the cell (DNA and RNA) can be easily damaged, resulting in impairment to the cell's control mechanism. With the control mechanism for growth now impaired, the cell rapidly duplicates and grows out of control as a cancer cell.

4. Various cell enzymes are also completely changed in the acid medium of the anaerobic cell. Lysosomal enzymes are changed into toxic compounds, which kill the cells in the main body of the tumor mass. (A tumor therefore often consists of a thin layer of rapidly growing cells surrounding a dead mass.) The acid toxins leak out from the tumor mass and poison the host. This is also the source of much of the pain associated with cancer. These acid toxins can then act as carcinogens on other healthy cells, in part by lowering the extracellular pH of normal healthy tissues to the point where that environment becomes oxygen deficient as well.

The above sequence of steps is how Dr. Brewer theorized that a normal cell becomes a cancer cell. His concept of how cesium can then be used therapeutically to *treat* cancer is based on the fact that cesium is the most alkaline (and most alkalizing) of all elements. In fact, when taken up by cancer cells, cesium is able to radically raise the intracellular pH of the cancer cells to the very alkaline range of 8.0 to 9.0. In this range, according to Dr. Brewer, the life of the cancer cell is short—a matter of days at most. The cancer cell soon dies and is absorbed by the body fluids and eliminated from the system.

It is important to realize that, when a cancer patient alkalizes his or her body through diet changes and the use of supplements other than cesium (or rubidium), the effect on the cancer cell is not nearly as profound. It is widely accepted that cancer cells thrive best in acidic extracellular fluids and do not thrive as well when their fluid environment is optimally alkaline. (See Chapter 18 for more details.) However, in most alkalizing programs that use diet and supplements, it is the *extracellular* environment of one's cancer cells that is being influenced the most. But what many people don't realize is that tumors create their own local acidic environments by their excretion of lactic acid as a by-product of anaerobic functioning (glycolysis). Thus, many alkalizing programs will have a difficult time fully alkalizing the area around a tumor, and the tumor will still be able to thrive in its own little acidic environment even if a person's attempts at alkalizing are having a positive effect on the rest of their body.

With the use of cesium or rubidium, a person is able to bypass the external environment of their tumor or tumors and impact the *internal* pH of their cancer cells so powerfully that the cancer cells quickly begin to die off. And cesium is able to limit the transport of glucose across the cancer cell's membrane. This causes an immediate decrease in fermentation and a resultant decrease in lactic acid formation. Since a large part of the pain associated with cancer is due to lactic acid build-up, cancer patients using cesium often find their pain subsiding within about 12 to 24 hours.[2]

Dr. Brewer also determined that there were some other key nutrients that, when administered in conjunction with high pH therapy, enhanced the cellular uptake of the cesium. These are vitamin A, vitamin C, zinc, and selenium. And he suspected that the administration of Laetrile would also greatly enhance the uptake of cesium by the cancer cells. According to Dr. Brewer:

> The therapy I am proposing is one of changing the pH of the cancer cell from acid to alkaline. This is entirely possible since as already stated, the cancer cells have lost their pH control mechanism. . . . There are areas of the earth where the incidences of cancer are very low. An analysis of the foods in these areas shows them to be very high in cesium and rubidium. It is these elements, which are absent in modern commercial foods, that prevent cancer growth. I am convinced that it is food that causes cancer, but it is the food we don't eat and not the food we do eat.[3]

Early Clinical Results

As mentioned earlier, Dr. Brewer reported on 30 cancer patients who were treated with cesium in the early 1980s. In his summary of these cases, Dr. Brewer stated, "In each case the tumor masses disappeared. Also all pains and effects associated with cancer disappeared within 12 to 36 hours; the more chemotherapy and morphine the patient had taken, the longer the withdrawal period."[4]

Another group of 50 patients was studied over a three-year period with similarly impressive results. These patients were treated by Dr. Sartori and written about in his book *Cancer—Orwellian or Utopian*. All of the 50 subjects were terminal cancer patients with metastatic disease. Forty-seven of the 50 had received maximal amounts of conventional treatment. Three of the subjects were comatose, and 14 were already suffering from previous treatment-related or cancer-related complications. After cesium treatment was started, pain in *all* 50 subjects disappeared within one to three days! Thirteen of the subjects died within the first two weeks, which was most likely due to the treatment simply coming too late for them. But, over the next three years, 50 percent of the original 50 survived.[5] This was an incredible survival rate given that all the patients were very late stage, had exhausted all conventional forms of treatment, and were all originally expected to die within weeks. Moreover, post-mortem examinations done on those subjects who died showed substantial shrinkage of those patients' tumor masses.[6]

Well-known German cancer researcher and physician, Dr. Hans Nieper, also conducted studies on cesium high pH therapy in Germany. Like the U.S. studies, Dr. Nieper's trials were extremely successful.

In Kathleen Deoul's revealing book, *Cancer Cover-Up*, Deoul presents the story of her husband, Neal Deoul, and his battle with the cancer industry's efforts to suppress effective natural and non-toxic cancer therapies. In 1996, Neal Deoul had provided financing which enabled a Maryland company, T-Up, Inc., to become a primary distributor of cesium and concentrated aloe vera, each sold as natural dietary supplements. (The form of aloe vera sold was found to have the ability to greatly stimulate the immune system and had proven to be very beneficial for both cancer and AIDS patients.) The cesium and aloe vera were obviously working for people because T-UP, Inc. had hundreds of testimonies on file from consumers who claimed life-changing beneficial results. T-UP also never received a single consumer complaint.

But "big business" was not interested in whether cesium or aloe vera were beneficial to T-UP's ailing customers. And even though Neal Deoul was *not* receiving profits from the sale of T-UP's products, he was targeted as a financier of the company and taken to court for bogus reasons.

Ironically, in January 1999 while Neal Deoul was battling his case in court, he himself was diagnosed with prostate cancer. Believing in T-UP's products, Deoul immediately started administering cesium high pH therapy to himself along with the aloe vera concentrate. By October of that same year, his PSA was down to normal levels and there were no more indications of cancer. Neal's complete story is presented in his wife's book, *Cancer Cover-Up*.

In *Cancer Cover-Up*, Kathleen Deoul describes one of the cases that Dr. Brewer reported in the following way:

> The patient [an individual suffering from lymphoma who arrived in a comatose state] had a massive tumor in his abdomen, as well as an enlarged liver and spleen. After three months of the High pH therapy, the tumor had been virtually eliminated, and the liver and spleen were returned to near normal size. Three years after the treatment the patient was still alive.[7]

Deoul states, "Clearly, the tests had shown that the High pH therapy kills cancer. But 'Big Medicine' ignored and continues to ignore these dramatic results."[8]

Form of Treatment

Until recently, the cesium used to treat cancer was a powdered form of cesium chloride, also referred to as cesium salts. (Which was the form that Neal Deoul used to cure his prostate cancer.) Usually given to patients in capsules, it was effective but somewhat risky to use. This was because the powdered form could build up to toxic levels in the body if taken for too long a period of time. It could only be safely administered under a doctor's care, and some doctors believed cesium in this form should not be used for longer than one or two months.

Although some cancer patients continue to successfully use the powdered form of cesium, the use of *liquid ionic cesium* is becoming more and more popular. When cesium is administered in liquid ionic form, it is thought to be more easily assimilated by the body and more quickly processed out so that it does *not* build up inside the body. Also, some experts believe that a smaller amount of the liquid ionic form of cesium can be used to achieve the same results as larger amounts of the capsule form.

An ionic mineral is an element that has a positive or negative electrical charge, meaning it has either too many or too few electrons. In this unstable state, the element bonds readily with water. Because the liquid ionic version delivers cesium in a form that is bonded to water molecules, it enters the bloodstream faster than the powdered form, which the body would have to dissolve in the stomach first. The liquid ionic form of cesium is also thought to penetrate cancer cell walls more easily, causing it to be more completely absorbed by the cancer cells. As to toxicity, a dose of 6 grams of liquid ionic cesium per day is only about 5 percent of the minimum toxic level. (One must remember, though, that extremely high doses of cesium could cause cancer die-off to occur too fast for the body to process, thus causing a detoxification crisis.)

The most important aspect about using cesium safely is making sure that enough potassium is supplemented along with it. James A. Howenstine, M.D. is an expert on cesium high pH therapy and author of the comprehensive book, *A Physician's Guide to Natural Health Products That Work*. On page 409 of his book, Howenstine explains why potassium must be supplemented along with cesium. He states:

> Any alkali therapy changes the pH of the body toward a more alkalotic state. This causes movement of potassium into cells, which may result in low serum potassium values. This movement of potassium into cells means that a person can become seriously depleted of potassium even if there is no diarrhea or vomiting.

Thus, taking high doses of cesium causes a lowering of serum potassium levels and a severe potassium deficiency can result if sufficient potassium supplementation is not also taken. The danger of potassium deficiency cannot be overstated, since severe potassium deficiency can result in death. The prime cause of death from this sort of deficiency is heart attack.

Any distributor selling liquid ionic cesium will also sell liquid ionic potassium, and this is the form of potassium supplementation preferred when using liquid ionic cesium. People using cesium (either in capsule or liquid form) should always have their blood potassium level checked on a regular basis to be sure they are getting enough potassium and not developing a potassium deficiency. For optimal effectiveness, cancer patients usually also make positive changes in their diets and take other supplements as well to enhance their overall health and immune system.

Even though this therapy is non-toxic when used correctly, cesium in the amounts required to kill cancer cells can cause stomach upset or nausea if taken on an empty stomach. The reason that cesium may cause nausea is because, as nature's most alkaline mineral, it reacts with anything that is highly acidic, including stomach acids. This type of discomfort is generally avoided by only taking cesium right after a meal.

Patients taking cesium may also experience some diarrhea and/or temporary numbness of the lips and tip of the nose for about 20 minutes after the intake of cesium. The numbness or prickling sensations in the skin on various parts of the body, however, are not indicative of long-term damage. They are simply a result of cesium being a mild nerve stimulant. Less common symptoms are vomiting, yellow vision, or a peculiar dark hue to the skin accompanied by cold hands or feet. If these less common symptoms occur, it is best to simply stop the therapy for 3 or 4 days or until the side effects subside, then start back up at one-half the previous dose for a while. People with high blood pressure or other heart conditions should be sure they are under the supervision of a physician while using cesium.

The following six real-life cases were recorded for this book from people who used cesium and potassium in the liquid ionic form.

Case Stories

Case Story #1—Lung Cancer Metastasized to Bones and Liver

In April 2003, at the age of 82, Olga was diagnosed with advanced lung cancer. She had such a large tumor in her lung that it could be easily felt from the outside around her ribs. She underwent chemotherapy and radiation. But these treatments were ineffective, and by June 2003, Olga's doctors proclaimed that her cancer had spread to every bone in her body as well as to her liver. The family was told she would be dead by September.

Because of her age and advanced state of illness, Olga was too weak to undergo any more conventional treatments. With no further treatment, her cancer began to progress quickly. Soon, Olga was having so much difficulty breathing due to the cancer in her lungs, she had to be hooked up to oxygen 24 hours a day, seven days a week. She was also on heavy pain medication.

Since the diagnosis, Olga's daughter, Trish, had been trying to find something else that could be done for her mother. Luckily, in late August 2003, when Olga's doctors thought she had only a few more weeks to live, Trish found out about cesium high pH therapy using liquid ionic cesium and potassium. She contacted someone who had experience and knowledge about how to use this approach safely and started her mother on it immediately.

Because Olga did not want to take too many different supplements, her treatment protocol was extremely simple. She just took 1 tablespoon of liquid ionic cesium and 1 tablespoon of liquid ionic potassium every morning right after breakfast and again every evening right after dinner. She simply stirred the liquid minerals into juice and drank them down. She also took a coral calcium supplement. Olga used no other treatments, but she did drink chocolate whey protein mixed into whole milk on a daily basis to make sure she was getting adequate protein and to help her gain weight. She also ate red beets every day to help support her liver.

When Trish started helping her mother with the cesium and potassium, she had to quickly lift the oxygen mask off her mother's mouth and nose to give it to her, then quickly put the oxygen mask back on. It was so difficult for Olga to breathe that she could barely get by without the oxygen long enough to take the minerals. But after just a few days of taking the cesium and potassium, Olga was not so desperate for the oxygen and could breathe without it for a few extra minutes whenever she took her minerals. Amazingly, only 10 days after starting the liquid ionic cesium and liquid ionic potassium, Olga was able to go off the oxygen altogether. Trish says, "It was like a miracle!"

Olga continued to feel better as she kept taking the cesium and potassium. Soon, she was out of bed walking around. Within a few months, Olga was back to being active and living her life almost normally. In mid-December 2003, another MRI was done. This time, only three-and-one-half months after starting on cesium high pH therapy, her MRI showed a very different picture. The cancer in Olga's lungs was gone, her liver was clear, and almost all of the spots on her bones had disappeared. It looked like her advanced, metastasized cancer was almost all gone, and the only problem she was experiencing was some severe bone pain that was either due to some bone fractures caused by the cancer or the fact that she may have still had a small amount of cancer in her spine that had not yet had enough time to go away.

Unfortunately, in February 2004, Olga contracted a bad case of the flu that quickly developed into pneumonia. She was rushed to a hospital and put on intravenous antibiotic treatment along with respiratory therapy. She showed signs of improvement, but after being sent home with oral antibiotics, she began to decline again. Her body just could not withstand the infection and she passed away. Olga's daughter, Trish, related the following, however, regarding her mother's cancer status when she passed. "They scanned Mom's lungs at the hospital, and her lungs were free of cancer and so was her brain."

Given that almost all of Olga's advanced metastatic cancer was gone, if she could have avoided the pneumonia somehow and been able to stay on the cesium therapy a little longer, it is reasonable to assume that she would have achieved a full recovery.

Case Story #2—Multiple Myeloma Metastasized to Bones

Jim was 57 years old when he went to a doctor because he was experiencing terrible pain in his neck. Tests revealed that he had a tumor on his C3 vertebra that had nearly destroyed the vertebra completely. More scans showed that he also had tumors on his pelvis, thigh bone, and a few other bones in his body. A bone marrow sample was then taken through the hip into the pelvis. This was biopsied, and the official diagnosis came back "multiple myeloma—IGG, stage III."

Multiple myeloma is a malignant cancer of the bone marrow, and this was considered the primary location of Jim's cancer, with metastases to other bone locations. The "IGG" is a particular type of multiple myeloma that is determined through a blood test, and his IGG count was high at 5,720. Jim's oncologist recommended radiation, chemotherapy, thalidomide, and a stem cell transplant. The doctor also told Jim, "We can't save your life; we can only prolong it. You have from a few months to a few years to live."

Understandably, Jim was not happy with his prognosis. He had already looked into coral calcium for another condition he'd had, so he knew about the importance of alkalizing the body. However, he also knew that taking the coral calcium had never been enough to keep his pH in the optimal range unless he took about nine capsules a day. He found out about cesium high pH therapy and was told that, as opposed to some of the old powdered forms of minerals, liquid ionic minerals do not build up to a toxic level in the body. Jim worked with someone who knew a lot about liquid ionic minerals, and he started the therapy using liquid ionic cesium and liquid ionic potassium. The only conventional treatment he did was one week of radiation right after his diagnosis. According to Jim, when he turned down all conventional treatment and started on the liquid minerals, it was much to the dismay of his oncologist.

Jim took the liquid ionic cesium and potassium three times a day. Besides the cesium and potassium, his protocol included a variety of other minerals in liquid ionic form such as germanium, sodium, silver, zinc, boron, and iron. He also supplemented with coral calcium, vitamin D, and a few other vitamins and enzymes. Before Jim was diagnosed, he drank only a glass or two of water each week, a lot of soda and coffee, and rarely ate fresh fruits or vegetables. When he started cesium high pH therapy, he cut out all soda and coffee and drank lots of good water instead. He avoided sugar and refined carbohydrates, and reduced his intake of red meat while eating more fish and chicken. He also greatly increased his intake of fresh fruit and vegetables and started juicing mostly green vegetables.

Unbelievably, just 24 hours after starting on the cesium, Jim's severe neck pain was completely gone. About four days into his program, he felt that he was already detoxifying dead cancer cells out his body. Some of his detoxing symptoms included a tired, weak feeling, loose stools, night sweats, and increased urination. But the symptoms were mild and not even as bad as flu symptoms.

Jim had started cesium high pH therapy in January 2003. Just two months later, he went back to his oncologist to be tested again. A blood test this time showed his IGG count to be down to 1,520 (from 5,720), which was actually in the normal range for a healthy person. His oncologist told Jim he was "blown away" by the test results. Jim told his doctor all the things he had done. The doctor said, "Well, I don't know why it's working, but keep doing it."

About a year after his cancer diagnosis of incurable multiple myeloma, Jim was back to living a normal life and his scans no longer revealed any cancer! He continued to take the liquid minerals and to maintain a healthy diet to keep the cancer from coming back.

Over the year that Jim was recovering through the use of cesium high pH therapy, he only experienced minor aches and pains, which he attributes to his bones rebuilding. He also felt a slight tingling in his neck and hips at times in the places where his tumors were, and he sometimes experienced a slight numbness in his lips and nose for about 20 minutes after taking the cesium. But all of these symptoms were easy to go through and simply a part of his healing process.

Jim says that, because he was going against the conventional establishment, he had to have faith that he was doing the right thing by following the alternative approach that he chose. He credits his ability to stay with the approach to his belief that God was guiding him and putting him in touch with the right method that could help him to fully heal!

Case Story #3—Non-Hodgkin's Lymphoma of the Stomach

LaVaughn had been a welder for an oil company for many years and breathing a variety of toxic substances on the job may have had something to do with the cancer he was diagnosed with in April 2002, at age 47. Before consulting a doctor, LaVaughn had started having excruciating pain in his stomach and was sometimes throwing up blood. LaVaughn and his wife, Cindy, thought he probably had a bleeding ulcer.

When his condition worsened, LaVaughn went to a doctor. Nothing abnormal showed up on the CT scan or the MRI, so an endoscope procedure was performed. With the endoscope, LaVaughn's doctor could visually see a huge tumor in his stomach. Right in the middle of the tumor mass was a bleeding ulcerated area about the size of a silver dollar. A sample of tissue was biopsied, and the diagnosis came back "non-Hodgkin's lymphoma of the stomach." It was considered to be of a medium to aggressive variety.

LaVaughn's doctors did not want to try to surgically remove the tumor because it involved too many large blood vessels and there was too high a risk that LaVaughn would bleed to death. He started himself on nutritional therapy immediately and began juicing and taking some herbs to strengthen and support his body. He felt better right away, as the pain left and his energy returned. However, the tumor continued to grow until it blocked the lower stomach. LaVaughn was now no longer able to eat and had to be put on intravenous feeding. His doctors started him on chemo in June, thinking that might cause the tumor to shrink enough so he could begin eating again. He knew that if he could eat again, he would then become more aggressive with the nutritional therapy.

Unfortunately, the chemo was not effective and on October 1, 2002, another endoscope procedure showed that the tumor was bigger than ever. It had been five weeks since the last chemo treatment, and LaVaughn was too weak to undergo any more chemo at this point. He was in terrible pain and had not been able to keep any food or drink down for 16 weeks. His oncologist suggested to LaVaughn that the only option was to *surgically remove his entire stomach*, then have his intestines attached to his esophagus.

LaVaughn did not want to undergo stomach removal surgery. Cindy had been searching for alternative options throughout his battle and finally found out about liquid ionic cesium and potassium. On September 29, 2002, just before the endoscope procedure, she had started LaVaughn on cesium high pH therapy. He was extremely weak and lethargic at this point, and his duodenum was completely blocked. Since nothing was going through his stomach, Cindy decided to spray the liquid minerals on his skin and let them absorb into his body that way. She sprayed the liquid cesium on his chest and back and sprayed the liquid potassium and some of the other minerals on his arms and legs. She did this four times a day for two days. By the end of these two days, LaVaughn's stomach had started gurgling and his vomiting had stopped. On the third day, Cindy was able to start carefully giving the liquid minerals to LaVaughn orally in juice, along with spraying them on him. It seemed like, each day after that, his stomach was able to handle more and more food and drink, and he gradually gained his strength back.

LaVaughn's treatment was focused around using liquid ionic cesium and liquid ionic potassium, as well as other liquid ionic minerals. After a while, Cindy also started him on Dr. Kelley's enzymes, Essiac tea, and a variety of other supplements. But he never stopped taking the liquid ionic cesium, potassium, and other minerals.

Incredibly, about six weeks after beginning cesium high pH therapy, LaVaughn felt well again. Two weeks after that, at the eight-week point, another endoscope procedure was done. It was the day before Thanksgiving, 2002. This time, the endoscope showed that the tumor was completely gone and the central ulcer part had shrunk down to the size of a pencil eraser. A biopsy accompanied the scoping, and the resulting pathology report stated that the cancer was now benign and no helicobacter pylori bacteria were present.

LaVaughn has not had any more endoscope procedures done, but he has continued to take the liquid ionic minerals and has continued to feel great. In fact, he now says he feels 15 years younger than he did before his diagnosis. In October 2003, he had a general physical and his doctor could not find anything wrong with him or any signs of cancer. Even the hernias that had developed because of the chemo were gone.

LaVaughn's treatment approach involved a three-to-one ratio of potassium to cesium at first. But he eventually switched to an even higher ratio of potassium to cesium to be sure he did not suffer any potassium deficiency. Although not everyone does this, LaVaughn also decided to follow the practice of taking the cesium for five days, then skipping it for two days every week. During the two days of not taking the cesium, however, LaVaughn would still take all his other minerals, including the potassium.

LaVaughn and Cindy believe that when a person is on cesium high pH therapy and starts to experience numbness or tingling in the mouth and nose, or a general disoriented, dizzy, or shaky feeling, it's an indication of low potassium. They believe that using the cesium "five days on, two days off" helps to avoid potassium deficiency and also gives the body time to detoxify or flush out the dead cancer cells. This may be a helpful dosing tip to others, though some people may decide *not* to incorporate the two days off per week until their cancer has been significantly reduced.

As of February 2004, LaVaughn is still feeling great, and as far as anyone can tell, is completely cancer-free. His wife, Cindy, is now a distributor of liquid minerals, and her contact information is listed at the end of this chapter.

Case Story #4—Non-Hodgkin's Lymphoma, Grade II

"Cheddy" is the nickname for a woman who was also diagnosed with a form of non-Hodgkin's lymphoma. Her diagnosis came in February 2002, when she was 70 years old. Cheddy had gone to her doctor because of a lump on her arm that had appeared and was about the size of a nickel. The lump was removed and biopsied. The resulting diagnosis was "non-Hodgkin's lymphoma, grade II." Cheddy was immediately referred to an oncologist who did more scans and tested her bone marrow to see if her cancer had metastasized. Luckily, these tests indicated that the cancer in her lymph system had not metastasized to other parts of her body. She was advised to have a small amount of radiation done on her arm for one month, which she did. After this, her doctor pronounced her clear of cancer.

Just three days later, however, the cancer reared its ugly head again as three new lumps appeared on her neck. Needle biopsies proved these to be the lymphoma, and it was obvious that the radiation had not fully gotten rid of Cheddy's cancer. Her oncologist wanted her to do chemotherapy. But Cheddy did not want to do chemo and told her doctor that she wanted to look into a nutritional approach instead. Her doctor gruffly replied, "I don't know anything about nutrition, and I don't want to know anything about it."

Cheddy pursued nutritional support on her own for about a year. She made major changes in her diet and took lots of supplements including liver capsules, CoQ_{10}, and garlic. Throughout the year, her approach seemed to be successful at keeping the cancer stable, but wasn't making it go away. She still had tumors on her neck and one inside her throat.

In mid-March 2003, Cheddy found out about liquid ionic cesium and potassium and started taking those. She also took other minerals in liquid ionic form, including germanium, trace minerals and selenium, plus an immune support supplement. After about six months of doing this, Cheddy's lumps started going down, so she patiently kept doing her program. Her persistence paid off as she saw the tumors go away, and she says she experienced very little in the way of side effects. She had no nausea, no numbness or tingling in the mouth or nose, was simply a little more tired initially, and had bowel movements that were a little looser.

By September 2003, all the lumps on her neck and in her throat were completely gone and she had no indication of cancer whatsoever. As of February 2004, she continues to feel great and show no further signs of cancer.

Case Story #5—Prostate Cancer

At age 56, Gerry was feeling so tired and depressed all the time, that he was contemplating early retirement. But he knew that if he gave up his job, he would need to get health insurance coverage from another source. So he decided to see if he could get medical coverage from a VA hospital. The application for coverage required a thorough medical exam. Gerry was checked for polyps and given an ultrasound to check his prostate gland. Unfortunately, the ultrasound showed a mass on his prostate, and Gerry was tentatively diagnosed with prostate cancer. This was in mid-November of 2002. About a month later, a needle-biopsy was performed on the tumor and Gerry's cancer was officially verified and classified as 7 on the Gleason scale. (However, even though Gerry definitely had prostate cancer, his PSA count was only 0.9, which shows that not all prostate cancer will cause a high PSA score. See Chapter 20 for more information on this issue.)

Gerry's oncologist suggested that they perform surgery to remove his entire prostate gland and to also remove any surrounding lymph nodes during the surgery, if it appeared necessary. But just about everyone in Gerry's family had died of cancer after going through conventional treatment, so he was extremely reluctant to go through it himself. Instead,

Gerry declined surgery and searched for alternative options. He found out about liquid ionic cesium and potassium and started taking those in January of 2003. When he told his oncologist about cesium high pH therapy, the doctor was appalled and actually mailed Gerry a letter urging him not to do it. In the letter, the doctor warned, "You are making a *big* mistake."

But Gerry was steadfast in his decision to decline conventional treatment. Along with the liquid ionic cesium and potassium that he began to take, he also took other liquid ionic minerals, including calcium, magnesium, germanium, sulfur, and vanadium. Plus, he used a "rebounder," which is a mini-trampoline that can be used for mild exercise indoors, and he started walking a lot outdoors. Gerry radically improved his diet and cut his bread and sugar intake to almost zero. He also bought a magnetic mattress pad for his bed.

About four months later, Gerry went back for another ultrasound, and this time *no tumor showed up at all*. As far as diagnostic tests were concerned, no cancer could be found. Gerry continued to eat well, exercise, and take liquid ionic minerals. After about six months, he was able to cut back on the amounts of the liquid minerals, continuing them at lower dosages. Gerry would have liked to continue to get ultrasounds and PSA tests to monitor his progress, but his doctors refused to do these tests on him anymore. They seemed to believe Gerry still had cancer and that more ultrasounds or PSA tests would not change their minds about this.

Gerry now realizes that the extreme tiredness and depression that had made him want to retire from his job early had been partly due to the cancer. About a month or two into his cesium high pH therapy, he began to feel a lot of energy and felt the depression go away. Now, at the beginning of 2004, he has so much energy that he jogs between 6 and 9 miles every day and is scheduled to run in this year's New York Marathon. He thinks his positive attitude and diet changes were very important to his healing, but he credits the bulk of his recovery to cesium high pH therapy and liquid ionic minerals.

Case Story #6—Ovarian Cancer

Sixty-one-year-old Merille (pronounced Marilee) had not been feeling well for some time when she went to her doctor in January 2002. A CT scan showed fluid in her lungs, and since one of the causes of this could be cancer, she was referred to a specialist at the Mayo Clinic. More tests at the Mayo Clinic revealed tumors on both of Merille's ovaries as well as in her lymph system. A blood test for the ovarian cancer marker CA-125 showed her to have a count of almost 800. (The normal, healthy range for the CA-125 is a count of around 34 or less.)

Merille was rushed into surgery to have her uterus and ovaries removed. After the surgery, biopsies were done on the tumors and the diagnosis came back "ovarian cancer, stage IIIC." At this point, Merille's oncologist recommended chemotherapy for the cancer in her lymph system, but told her there was no cure for her type of cancer. The implication was that conventional medicine would only be able to manage her cancer for a while, but they would not be able to cure it and she would eventually die from it. Merille did not know of any other option but to go with her doctor's recommendation, so she followed her surgery with six rounds of chemotherapy.

When the chemotherapy was completed, Merille's CA-125 had gone down to a count of 9 and she was pronounced in remission. But as often happens soon after chemotherapy, her count immediately started going back up. By March 2003, her CA-125 was up to 84 and her cancer was obviously still there and growing. Merille now had new tumors in her abdomen and also in her neck area around her collar bone. Her Mayo Clinic oncologist pronounced that "the chemo had failed." At this point, the doctors performed more surgery on Merille, but they could not remove all her cancer. They recommended more rounds of chemo, but at the same time told Merille that there was a significant risk that further chemo would damage her heart. Merille was forced to make a difficult decision and she decided to decline further chemo and to look into alternatives instead.

Merille's daughter found out about cesium high pH therapy and Merille was able to contact an experienced consultant and start on liquid ionic cesium and liquid ionic potassium immediately. She also began to take other supportive liquid minerals and supplements. Within three months, all her tumors disappeared and her cancer marker test had gone from 84 down to 23. Now her CA-125 was back in the normal range. Merille's doctor at the Mayo Clinic was amazed and wondered what she was doing. When she told him, he just said, "Keep doing what you're doing!"

Merille reduced her dosage of liquid minerals at this point, but her next CA-125 test three months later showed her marker results to be up another 10 points. So she went back on the full dose of cesium and other minerals and her marker numbers began to go back down again.

By January 2004, her CA-125 marker was all the way down to 12, and she had no clinical signs of cancer at all. The latest CA-125 test, taken in April 2004, was 6.4—the lowest it has ever been.

Merille did nothing other than the cesium high pH therapy while she was recovering from her metastasized ovarian cancer. To ensure that she stayed free of cancer, she continued to take the liquid minerals and supportive supplements. Merille says she took the cesium five days out of each week, followed by two days off. (During those two days, she continued the liquid ionic potassium and other supplements, though.) She took potassium four times a day and cesium twice a day with the overall ratio of potassium to cesium being five to one so that she could be sure to avoid potassium deficiency.

Merille also says that she felt very good during her treatment, with only mild detoxing symptoms and sporadic diarrhea. And she only experienced a little tingling and numbness around the nose and mouth at times. All in all, it was a truly easy and miraculous recovery!

Variations on Dosing

It appears that different practitioners or consultants suggest different dosing amounts. According to Dr. Brewer, the most common cesium dosing that Dr. Nieper and Dr. Sartori used on their cancer patients was 2 grams of cesium chloride three times a day after eating for a total of 6 grams of cesium each day. Along with the cesium, 5 to 10 grams of vitamin C and 100,000 units of vitamin A, along with 50 to 100 mg of zinc were also administered to each patient.[9]

It is also known that Dr. Sartori significantly increased the amount of cesium he gave to some of his extremely late-stage cancer patients— particularly those who only had been given two weeks to live. In some cases, Sartori administered up to 27 grams of cesium per day. The most common cesium dosing he administered, however, was from 6 to 9 grams daily, divided into three equal doses each day, given intravenously. Dr. Sartori also intravenously administered high doses of vitamin A, vitamin C, zinc, selenium, and Laetrile to his patients, but it was not clear how much potassium was given. Dr. Brewer also thought that the use of Laetrile could reduce problems with diarrhea in some patients.

But of course Dr. Sartori and other physicians Dr. Brewer consulted with were using the powdered form of cesium. Some people believe that the *liquid ionic* form, which was used in the case stories of this chapter, is actually more effective and easier for the body to assimilate as well as process out. Even so, various sources recommend variations on dosing. Dr. Jim Howenstine regularly recommended a 1:1 ratio using 3 grams per day of cesium and 3 grams of potassium divided into 2 equal doses of 1½ grams each twice a day. (He did not recommend taking the 2 days off from the cesium each week, but simply suggested taking a few days to a week off if strong symptoms of potassium deficiency occurred.) Olga in Case Story #1 also used a 1:1 ratio, but only 2 grams of cesium and potassium each day. LaVaughn in Case Story #3, on the other hand, started with a 3:1 ratio of potassium to cesium, then increased to a 5:1 ratio later on.

The tricky thing about trying to figure out dosing ratios is that some people will compare grams to grams, while others may compare the number of tablespoons or ounces of the liquid they use. This is a problem since the number of grams of liquid cesium in a tablespoon may be different than the number of grams of liquid potassium in a tablespoon. Thus, for clarity, it is best to only compare the number of *grams* of cesium used per day to the number of *grams* of potassium used per day. Most liquid ionic cesium products provide 1½ grams of cesium per tablespoon, and a common way of dosing is one tablespoon of the liquid cesium in the morning and one tablespoon in the evening. That comes to a total of 3 grams per day. But the number of grams of potassium per tablespoon may be different. So, comparing grams to grams to understand your dosage ratio is important.

Also, at least one liquid ionic product provides both cesium *and* potassium in the same liquid. This type of product can work out well and be easier for some people, but the downside is that the ratio of potassium to cesium cannot be altered when needed. So, those who are trying a combination cesium/potassium product for the first time may want to have some extra liquid ionic potassium on hand in case they feel they need more potassium at any point.

Dr. Brewer also wrote that, while dealing with active tumors, a person should never take *less* than 3 grams of cesium per day.[10] His reasoning for this was that several physicians observed that the administration of 0.5 grams per day (half a gram) will actually *enhance* the growth of the cancer. According to Brewer, "This is to be expected, since this low amount is sufficient only to raise the cell pH into the high mitosis range."[11] He felt, however, that clinical findings proved a quantity of 3 grams or more per day to be effective against cancer. On the other hand, it is fairly well accepted that once a cancer patient is in remission (no more tumors or diagnostic evidence of cancer) then a daily dose of half a gram of cesium per day can be used as a maintenance amount.

Brewer also stated, "The material comprising the tumors is secreted as uric acid in the urine; the uric acid content of the urine increases many fold."[12] Thus, people testing their urine pH may find it more acidic as their tumors are breaking down. Measuring the uric acid content in urine might also be an area for future research as a way to measure how much cancer breakdown is occurring.

Unfortunately, the FDA is making it more and more difficult for companies to sell cesium. And cesium distributors cannot legally give out advice for using cesium to treat cancer. They can only legally give out advice for using cesium to alkalize the body and support overall health.

(**NOTE:** If you come across a cesium distributor advertizing that cesium does *not* kill cancer, keep in mind they are probably saying that to avoid being shut down by the FDA/FTC for claiming cesium as a cancer treatment.)

Many people obtain their cesium, potassium, and other liquid minerals from www.essense-of-life.com. It may be that the use of some other liquid minerals, such as germanium and selenium, can aid in the success of cesium high pH therapy and, as Dr. Brewer hypothesized, it may be that B_{17} also can aid in the success of cesium high pH therapy.

It is very difficult to find practitioners who administer cesium intravenously these days. However, one clinic in Reno, Nevada, is currently providing intravenous cesium for cancer patients who are able to attend their clinic for the first 3 weeks of their treatment. Then, they give them supervision on self-administering the cesium and potassium at home until the patient's body becomes saturated. (See "Reno Integrative Medical Center" in the Resources section at the end of this chapter.)

The Reno Integrative Medical Center has a long and successful history of treating cancer through alternative methods and they have many modalities at their disposal. For instance, Mistletoe, B_{17} and DMSO are also given intravenously along with the cesium. Potassium blood levels are monitored and German New Medicine is offered as well for resolving any possible emotional roots of the cancer. This clinic is highly recommended and worth looking into for anyone interested in cesium who wants to be supervised by a physician.

The real-life experiences of people who have used cesium high pH therapy show that, when administered correctly, it is safe and non-toxic.

But like other alternative, non-toxic approaches, it is not approved by the FDA as a cancer treatment. Thus, it cannot be legally prescribed by most physicians. Also, distributors of cesium are not legally allowed to advise people of its use as a cancer treatment. However, they *can* advise people as to how to use cesium and other minerals for raising one's pH levels.

For those people who choose to use cesium high pH therapy, seeking the guidance of a qualified practitioner or consultant to find out how to use it safely and effectively is advised. Taking precautions to not become potassium deficient is the only serious concern and because of that, it is *always* advised to get regular blood tests to check your potassium blood serum levels. If you have any type of heart condition, you should be under a doctor's supervision while using cesium.

As long as one is getting adequate guidance, this is an easy and extremely effective approach to self-administer at home. Overall, it is certainly one of the most impressive approaches for "outsmarting" cancer available today.

Resources:

Distributors of Liquid Ionic Cesium and Potassium:

(888) 336-4972. Knowledgeable distributors of liquid ionic minerals and other supplements. Ask for Cindy, or email Cindy at: Lcyordy@ swbell.net

(888) 476-9414. www.floridaherbhouse.com Email: Info@Florida HerbHouse.com

Cost of self-administered cesium high pH therapy: This varies, depending on how many other liquid minerals or supportive supplements are used along with the cesium and potassium. The cost ranges from approximately $200 per month for just cesium and potassium, to up to about $650 per month when a variety of other minerals and supplements are added. For cost of intravenous treatments or guidance by a medical professional, contact that clinic or practitioner.

For Intravenous Cesium Treatment:

Reno Integrative Medical Center   (775) 829-1009
6110 Plumas, Suite B   www.renointegrative.com
Reno, NV 89509

Books

Kathleen Deoul. *Cancer Cover-Up*. Baltimore: Cassandra Books, 2001.

H. E. Sartori, M.D. *Cancer Orwellian or Utopian?* Life Science Universal Inc., 1985.

Booklets Written by Dr. A. Keith Brewer (available from the Brewer Library listed below):

"High pH Cancer Therapy with Cesium"
"Cancer: Its Nature and a Proposed Treatment"

A. Keith Brewer International Science Library (608) 647-6513
325 N. Central Avenue
Richland Center, WI 53581

Websites

www.mwt.net/~drbrewer/brew_art.htm

www.cancer-coverup.com

www.essense-of-life.com

www.advancedhealthplan.com/2cesiumchlorideforcancer2.html

www.thewolfeclinic.com/cesium.html

http://cesium.alternative.cancer.cure.googlepages.com/home

17

Ten More Treatment Options

This chapter highlights ten *more* excellent options for treating cancer that are safe and non-toxic. Though discussed more briefly than previous approaches in this book, that does *not* mean they are less effective. In fact, for some people, one of the methods presented here could be their *best* option for a complete cure—or, when used adjunctively with another compatible approach, may help to bring about recovery. They are:

1. Poly-MVA — Liquid Formulation

2. The CAAT Protocol — Controlled Amino Acid Therapy

3. LifeOne Formula — Liquid Formulation

4. German New Medicine — New Paradigm for Cancer

5. Low Dose Naltrexone — Non-Toxic Pill by Prescription

6. Lapacho/Pau D'Arco/Taheebo — Rainforest Herb in Tea or Capsules

7. N-Tense — Graviola-Based Herbs in Capsules

8. Mexican Cancer Clinics — Multiple Combined Approaches

9. German Cancer Clinics — Multiple Combined Approaches

10. Ellagic Acid — Compound from Red Raspberries

1. POLY-MVA

Though it only became available to the public in the late 1990s, Poly-MVA has quickly become one of the more widely used alternative cancer treatments in the U.S. today. Unlike some of the more obscure alternative methods, Poly-MVA has ample information in print and on the Internet about it, and many medical practitioners are recommending it. Like Protocel®, Poly-MVA is a dark liquid formula that targets anaerobic cells. But that is where the comparison ends. The ingredients in Poly-MVA are completely different from those in Protocel® and the two products target anaerobic cells in different ways. One drawback is that Poly-MVA is more expensive than Protocel®. On the other hand, a positive aspect is that it is not as restrictive a treatment as Protocel® in that most other cancer-fighting and health-supporting supplements are compatible with it. Thus, many people using Poly-MVA can enjoy taking a variety of other health supplements at the same time to support their recovery.

Poly-MVA is classified as a nutritional or dietary supplement and is made up of all natural ingredients. Technically, it is a patented type of palladium lipoic complex, where the mineral palladium is bonded to alpha lipoic acid and specific minerals, vitamins, and amino acids have been added to the formula to enhance its action. (The "MVA" in Poly-MVA stands for minerals, vitamins, and amino acids.) This liquid formula was developed over about a 40-year period by Dr. Merrill Garnett, a research chemist and dentist who headed the Garnett McKeen Laboratories of Islip and Bohemia, New York. Dr. Garnett wrote a book called *First Pulse: A Personal Journey in Cancer Research* which, though highly technical, is only 117 pages and worth reading for anyone interested in the history and science behind this approach.

The story of Poly-MVA began in the late 1950s when, after finishing his work in the military as a naval dentist, Dr. Garnett was drawn to medical research and returned to graduate school to study molecular biology. His specific interest was cancer research. At that time, genetics was the most exciting focus in biology, but Garnett felt that the genetics paradigm for cancer was incomplete. He also believed that the conventional mode of treating cancer through toxic poisoning was not the best solution. He wanted to discover *why* cancer cells did not differentiate (form tissues and organs) and felt they lacked a certain signal that made healthy cells behave normally. In his search for that signal, Garnett focused his research on the differences between the energy pathways of normal cells and cancer cells. To do this, he needed to look more closely at electron transfer. In *First Pulse*, Dr. Garnett wrote,

> I felt that I had a grasp of the literature, but that the ability to manipulate the electron transfer resided in compounds I didn't have at my disposal. These were industrial-type compounds containing metals. I came to believe that metals were the catalyst of electron transfer. I would have to study metals and metallo-organic chemistry.[1]

After more than 20 years of laboratory study and testing on more than 20,000 compounds, Dr. Garnett finally developed a compound using palladium combined with lipoic acid, B_{12} and thiamine that could effectively target anaerobic (cancer) cells and leave normal cells unharmed. In *First Pulse*, Dr. Garnett describes how he tested this first palladium-lipoic compound by injecting 12 mice with a nasty type of cancer called Ehrlic carcinoma. This type of cancer usually kills mice in less than two weeks after injection. Then, Garnett administered the palladium-lipoic compound to 6 of the mice after waiting four to five days to let the cancer develop. The other 6 received no treatment and were the control group.

Dr. Garnett couldn't believe the results. In just 12 days, the mice that had not received treatment were all dead from the cancer but the mice he had treated with the palladium compound were all running around acting normally. In his book, Dr. Garnett related the following experiences with that first trial of the palladium-lipoic complex:

> . . . So 30 days later I've still got the six mice and I'm doing cage cleaning and feeding. The results were undeniable. This was a real drug.
>
> Six months later, I repeated the experiment and had about two dozen mice that were still alive. There was some recurrence in the inguinal region. Most of the tumors disappeared. Some did not, but set up in the lymph nodes and about two months later I found solid tumors in the inguinal region. That was also treatable; I was able to make those break down as well. I had these mice around for a year and a half, and I was tired of cleaning cages. So I had to let them go. I have a rule in the lab. If you cure a mouse you have to let it go. You can't give it the tumor again. I had to find secret haunts for them. I don't believe in double jeopardy. I hope those first mice to be cured of the Ehrlich carcinoma lived a long life.
>
> Then we developed a program. We treated dogs and cats. I started palladium research in 1990. In 1993 I filed for a patent. Two years later, October 31, 1995, it issued. Then, two more patents were granted.[2]

As to how Poly-MVA gets rid of cancer, there appears to be some conflicting information in the literature. According to Dr. Garnett's book, his goal was to find a way to *normalize* cancer cells by restoring normal aerobic functioning. Dr. John Diamond et. al support this description in their highly regarded book, *An Alternative Medicine Definitive Guide to Cancer*, where they write,

> The thinking behind PolyMVA is gene repair. Molecular biologists point to altered DNA (under the negative influence of a carcinogen or contributing cause) as a factor in the development of tumors. Altered genes in turn produce protein substances that are abnormal. 'A major factor in the success of PolyMVA has been to provide an electron energy transfer mechanism from normal metabolic hydrogen carriers to nucleic acids,' Dr. Taylor explains. 'Nucleic acids are the main constituents of DNA. Poly-MVA induces energy-dependent changes in the shape of DNA or RNA as a result of the new reduced state it induces in the nucleotides.' Simply put, PolyMVA is a DNA nutrient.
>
> Although the concepts underlying PolyMVA are couched in complex chemical and genetic terms, the essence of its action is simple: it repairs the abnormally altered gene that is believed to set the cancer mechanism in motion.[3]

According to Robert D. Milne, M.D., author of *Poly-MVA: A New Supplement in the Fight Against Cancer*, what Dr. Garnett developed was "a synthetic enzyme that could facilitate a sort of 'selective electrocution' of tumor cells by shuttling electrons into the mitochondria and DNA."[4] Possibly the best website about Poly-MVA, www.polymvasurvivors.com, supports Dr. Milne's description of how Poly-MVA works by explaining it as follows:

> Cancer cells lack the electrical pathways necessary to redistribute electrical current. The electrical current damages the mitochondria which initiates the release of Cytochrome c. The release of Cytochrome c inside the cell is the first step to apoptosis (programmed cell death). Caspase-3 enzymes are activated which results in the membrane rupture.

Thus, there may be more than one mechanism by which Poly-MVA gets rid of cancer—by sometimes normalizing cancer cells, and by sometimes electrocuting them to death.

Of course, the proof is in the pudding and Poly-MVA has already shown an impressive track record for treating people with many types of cancer, including multiple myeloma, breast, prostate, colon, lung, stomach, ovarian, and brain cancer. It has also been effective against psoriasis, lupus, viral conditions, and stroke. An impressive array of cancer recovery testimonials can be found online, particularly at www.polymvasurvivors.com and in the books by Dr. Robert D. Milne and Michael L. Culbert. Poly-MVA was developed to be taken orally and most people self-administer this approach at home. However, a few doctors administer Poly-MVA intravenously to their patients for the first few weeks, then allow them to continue to take it orally at home. Doctors and other medical practitioners who oversee patients using Poly-MVA can be found online and a very helpful "Practitioners List" is available on the www.polymvasurvivors.com website.

One clinic that is particularly experienced in the use of Poly-MVA is the Cancer Screening and Treatment Center of Nevada, located in Reno. James W. Forsythe, M.D., the director of the clinic, offers Poly-MVA both intravenously and orally as part of his integrative cancer treatment approach. Intravenous administration is generally done for the first few weeks or so, then instructions for oral administration are given to the patient so they can continue taking the Poly-MVA at home.

Dr. Forsythe is the only licensed medical oncologist in the U.S. who is also board certified in Homeopathic medicine, and he integrates both disciplines. His clinic offers 3 treatment options for cancer patients:

1. Conventional chemotherapy alone

2. Poly-MVA alone

3. Poly-MVA with low-dose chemotherapy

The low-dose chemotherapy is administered either in the form of IPT (insulin potentiated therapy) or as fractionated chemo given weekly or for several days in a row. According to Dr. Forsythe, the cancers which appear to respond *best* to Poly-MVA are prostate, breast and lung cancer. (Which is fortunate because these are the three most common types of cancer.) And he has observed a number of complete remissions through the use of Poly-MVA along with other natural supplementation *without* the use of chemotherapy. Dr. Forsythe and his clinic can also be seen on the DVD called "Cancer Conquest," listed at the end of this section. Though the focus of the DVD is not on Poly-MVA, it does show interviews of Dr. Forsythe and patients at his clinic.

Dr. Forsythe is one of the few physicians who has conducted clinical studies on the use of Poly-MVA for cancer. All of the patients in his studies were stage IV cancer patients which conventional medicine in general has a very poor track record with. One was a 5-year clinical outcome based study on 225 patients. In this study, patients were given either Poly-MVA alone or combination therapy. The combination therapy involved Poly-MVA along with other natural supplements and/or low-dose chemotherapy. 35 percent of the patients in the combination group did the best and are still alive and doing well today (past the completion of the 5-year study.) This is an excellent result given that all subjects were stage IV cancer patients and given that conventional chemotherapy can only offer an overall survival rate of 2.1 percent after 5 years.

Dr. Forsythe then conducted another study, this time involving 300 stage IV cancer patients. In this study, *all* patients were given a natural homeopathic substance in conjunction with Poly-MVA and low-dose chemo. Results after 40 months (almost 3½ years) were excellent with a 68 percent overall survival rate for all cases. When broken down into cancer types, this study showed an 87 percent survival rate for prostate cancer, an 80 percent survival rate for breast cancer, and a 56 percent survival rate for lung cancer. Again, these were all considered late-stage cases.

Needless to say, the Cancer Screening and Treatment Center of Nevada is well worth considering for high quality care, especially for those looking for a doctor-supervised alternative or integrative approach.

For those people who can't attend Dr. Forsythe's clinic, or who only wish to self-administer Poly-MVA for other reasons, instructions on dosing are offered on the main websites listed below. In general, though, most adults take between 8 and 16 teaspoonfuls of Poly-MVA per day, divided into 4 equal doses. The dose amount varies according to severity of disease and how much the patient can afford. Some sources indicate that the 4 doses should be taken with each of the three daily meals and then at bedtime. Other sources indicate that the four doses should be taken six hours apart which would mean taking a dose in the middle of the night. People have also used Poly-MVA successfully to cure their pets of cancer.

For detailed instructions on self-administering Poly-MVA in the most effective way, including instructions for children and pets, please refer to the websites and books listed below or contact a practitioner who recommends it. There appears to be no contraindication to using this product at the same time as chemotherapy and/or radiation and evidence points to increased energy and a feeling of well-being for most people who use it.

Websites

www.polymvasurvivors.com

www.polymva.org

www.firstpulseprojects.com

www.facr.org

Dr. James W. Forsythe	(877) 789-0707
Cancer Screening and Treatment	or (775) 827-0707
Center of Nevada	www.drforsythe.com
521 Hammill Lane	
Reno, Nevada 89511	

DVD

"Cancer Conquest," by Burton Goldberg. 2-hour video for $39.95. Buy from Amazon, www.burtongoldberg.com or by calling (800) 597-9250.

Books

Dr. Merrill Garnett. *First Pulse: A Personal Journey in Cancer Research, 2nd Ed.* New York: First Pulse Projects, Inc., 1998.

Robert D. Milne, M.D., & Melissa L. Block, M.Ed. *Poly-MVA: A New Supplement in the Fight Against Cancer.* North Bergen, NJ: Basic Health Publications, Inc., 2004.

Michael L. Culbert, ScD. *Fire in the Genes: Poly-MVA—the Cancer Answer?* Foundation for the Advancement of Medicine, 2000.

Ingredients: Poly-MVA is a proprietary formulation containing palladium, alpha-lipoic acid, vitamins B_1, B_2, and B_{12}, the amino acids formyl-methionine and acetylcysteine, and trace amounts of the metals molybdenum, rhodium, and ruthenium.

2. THE CAAT PROTOCOL

The CAAT Protocol is a powerful nutritional/dietary approach that cancer patients have been using since 1994 with great results. Many have been patients with very advanced cancer who have used this approach along with conventional chemotherapy and/or radiation, others have used it by itself as a non-toxic alternative to conventional treatment.

CAAT stands for "Controlled Amino Acid Therapy" and is a method that was developed by molecular biologist and cancer researcher, Angelo P. John. Angelo P. John was a cancer scientist and theorist for more than 40 years before passing away in 2006. He founded the A.P. John Cancer Institute in Connecticut in 1978. This institute is a non-profit organization and still provides the CAAT Protocol today. The program involves taking a special scientific formulation of amino acids, a strict dietary plan, and certain key phytochemicals. The avoidance of certain foods and supplements that help cancer form and thrive are also an important part of the protocol. With CAAT, the goal is to starve existing cancer cells to death and prevent new cancer cells from forming in the body. Basically, it is seen as an amino acid and carbohydrate deprivation cancer therapy. The protocol is tailored to each individual and is generally followed for 6 to 9 months.

The CAAT protocol is quite unique and detailed and a good general overview is provided by the CanCure organization. According to their website, www.cancure.org,

> The treatment attacks cancer cells in four ways: (1) It helps to prevent new blood vessel formation, which is necessary for the growth of solid cancers; (2) It interferes with the cancer cells ability to produce energy by blocking a process called glycolysis in cancer cells; (3) It reduces the ability of the body to produce growth factors that stimulate cancers to grow; and (4) It interferes with the production of specific amino acids that are necessary for DNA replication in cancer cells.
>
> The diet is quite strict and is low in both carbohydrate and protein. Fat intake is moderate and involves specific fats. The amino acid blend reduces certain amino acids (such as glycine, valine, leucine and isoleucine) and increases others, resulting in the reduced production of the protein elastin, which is necessary for new blood vessel formation (angiogenesis).[5]

Though some of the supplements can be purchased at one's local health food store, guidance and the proprietary blend of amino acids are available only through the Institute. A free consultation can be obtained through the www.apjohncancerinstitute.org website and there is information on the website for doctors to read regarding the protocol. A strict adherence to the program is required for best results.

The CAAT protocol is based on sound science and also has an impressive record. To read about some remarkable cancer recoveries, go to the "Case Histories" section of the A.P. John Cancer Institute website (www.apjohncancerinstitute.org/case.htm). Many of these cases relate how people used the CAAT protocol along with conventional treatment, but some show how people used it successfully alone. Either way, it can provide a powerful path toward recovery.

A.P. John Institute for Cancer Research   Phone (877) 260-1588
16 Northwater Street Greenwich, CT 06830

Websites

www.apjohncancerinstitute.org

www.cancure.org/CAAT/htm

3. LIFEONE FORMULA

"LifeOne" is a liquid formula that is another recent development in non-toxic cancer treatment. It is also particularly effective at treating HIV/AIDS. This product consists of powerful herbs, flavonoids, medicinal mushrooms, phyto-chemicals, lecithin, phosphatidyl choline, resveratrol and organic selenium, among other substances. The company producing it claims to have developed an efficient liposomal delivery system that allows for higher cellular uptake of the formula and increased effectiveness.

LifeOne is a powerful nutritional product that can literally normalize a person's immune system. Its synergistic ingredients also kill viruses, help balance hormones, and improve cell functioning on a number of different levels. Dr. James A. Howenstine is an expert on LifeOne Therapy, and in his book, *A Physician's Guide to Natural Health Products that Work*, he states:

> LifeOne has been able to cure an extremely wide variety of cancer cell types. In vitro testing has shown it to be effective on 7 out of 7 cancer

cell types tested. They included two types of breast cancer, colon cancer, prostate cancer, cervical cancer, ovarian cancer and acute Promyelocytic leukemia. Clinical cancer and AIDS trials in Venezuela have led to negotiations to purchase the product for use in cancer and AIDS patients. Therapeutic failures in treating cancer have occurred when therapy was discontinued prematurely or the patient died from organ failure due to earlier chemotherapy and or radiation therapy complications.[6]

LifeOne is an easy formulation to take. The standard recommended dose is two tablespoons three times a day for the first month, then one tablespoon three times a day for the next 11 months. People who have not undergone chemotherapy or radiation usually have the quickest responses and the most effective use of this formulation may be as a stand-alone treatment. However, patients who choose to use LifeOne while getting chemotherapy usually experience fewer side effects from the chemo. Natural supplementation of Vitamins C and E and a multiple B-complex may also help.

People interested in learning more can go to the main website, www.LifeOne.org, and click on "Clinical Trials" or "User Feedback" to read about how successful LifeOne has been for others. There is also a protocol page that gives usage instructions. According to Dr. Howenstine, "The response is made more effective and quicker by dietary restriction of sugar intake and elimination of high glycemic foods (sugar foods, rice, wheat, white potatoes, corn, bananas, pasta) from the diet."[7]

Though this formulation works best when people have not done chemo or radiation, there is no reason to believe that it could not be combined with many of the other natural therapies that are presented in this book and elsewhere. For those wishing to do everything they can to recover from cancer, adding LifeOne to one's alternative treatment plan (provided the different approaches do not conflict) might provide the added boost needed for full recovery.

Websites

www.LifeOne.org

www.lifeonesales.com   (407) 349-2241

4. GERMAN NEW MEDICINE

German New Medicine, abbreviated as "GNM," is one of the most fascinating approaches to cancer ever developed. This innovative approach focuses on the brain's response to unexpected psychological/emotional shocks and how the brain then sends signals to various parts of the body in an attempt to correct the problem. These signals are meant to help the body survive, but often end up instigating a disease process (such as cancer) instead. German New Medicine goes into great detail in explaining a new way of looking at the mind/body connection and literally proposes a *paradigm shift* in how we view cancer in every way—how cancer starts, how cancer metastasizes, and how to treat cancer. And since German New Medicine also explains the development of many other disease processes, it could well become a primary medical paradigm in the future.

German New Medicine was developed in Germany by Ryke Geerd Hamer, M.D. In August of 1978, Dr. Hamer was head internist at the oncology clinic of the University of Munich when he received the shocking news that his son, Dirk, had been tragically wounded in a shooting accident. For months, doctors performed medical procedures on Dirk to try to save his life. But, unfortunately, Dirk died in December of that year. Just a few months later, Dr. Hamer himself was diagnosed with testicular cancer. This was very unexpected, since Dr. Hamer had not been ill nor had he experienced any indications he was becoming ill. While still dealing with his own grief, Dr. Hamer wondered if his cancer might in some way be related to the loss of his son that had occurred only months before.

Being an oncologist, Hamer decided to investigate the personal histories of his own cancer patients. Not only did he find that all of his patients had experienced some form of emotional trauma (or "conflict shock" as Hamer called it) prior to the development of their disease, but he also discovered that evidence of this conflict shock could be seen *physically* on the scans of his patients' brains! This was something medical experts had never identified before and was no less than groundbreaking. What Hamer found were small rings, and sometimes rings around rings, that showed up in certain areas of the brain. Many times these concentric rings looked like the radiating rings in a pond where a pebble has been dropped. He then learned that the areas of the brain showing a ring or sets of rings would invariably correlate with a particular organ or system of the body in which a disease process had started. No other doctor, oncologist or radiologist had ever been trained to see what Hamer could see on a brain scan. Yet Dr. Hamer became so good at it that in medical conferences he would offer to diagnose a patient based on the person's brain scan alone, having no prior knowledge of the patient's history or diagnosis.

Interestingly, Hamer discovered that the new principle of disease formation that he was developing applied to virtually *all* diseases, not just cancer. Moreover, he could often tell what stage of development or recovery the illness was in. An impressive example of just how well Dr. Hamer could see evidence of disease in the brain was reported in the following account he gave during a 1992 interview:

> After I gave a lecture in Vienna in May 1991, a doctor brought to me a computer tomogram (CT) of a patient's brain. He asked me on behalf of the other 20 colleagues in attendance, among whom were many radiologists and computer tomography specialists, to say what conditions the patient had in his body and the conflicts corresponding to those. So only one level was presented to me, namely the brain level, and from this I was supposed to derive facts about the other two levels. I diagnosed from the CT a freshly bleeding bladder carcinoma in the healing phase; an old prostate carcinoma, a diabetic condition, an old bronchial carcinoma, and a sensory paralysis of a certain area in the body—and for each of these the corresponding conflicts that the patient must have experienced. At this point, the doctor stood up before all his colleagues and said, 'Dr. Hamer, congratulations! Five specific claims— five successes. The patient had exactly what you say. And you can even differentiate what he now has from what he had earlier.'[8]

So, according to Hamer's German New Medicine, a physical mapping, so-to-speak, of a person's various disease conditions is imprinted in the brain and can literally be seen by the trained eye on brain scans. When Dr. Hamer taught other physicians how to read the mapping signs, *they* could see them as well. Since the 1980's many different tests of Hamer's principles have been carried out at conferences or in private practices and more and more medical practitioners began seeing the little rings and other signs of disease that showed up on the brain scans of their patients. Moreover, at least 30 different official investigations into Hamer's principles proved his ideas to be scientifically verifiable.

Seeing the signs of cancer and other illnesses on brain scans, however, is only part of what GNM is all about. After examining thousands of brain CT scans and observing the progress of disease in countless patients, Dr. Hamer developed a whole new theory about how disease develops and how it can be resolved. He proposed that virtually all disease originates from an original emotional trigger or conflict shock, which he named the "DHS" (Dirk-Hamer-Syndrome) after his son. He then called the brain's response to this shock the "Meaningful Special Biological Program" (MSBP). According to the principles of GNM, the brain responds to a conflict shock by either *removing* cells from a specific part of the body, by *adding* cells to a specific part of the body, or by *changing* a specific part of the body in some other way. The MSBP is what ends up instigating the development of disease if the perceived conflict is not adequately resolved over a reasonable period of time. Dr. Hamer even identified specific *areas* of the brain that would typically respond to specific *types* of conflict shocks. In other words, the GNM paradigm explains that the brain tries to correct the problem posed by the conflict shock by somehow altering a part of the body that is *linked* to the resolution of that type of conflict shock in some way.

Hamer observed that the MSBP pathways between the brain and the body involved layers of embryology. It has long been understood that every cell and organ of our body develops from one of three embryological cell layers: the endoderm, mesoderm, or ectoderm of the embryo. According to Hamer, each organ is controlled by a part of the brain that is linked to the specific embryological layer which that organ developed from. Amazingly, Hamer was able to show scientific correlation between a specific type of conflict that would show up as rings in a specific physical area of the brain and would then result in a specific type of disease in a specific organ.

Hamer also discovered that every disease has a two-phase pattern it would go through in the body's attempts to heal itself. He called these (1) the *conflict-active phase* and (2) the *reparative phase* that occurred once the conflict was resolved. The reparative phase is the part of the natural healing process where tumors develop, and Dr. Hamer discovered that if a person could successfully resolve the emotional conflict, the tumors would play their role in healing and then resolve themselves on their own. However, if the conflict in the psyche was *not* resolved, the tumors would continue to grow out of control and, in some cases, become life-threatening cancer.

Many new ways of understanding cancer are explained by Hamer's theories, including the role of microbes in cancer development and resolution. According to Hamer, at least some of the microbes in the body are actually *directed by the brain* as part of the healing reparative phase. He also explains why and where metastases occur in a completely different way from conventional medicine. Though GNM is often done along with either conventional or alternative medicine, Hamer's unusual understanding of metastases has allowed many cancer patients to resolve their disease-associated conflicts to the point where their metastasized cancer regresses and finally disappears without any conventional treatment at all.

The important thing is that Dr. Hamer not only discovered the physiological connection of disease to the brain, but he also developed ways for patients to *use* this knowledge to resolve their own conflict shocks and bring about recovery for themselves. This is an area where different GNM practitioners may use different techniques, but the important thing is to identify the conflict shock or shocks behind the disease and resolve them. Through helping his own patients to do this, Hamer claimed to have a cure rate of 95 to 98 percent for cancer patients who had never been given conventional treatments. (In other words, they hadn't been *damaged* by conventional toxic treatments yet.) Unfortunately, in 1986, Dr. Hamer's medical license was taken away because he would not conform to accepted medical practices. As is common, medical dogma was given precedence over medical results. Yet Hamer continued his scientific research.

Were Hamer's amazing results *real*? A revealing event occurred that helps answer this question. In 1997, Hamer was finally arrested for giving 3 patients medical advice though he no longer had a license to practice. The police confiscated his patient files and a court trial ensued. After official analysis of the patient files, it was revealed that Hamer's results *were* extremely impressive. Though not all his cancer patients had been free from conventional treatment, which brought the cure rate down, after five years of treating cancer patients with German New Medicine, 6,000 out of 6,500 were still alive! By comparison, a meta-analysis of 155,000 cancer patients in the U.S. who were treated with chemotherapy for all types of cancer showed that after 5 years only 2.1 percent were still alive.

Nevertheless, Dr. Hamer was sentenced to jail. But other doctors are learning his theory of disease formation and treatment. One of those doctors is David Holt, D.O., HMD, of the Reno Integrative Medical Center in Nevada. Dr. Holt has been interviewed about his success with German New Medicine. Some of his interviews can be found on YouTube.com.

More details of German New Medicine are explained in the articles, books, and websites listed below. The concepts of GNM may seem quite "out there" at first, but it just may be that this will become a foundation of cancer treatment in the future.

Websites

www.newmedicine.ca

http://germannewmedicine.ca

Articles

http://germannewmedicine.ca/documents/Explore%20GNM%20Website%20Update.pdf

Books

Hamer, Ryke Geerd, M.D. *Summary of the New Medicine.* Amici di Dirk, 2000.

Taddei, Andrea. *The 5 Biological Laws and Dr. Hamer's New Medicine.* CreateSpace Independent Publishing, 2012.

5. LOW DOSE NALTREXONE

Another new way of dealing with cancer that has produced some astounding results is a non-toxic drug called low dose naltrexone. Since low dose naltrexone, or LDN, simply involves taking one small pill at bedtime, it may be the easiest cancer treatment ever developed. It is also incredibly inexpensive, costing only about $30 to $45 per month.

To understand the history of this approach, one has to go back a few decades to when Naltrexone became an FDA-approved prescription drug in 1984. The official approval was in 50 mg doses for the treatment of heroin or opium addiction. Because naltrexone is an opioid blocker, it is quite helpful in treating these types of addiction. When used in high doses (100 and 300 mg per day), it is able to block the opioid receptors in the body to the point where it effectively blocks the "high" or euphoria that an addict feels if they take heroin or opium. It has also been used to some extent for the treatment of alcohol addiction.

Ian S. Zagon, Ph.D., is a professor of neural and behavioral sciences at Pennsylvania State University who has spent over two decades conducting laboratory research on endorphins and on the use of LDN for certain diseases. However, Bernard Bihari, M.D. of New York City (now retired) was the main medical practitioner to pioneer the use of low dose naltrexone in humans. Dr. Bihari knew that scientific study showed endorphins to be highly involved in the regulation of immune function. He also knew that the administration of a very *low dose* of naltrexone once a day could actually *increase* the body's production of endorphins.

The theory behind this is that a very low dose of naltrexone, usually only 3 to 5 mg at bedtime, will block a person's endorphin receptors for just a few hours overnight. This is not enough to cause a person problems, but it is enough to cause endorphins in the body to fail to attach to their receptors for a short period of time. This signals the body to compensate by creating *more* endorphins, particularly in the pre-dawn sleeping hours when endorphin production tends to be highest. (Ninety percent of the day's endorphins are produced by the pituitary and adrenal glands between 2 a.m. and 4 a.m.[10]) Research has shown that this brief blockade of opioid receptors specifically stimulates the body to produce a significant increase in the beta-endorphins, including enkephalin and metenkephalin.

At first, Dr. Bihari hoped that by using LDN he might be able to stimulate the immune system of people with HIV, so he began trying it on his own HIV/AIDS patients in 1985. The results were extremely positive. In fact, over a period of 4 years, 85 percent of his patients on low dose naltrexone showed no detectable levels of the HIV virus when LDN was used in conjunction with accepted AIDS therapies. And a large number of his HIV/AIDS patients lived symptom-free with absolutely no disease progression for many years by taking LDN alone (without any other AIDS medications.)[11]

Research had shown that heroin slows the growth of some tumors and that metenkaphalin prolongs the life of mice with leukemia, melanoma, and other cancers. So Dr. Bihari decided to try low dose naltrexone on his cancer patients as well. He started with a woman who had recurrent non-Hodgkin's lymphoma and had refused further chemo treatments. Within 3 months, the woman's large groin tumors regressed and she remained in remission until 4 years later when she died of an unrelated cause.[12] Presumably, this amazing recovery was from using LDN alone. Bihari then went on to use LDN for a variety of cancers in his clinical practice. (Since naltrexone is an FDA-approved prescription drug, it is perfectly legal and ethical for any physician to prescribe it for off-label purposes. But because it is not officially approved as a treatment for cancer by the FDA or any facet of the medical establishment, it is currently considered an alternative cancer treatment.)

Dr. Bihari's results with other cancer patients were impressive as well and are posted on a number of different websites, including some listed at the end of this section. The cancers thought to be *most* responsive to LDN are those that originate in tissues with high densities of opioid receptors, particularly lymphomas and pancreatic cancer. Overall, positive responses have been observed for non-Hodgkin's lymphoma, Hodgkin's Disease, chronic lymphocytic leukemia, myeloid leukemia, multiple myeloma, pancreatic cancer, glioma, astrocytoma and glioblastoma brain cancers, head and neck squamous cell carcinoma, cancer of the small intestine, lung cancer, neuroblastoma, breast cancer and prostate cancer.

David Gluck, M.D. is the editor of the most informative website on low dose naltrexone. This website can be accessed at www.ldninfo.org. It is a comprehensive site that presents the history, theory, and science behind LDN, plus impressive cancer recovery cases, other types of illnesses LDN can be used for, and news about LDN conferences. On his website, Dr. Gluck also presents a pie chart that describes the success that Dr. Bihari had using LDN for cancer. By March of 2004, Dr. Bihari had prescribed LDN to about 450 cancer patients, many of whom had exhausted conventional treatments and the pie chart shows the following:

out of 450 patients, 19 percent died (usually within the first two or three months because they were just too ill to recover or too damaged by previous toxic treatments) and Bihari was not able to follow up on another 21 percent. 11 percent were people who'd only been on LDN for less than 6 months, so they were cases that were still undetermined. However, of the rest of the patients whom Bihari was able to follow and keep on LDN for 6 months or more, 19 percent went into full remission, 28 percent had stabilized (no growth or spread of tumors), and 2 percent had not stabilized. Given that this was through the use of just one pill at bedtime, these results are astounding!

According to Dr. Gluck, out of the 450 cancer patients discussed above, the remissions included: 2 children with neuroblastoma, 6 patients with non-Hodgkin's lymphoma, 3 with Hodgkin's Disease, 5 with pancreatic cancer that had metastasized to the liver, 5 with multiple myeloma (bone marrow cancer), 1 with carcinoid, 4 with breast cancer metastasized to the bone, 4 with ovarian cancer, 18 with non-small cell cancer of the lung, 1 with small cell cancer of the lung, and 5 with prostate cancer (in men with no previous hormone-blocking drug usage.)[13] Virtually all of the these patients would be considered incurable by conventional methods. Dr. Bihari also had some success using LDN for cancer in the brain. In fact, he reportedly treated a patient suffering from melanoma that had metastasized to the brain. As of the last report, the patient had been in remission for 12 years!

Dr. David Gluck presents one of the clearest explanations of how low dose naltrexone works for cancer on his website www.ldninfo.org. He states that it may exert its effects on tumor growth through a mix of three possible mechanisms:

1. By inducing increases of metenkaphalin (an endorphin produced in large amounts in the adrenal medulla) and beta endorphin in the blood stream;

2. By inducing an increase in the number and density of opiate receptors on the tumor cell membranes, thereby making them more responsive to the growth-inhibiting effects of the already-present levels of endorphins, which induce apoptosis (cell death) in the cancer cells;

3. By increasing the natural killer (NK) cell numbers and NK cell activity and lymphocyte activated CD8 numbers, which are quite responsive to increased levels of endorphins.[14]

The fact that low dose naltrexone is able to stimulate the immune system accounts for why it is so effective as a treatment for so many different types of disease. For instance, besides HIV/AIDS and many types of cancer, Dr. Bihari found that LDN showed beneficial effects for multiple sclerosis, Crohn's disease, ALS, Parkinson's, psoriasis, Rheumatoid arthritis, fibromyalgia, and other immune disorders. And some of the improvements in MS and Crohn's cases are nothing short of miraculous! The fact that LDN is often able to bring about remarkable improvements in people suffering from auto-immune disorders also contradicts the common conventional belief that auto-immune disorders are caused by an overactive immune system. Clinical results with LDN indicate the cause of these disorders to be immune deficiency, not immune system overactivity.

In high doses of around 300 mg per day, naltrexone has been shown to carry some risk of damage to the liver and may cause other negative side effects as well. However, treatment using 100 mg per day has shown no significant side effects or damage to the liver. And at the very low doses of just 3 to 5 mg per day, Naltrexone is completely safe and non-toxic. Any physician can legally prescribe low dose naltrexone, however many have no experience using it for cancer or auto-immune disorders. If you are interested in having your physician prescribe LDN to you, referring him or her to the websites and books below, as well as the annual conferences on low dose naltrexone, could be helpful.

Dr. Bihari observed that the patients who were most likely to have significant movement towards remission were those who had never done chemotherapy. Though some patients who have undergone chemo may still respond positively, it is difficult to know who those will be. Since most of the endorphins of the body are produced by the pituitary and adrenal glands, it is possible that those who will respond to this approach are those people who have *not* suffered damage to their pituitary or adrenals through the use of chemo or other toxic treatments such as radiation. Bihari also found that, although LDN worked very well for men with previously untreated prostate cancer, it did not work at all for those men who had received testosterone-blocking drugs such as Lupron, Casodex or others (even if they stopped the hormone-blocking drug before starting the LDN.) It is also possible that LDN therapy may not work as well for patients who are on steroids in doses that suppress immune system functioning.

Some patients do not respond to just 3 mg at bedtime, but do respond when that dose is increased to 4.5 mg at bedtime. Also, LDN should *not* be used at the same time as any narcotic medication that is an opioid agonist (such as morphine, Percocet, Ultram, the Duragesic patch, or codeine-containing medications.) Thus, it is important to work with a practitioner who is familiar with the most effective way to use low dose naltrexone whenever possible. Because LDN is such an easy and inexpensive non-toxic treatment, it may be a perfect adjunctive treatment for many cancer patients. It is also unlikely to interfere with most other non-toxic approaches. It may not work for every type of cancer or every cancer patient, but for those who do respond, it has been called a "Wonder Drug."

Websites

www.ldninfo.org

www.ldninfo.org/ldn_and_cancer.htm

www.ldners.org

www.ldnresearchtrust.org

www.elaine-moore.com

www.youtube.com/watch?v=DAZ1fQKdOC8 (To View U-Tube Video)

Books

Moore, Elaine, A. and Samantha Wilkinson. *The Promise of Low Dose Naltrexone Therapy: Potential Benefits in Cancer, Auto-Immune, Neurological and Infectious Disorders.* McFarland & Co., 2008.

Bradley, Mary Anne Boyle. *Up the Creek With a Paddle: Beat MS and Many Auto-Immune Disorders With Low Dose Naltrexone (LDN).* PublishAmerica, 2005.

6. LAPACHO / PAU D'ARCO / TAHEEBO

It is common to hear about scientists searching the Amazon jungle for exotic botanicals that can cure cancer. What is *less* common is to hear about are cancer-curing botanicals that have *already* come out of the rain forests and are already well-known. (Maybe because these were discovered by the indigenous people of the area long ago and not by modern scientists.) One of the best examples of these is a tea made from the inner bark of a tree that grows in the rain forests and mountains of Brazil, Argentina, and Paraguay. The tree is well-known as the Lapacho tree and belongs to the genus Tabebuia, but it also has many other common names. One commonly known tribal name for the tree is Taheebo and the Portuguese in South America called the tree Pau D'Arco. Thus, Lapacho, Taheebo and Pau D'Arco (as well as Ipe Roxo) all refer to the same tree and the same medicinal tea preparation. The Guarani, Tupi and other tribes call it Tajy, meaning "to have strength and vigor," or simply, *the Divine Tree.*

The Lapacho is a huge evergreen canopy tree that can grow 30 meters high with a base of 2 to 3 meters in diameter. Nearly 100 species of trees in the Tabebuia genus are known, however only a few species are sought after for their medicinal value. The Tabebuia impetiginosa is probably the most prized for its healing powers and is referred to as purple Lapacho because of its purple flowers. Red Lapacho is the next most commonly used. The native people of South America have used Lapacho for many hundreds of years to treat a wide variety of ailments. (Some evidence points to it being used even before the Incas.) The broad variety of healing uses may be accounted for by the fact that Lapacho Tea has been shown to have astringent, analgesic, sedative, decongestant, antioxidant, anti-inflammatory, antibacterial, anti-fungal, anti-viral, anti-microbial, anti-cancer, diuretic and hypotensive properties. It is also a powerful treatment for stimulating the production of red blood cells, and now is an accepted treatment for leukemia in many South American hospitals. Scientific studies on Lapacho's healing properties have been carried out in South America, Europe, the U.S. and Asia, and one of the key active ingredients in this tea has been named "lapachol." Lapachol is a type of plant substance known as napthaquinones or N-factors.

In a South American study, pure lapachol was given in 250 mg capsules with meals to 9 patients who had varying types of cancer. (These included liver, kidney, breast, prostate, squamous cell, and uterine cancer.)

The result was that 3 of the 9 patients went into complete remission; all of the patients experienced tumor reduction; they all reported reduced cancer-related pain; and none of the patients experienced any negative side effects.[15]

But one of the problems with western medicine is that it is always trying to break herbal treatments down into their single most healing constituents, so that these can then be reproduced (preferably with some patentable alteration) and treated as drugs. Physicians in South America and other places around the world who have studied or prescribed Lapacho Tea in its whole form have achieved much better overall results with cancer than the studies that have singled out lapachol. As with other herbal medicines, the indigenous preparations preserve many different biologically active ingredients that work together synergistically for optimum effect. For instance, in addition to N-factors, anthraquinones (called A-factors) are also a type of healing plant compound and the Lapacho tree is one of the few plants in the world where both N-factors and A-factors occur together. This may account at least in part for its powerful ability to heal. Also present in Lapacho are quercitin, xloidone and other flavonoids.

Lapacho tea was first studied in the west in the late 1800s. But it didn't gain notoriety until around 1960 when a physician, Dr. Orlando de Santi of the Brazilian municipal hospital of Santo Andre, heard about a young girl who was quickly cured of leukemia through the use of Lapacho tea. He decided to try it on his own brother who was dying of cancer and his brother had a complete recovery as well. Dr. de Santi then began to use it on his patients with cancer and had some astounding successes. Seeing the great results, other doctors at the same hospital began using it on their cancer patients and soon Lapacho for cancer became a phenomenon in Brazil. Reports of miraculous cures were coming out and some patients were going into remission in as little as four weeks![16] Media reports were producing such a public frenzy that the Brazilian government ordered a blackout of any more public statements by doctors using Lapacho until further studies could be done. Since then, Lapacho has been a standard form of treatment in Brazil for some types of cancer and all kinds of infections.

More study needs to be done on the whole Lapacho tea (as opposed to just one or more of its components) to understand all the ways that this herbal preparation kills cancer. However, preliminary research points to the premise that Lapacho works like other benzoquinones, in that it uncouples mitochondrial oxidative phosphorylation that occurs during anaerobic respiration.[17] (Since normal healthy cells use aerobic functioning, they are left unharmed.) Other scientific indications are that Lapacho inhibits the proper functioning of ATPase, an enzyme that is critical for the final step in ATP production,[18] and that beta-lapachone, a similar compound to lapachol in Lapacho tea, works by disrupting DNA replication in cancer cells.[19] Another isolated compound found in Lapacho is called "Quechua" which has powerful antibiotic and virus-killing properties.

The most common type of cancer Lapacho is used for in South America is leukemia. But many forms of cancer have responded as well, including lymphoma, brain cancer, prostate cancer, and others. Unfortunately, most of the scientific and clinical reports by physicians are in Portuguese or Spanish and sample cancer cases in English are hard to find, especially with the current crackdown by the FDA on websites posting cancer recovery testimonials. But some cases are reported in the books and websites listed at the end of this section.

Most people using Lapacho have taken it in the traditional tea form, though some distributors also offer it in capsule or tincture form. It is very important to be sure to get this product from a legitimate source. Some companies selling to the United States have produced products that are not properly harvested or prepared, so it is important to make sure to get Lapacho, Pau D'Arco, or Taheebo from a reputable company that harvests the Lapacho and prepares it in the traditional way.

One company that claims to produce a high-quality medicinally active form of Lapacho in capsule form is Vibrant Life Vitamins. Their product, called "Taheebo Life Tea" has produced some impressive testimonials. Each concentrated capsule supposedly contains the equivalent of 6 or 7 cups of the tea and 2 to 5 capsules per day are recommended for prevention of minor ailments. For serious diseases, however, a much higher dose should be taken. For cancer, the recommended dosing for this capsule form of Taheebo is to take 5 capsules upon awakening in the morning and then take 2 capsules every hour throughout the day and evening and another 5 capsules at bedtime. This is a lot of pills and is somewhat expensive at first, but the claim is that with this high a dose a person with cancer will either see impressive results within the first 3 weeks or no results at all. If tumors reduce in size in the first few weeks, it is best to keep taking the high doses of capsules until the tumors are completely gone, then gradually reduce to a lower maintenance dose. If no results are seen within a few weeks, one can stop the Taheebo and try something else.

Though not much information is available regarding dosing for animals,

Taheebo has been given to pets with cancer and shown some remarkable results. And some sources recommend that Lapacho, Pau D'Arco or Taheebo be taken along with Graviola and Cat's Claw for cancer. For people who want to consider this, the product "N-Tense" might be a good adjunct along with Lapacho, Pau D'Arco or Taheebo.

Websites

www.organicgermanium.net

www.paudarco.com

www.pau-d-arco.com

www.pau-d-arco.com/Dr. Mowry.html

Books

Luebeck, Walter. *Healing Power of Pau D'Arco.* Lotus Press; 1998.

Jones, Kenneth. *Pau D'Arco: Immune Power From the Rain Forest.* Healing Arts Press; 1995.

Elkins, Rita. *Pau D'Arco: Taheebo, Lapacho (The Woodland Health Series).* Woodland Publishing; 1997.

7. N-TENSE

N-Tense is an herbal formulation made up of 7 powerful botanicals from the South American rainforests. Its main ingredient, which comprises 50 percent of the formula, is Graviola. The other 7 botanicals are Guacatonga, Bitter Melon, Espinheira Santa, Mullaca, Vassourinha, Mutamba, and Cat's Claw. This formulation is produced solely by Raintree Nutrition, Inc., a well-respected company with high quality products and reasonable prices.

Though Raintree Nutrition makes no claims as to the effects of N-Tense upon cancer, anecdotal cases have shown it to work on virtually every type of cancer. (However, because some of the ingredients are slightly estrogenic, it is *not* indicated for estrogen-positive breast cancer.) The most independently researched ingredient is Graviola, which has been shown to kill cancer cells in at least 20 different laboratory studies. Unfortunately, these tests were all *in vitro* and no large clinical (human) studies have been done. Rumor has it that a leading multi-billion-dollar drug company spent seven years studying Graviola in the effort to isolate one or more compounds that could be synthetically altered and patented for use against cancer. The drug company finally gave up, likely due to the fact that the compounds in Graviola were only effective in their natural state and in combination with other compounds in the plant. And since natural compounds cannot be patented, the drug company abandoned their work on Graviola after 7 years of research and declined to share the information they learned about it with the world.

The cancer-killing ingredients within Graviola that have been primarily focused on are various forms of compounds referred to as "acetogenins." One of the methods of action of acetogenins is that they are inhibitors of ATP production in anaerobic cells. Thus, it may be a good idea for anyone using N-Tense to avoid taking ATP *promoting* substances along with it such as vitamin C, CoQ_{10}, vitamin E, L-Carnitine, Alpha-Lipoic Acid, and IP6, to name just a few—though this is just theoretical. N-Tense can also be used on dogs with cancer. For more information about using it for dogs, please visit www.annieappleseedproject.org/grandcaindo.html.

Raintree Nutrition, Inc.   (800) 780-5902 or (775) 841-4142
3579 Hwy. 50 East, Suite 222
Carson City, NV 89701

Websites

www.rain-tree.com

www.hsibaltimore.com/articles/hsi_2001ds/hsi_200101_awb9.html

www.annieappleseedproject.org/grandcaindo.html

8. MEXICAN CANCER CLINICS

Most people in the U.S. have heard about Americans going south of the border to be treated for cancer. But because of an old stigma associated with Tijuana and foreign hospitals in general, many Americans sadly do not even consider seeking treatment in Mexico. For most of the Mexican cancer clinics, this stigma is completely unwarranted. High-quality evidence-based medicine with a wide variety of treatments has been carried out in these clinics for decades by skilled and highly respected doctors. And the results in general have been far better than what conventional medicine in the states is able to achieve for cancer patients. Americans who do go to Mexico for treatment are often surprised at how professional yet friendly the clinics are and are very glad they went there once they see the treatments working for them. Indeed, some of the *best* cancer treatment doctors in the world and many of *the most cutting edge treatments* can be found in Mexican cancer clinics.

In essence, it has largely been the suppression of good non-toxic approaches in the U.S. that created the Mexican cancer clinic phenomenon in the first place. Due to U.S. legal restrictions, many American physicians have moved their practices out of the U.S. and joined up with doctors south of the border so that they could practice good medicine. Due to the high number of Americans who need cancer treatment and have the money to pay for it, many cancer clinics in Mexico have been set up to be a short, easy drive across the border for cancer patients living in the U.S. Most of the clinics are located in the Tijuana area for its proximity to San Diego, but some are in other locations. For instance, one excellent clinic, St. Joseph Medical Center, is located over the border from Del Rio, Texas (southwest of San Antonio.)

A vast array of treatments are available in Mexican cancer clinics, including: intravenously administered Laetrile, DMSO and vitamin C; hyperbaric oxygen; hyperthermia; cancer vaccines; ozone; UV light; IPT (insulin potentiation therapy); Iscador and other herbal treatments; detoxification; nutritional supplements and diet changes. The clinics are friendly and many have non-chlorinated swimming pools for recreation that are treated with either ozone or hydrogen peroxide. Surgery and/or small amounts of radiation or chemo are administered in some clinics, but only when absolutely necessary and always in smaller amounts than would be given in the states. All the good Mexican cancer clinics offer compassionate personalized care on a case-by-case basis.

Fortunately, several organizations offer bus tours out of San Diego for Americans who wish to visit and evaluate a variety of clinics before they decide on where they want to go for treatment. These tours can be particularly helpful and anyone can call one or more clinics they are interested in to see which tours go to that particular clinic. An eBook called *The Amish Cancer Secret* by Frank Cousineau and Andrew Scholberg is also very helpful and costs just $19.95. This eBook discusses a variety of

Mexican clinics in detail and presents contact information for up to 20 reputable cancer clinics in the Baja area along with valuable travel tips. The author offers tours as well and a consultation service for help regarding cancer treatment in Mexico.

Two of the smaller clinics not mentioned in Cousineau's book are worth mentioning here because they restrict their patient load to small numbers and offer *particularly* close attention to each patient. They also use *only* natural non-toxic methods for treating cancer (no chemo or radiation, even in low doses).

The first is an in-patient facility in Tijuana called the Hope4Cancer Institute. Also referred to as the Rapha Clinic, this highly professional yet small treatment center is conveniently located just 10 minutes south of the San Ysidro border crossing and only 30 minutes from the San Diego International Airport. The clinic provides a shuttle bus from San Diego to the Hope4Cancer Institute. It is also right on the beach and patients can enjoy walking on the sand and watching the ocean just outside the clinic. The medical director and founder of the clinic is Antonio Jimenez, M.D., who is affectionately referred to as "Dr. Tony" at the clinic.

Dr. Tony Jimenez has about 20 different treatments and therapies to offer his patients depending on their situation, including hyperthermia, ozone, detoxing methods, electromagnetic therapy, intravenous Poly-MVA, infra-red sauna, stem-cell therapy, and nutritional supplementation. Three special treatments offered that are unique to this clinic are: (1) a powerful cancer injection called "Rapha-El" that is an advanced non-toxic botanical formula. All types of cancer appear to respond to it, but the *fastest* responders may be lung, breast, colon, and liver cancer; (2) Sono-Photo Dynamic Therapy (SPDT). For more details, go to www.sonophoto dynamictherapy.com; and (3) A proprietary cancer-killing formula derived from yeast and developed in Russia called "PriMed," which is also very effective at boosting the immune system and accelerating healing.

Cancer patients can stay at the Rapha Clinic as in-patients for varying lengths of time, but it is also sometimes possible to visit the clinic for just a few days to learn how to take some of the treatments (including the Rapha-El injection) home to self-administer them. This can be very helpful to those people who cannot afford to be away from home for a long time. Very impressive recovery testimonials can be viewed at www.hope 4cancer.com.

The second clinic is an out-patient facility called St. Joseph Medical Center just south of the border from the small town of Del Rio, Texas.

People can either take a short flight from Houston to Del Rio, or they can drive 2½ hours from San Antonio to Del Rio. Patients stay in hotels in Del Rio on the U.S. side and St. Joseph Medical Center provides a bus that takes only 5 minutes to shuttle them across the border from Del Rio to the clinic in Mexico.

Since Mexican cancer clinics often involve in-patient care for at least a few weeks and may involve daily intravenous or infusion-type treatments that are expensive, the overall cost can sometimes be quite high. It is not uncommon for an American to end up paying between $25,000 and $40,000. One of the advantages of seeking treatment at St. Joseph Medical Center is that it is one of the few Mexican clinics to offer a flat-rate for treatment. Cost of treatment for everyone at St. Joseph's is $10,800 and people usually get daily treatments for at least 10 weeks. If you continue receiving treatment for as long as it takes to go into remission, which could be months, the cost is still no more than $10,800 no matter how long it takes. However, if you start treatment there and stop for a while, then come back, it is not considered continuous treatment and more charges will then be involved. For more information about St. Joseph Medical Center or to request a free brochure, call (877) 943-4673. Recovery testimonials on audio and video are available at www.doctorofhope.com.

Two other clinics in the Baja area that are highly respected and worth looking into are Ernesto Contreras's clinic called Oasis of Hope and the Issels treatment center that carries on the legacy of the famous Dr. Issels of Germany. These clinics may suggest low-dose chemo or radiation for a few cases, but they also offer a wide array of alternative, non-toxic approaches. Though not everyone who goes to a Mexican clinic for treatment will get well, many Americans may be pleasantly surprised after visiting the various clinics' websites and reading their impressive treatment descriptions and cancer recovery testimonials.

It is worth noting that many American health insurance companies often *will* pay for certain aspects of treatment outside the country. But it is important to know just how to bill them for international services. One company, Global Billing Service in Houston, is set up for this purpose alone. All they do is file foreign insurance medical claims to American health insurance companies and they work on a commission basis. Thus, they only take a small percentage of what they are able to get your insurance company to pay. Their website is www.GlobalBillingService.com and you can contact them by calling (832) 615-3531 if you would like to find out more about how they can help you. This service works for cancer treatments obtained in Mexico as well as other countries such as Germany, Switzerland, and the Bahamas. They will *not* bill for alternative treatments that are not FDA-approved. However, they *can* bill for localized hyperthermia, for certain types of intravenous treatments, for hospital inpatient fees and often for many other medical charges that one wouldn't always think about. This can often alleviate the cost of getting treatment outside the U.S. and is well worth looking into.

Hope4Cancer Institute   (619) 468-9209
482 W. San Ysidro Blvd., #1589
San Ysidro, CA 92173   www.hope4cancer.com
(Call for Information about Tours)

Saint Joseph Medical Center   (877) 943-4673
South of Del Rio, Texas   www.doctorofhope.com
Patient Coordinator: Marla Manhart   (941) 929-7317

Oasis of Hope Clinic   (888) 500-4673
Tijuana, Mexico   www.oasisofhope.com
(Dr. Ernesto Contreras's Clinic)

Issels Treatment Center   (888) 447-7357
Tijuana, Mexico   www.issels.com

Global Billing Service   (832) 615-3531
Houston, TX

Websites

www.hope4cancer.com

www.doctorofhope.com

www.cancerdefeated.com

www.consumerhealth.org/links/clinics.html

www.cancure.org/directory_mexican_clinics.htm

www.healthtours.com

www.sonophotodynamictherapy.com

eBook

Cousineau, Frank with Andrew Scholberg. *The Amish Cancer Secret.* Online Publishing & Marketing, LLC. Virginia: 2012. A 53-page eBook about clinics in Baja which can be ordered from www.cancerdefeated.com for $19.95. ($7.95 S/H added for printed copy sent through mail.)

9. GERMAN CANCER CLINICS

For those people who prefer a European environment, Germany is a common destination for alternative cancer treatment. Full of highly acclaimed clinics, or "Kliniks," as they are referred to in Germany, many Americans have enjoyed being treated there—often in quaint small towns rimmed by the Alps. German doctors are masters of hyperthermia for treating cancer, and most of the clinics offer that. Other treatments include intravenous vitamin C and other nutritional support, IPT (Insulin Potentiated Therapy), Mistletoe, oxygenation therapies, homeopathy, magnetic field therapy, dendritic cell cancer vaccines, and fever therapy (in which a fever reaction is induced by injection).

One advantage to the cancer clinics in Germany is that many of them are located in spa towns, which are towns that have natural mineralized waters. Patients can soak in these waters and also drink them to enhance their recovery. Another advantage to the cancer clinics in Germany is that the costs are quite reasonable compared to other clinics around the world that offer in-patient care. For detailed written information on these clinics, I recommend a well-written eBook called *German Cancer Breakthrough* by Andrew Scholberg. This 50-page eBook costs just $19.95 and is available at www.germancancerbreakthrough.com. It not only describes a variety of German clinics and the types of treatments they offer, but it also gives valuable information about travelling and how to go about contacting the clinics.

There is also a very informative DVD about new German cancer therapies and diagnostic techniques called "Cancer Conquest." It was produced by Burton Goldberg, founder and former editor of *Alternative Medicine Magazine.* This DVD does not focus on showing the different alternative cancer treatment clinics and what each of them has to offer, the way Scholberg's eBook does, but it presents some very interesting information about cutting edge cancer therapies and diagnostic techniques being pioneered in Germany. The focus is on "integrative" medicine, which means using the best from alternative as well as conventional methods. This

DVD also highlights a cutting-edge blood test that looks at the DNA of cancer cells and their resistance factors to be able to tell which chemo will work best for any particular cancer patient. The premise is that each person's cancer is unique to some extent and that metastatic cancer cells and primary tumor cells within the same person may even respond differently to a particular treatment. (In other words, one chemo drug may work for a primary tumor, but not for the metastatic cancer within a particular patient.) The German doctors also have no legal restriction on which drug they can use as doctors in the U.S. have. Thus, one man had advanced prostate cancer but his DNA blood test showed that the best chemo for him was one commonly used for ovarian cancer. The doctors used this drug on him with great success—something doctors in the U.S. would not be allowed to do.

(**NOTE:** The use of hyperthermia alone for cancer is not legal in the United States unless a small amount of low-dose radiation is given at the same time. One very reputable clinic that has specialized in doing this is "The Valley Cancer Institute" in Los Angeles. Hyperthermia treatment is administered there by M.D.s and covered by most insurance companies. For more information, go to www.vci.org or call (310) 398-0013 for a consultation.)

eBook

Scholberg, Andrew. *German Cancer Breakthrough: Your Guide to Top German Alternative Clinics.* Online Publishing & Marketing, LLC. Virginia: 2008. A 50-page eBook about cancer clinics in Germany which can be ordered from www.germancancerbreakthrough.com for $19.95. ($7.95 S/H added for printed copy sent through mail.)

Websites

www.germancancerbreakthrough.com

www.cancertutor.com/Cancer03/GermanClinics.html

DVD

"Cancer Conquest," by Burton Goldberg. 2-hour video for $39.95. Buy from Amazon, www.burtongoldberg.com or by calling (800) 597-9250.

10. ELLAGIC ACID

A natural anti-cancer compound that has been used by itself to cure cancer and can also be an excellent adjunct to just about any cancer therapy is ellagic acid. Good natural sources of ellagic acid are strawberries, blackberries, walnuts, pecans, pomegranates, blueberries and cranberries, but the highest density occurs in red raspberries. In fact, red raspberries have been found to have up to 6 times more ellagic acid than any other food source.

Actually, to be accurate, ellagic acid comes from ellagitannins, which are phenolic compounds found in at least 46 different fruits and nuts. Thus, the way this substance occurs first in nature is in the form of ellagitannins. When we eat the fruits, seeds or nuts that contain ellagitannins, our bodies then *convert* the ellagitannins into ellagic acid. (Much the same way our bodies convert beta-carotene into vitamin A.) The terms "ellagic acid" and "elagitannins" are often interchanged when supplement companies refer to their products or to research studies, but most sources use the term ellagic acid.

Many scientific studies on the benefits of ellagic acid were carried out and published in the 1970s and 1980s. But the best research on its anti-cancer action was done in the 1990s by Dr. Daniel Nixon at the Medical University of South Carolina's Hollings Cancer Institute. Dr. Nixon's research showed that about 40 mg of ellagitannin per day (equivalent to ingesting about one cup of red raspberries) can prevent the development of cancer cells. For people who already had cancer, less than 40 mg per day proved to only slow the growth of cancer in the cervix, colon, breast, pancreas, prostate, and esophagus. Higher amounts than that were able to induce normal cell death in cancer cells. A number of other studies have supported Dr. Nixon's research and also shown ellagic acid to be effective against colon, cervical, breast, prostate, lung, esophageal and pancreatic cancer, as well as melanoma and leukemia.

So, how does ellagic acid work? It is commonly known that one of the characteristics common to all cancer cells is uncontrolled growth. Ellagic acid has been scientifically proven to be able to stop or slow the uncontrolled growth of malignant cancer cells in two ways:

1. By supporting the P53 gene so that it can induce "apoptosis" (normal cell death), and

2. By inducing "G-arrest," which means that it stops the process that

causes cancer cells to mutate and start dividing out of control in the first place.

In fact, Dr. Nixon at the Hollings Institute was able to induce G-arrest within 48 hours and apoptosis within 72 hours for breast, pancreatic, esophageal, skin, colon and prostate cancer. Other ways that ellagic acid can help fight cancer that even the American Cancer Society admits to are the following: By activating detoxifying enzymes in the liver; by preventing the binding of carcinogens to cellular DNA; by being an antioxidant and helping to clear away free radicals; and by stimulating the immune system. Ellagic acid has antibacterial and anti-viral action as well.

Quite a few sites on the Internet have cancer recovery testimonials posted from people who have used an ellagic acid or ellagitannin supplement. Some of them report the reversal or complete elimination of colon, prostate, breast, cervical, skin, or pancreatic cancer. And a significant number of people have helped their dogs recover from cancer or non-malignant fatty tumors using ellagic acid.

The Meeker variety of red raspberries is thought to be the single best source of ellagic acid producing ellagitannins. This is the variety of red raspberries that the Hollings Institute used in their studies. Even though most ellagic acid supplements claim to use Meeker red raspberries, there is still a wide range of quality when it comes to the production of ellagic acid supplements. For instance, one company was found to be using red raspberry extract that had been sitting on warehouse shelves for years and had seriously degraded before being processed into supplement form. Thus, it is important to find a good quality product from a company with integrity.

One highly reputable source for ellagic acid in either pill form or as bulk powder for mixing into juice or smoothies is www.Raspberry Gold.com. Dr. Jim Webb is a naturopath and Ph.D. nutritionist who heads this company, and he was involved with the original group that conducted research on ellagic acid at the Hollings Institute. Dr. Webb sells the same high quality ellagic acid product that Dr. Nixon used to achieve his excellent results with cancer. The Raspberry Gold products are also endorsed by Dr. Russell Blaylock, a well-known neurosurgeon who has led the way in the fight against excitotoxins in our foods and has written up his endorsement of www.RaspberryGold.com more than once in his wellness reports. (To order Dr. Blaylock's reports or newsletter, go to www.blaylockreport.com.) Dr. Webb offers reasonable prices and a "no questions asked" money back guarantee on all his products. Moreover, he is happy to spend his time over the phone at no charge answering questions about ellagic acid and helping people understand how to use it for best results.

Another high quality product is Ellagic Insurance Formula from Greenwood Health. This is not a pure ellagic acid product because it also contains graviola, vitamins A, C, and E, selenium and enzymes, but it is an option for anyone interested in a good combination product. One website that offers a powerful cancer-fighting protocol based around the use of Ellagic Insurance Formula is www.HopeforCancer.com. (Remember, though, that vitamins C, E, and selenium should be avoided in supplement form by anyone using Protocel®, so Ellagic Insurance Formula should not be used at the same time as Protocel®.)

Ellagic acid is yet another great cancer-fighting compound that is relatively inexpensive and easy to take. Anyone dealing with cancer should know about it, whether they are using alternative or conventional treatment methods.

Websites

www.RaspberryGold.com
For pure ellagic acid products and bulk powder   (928) 758-3091

www.HopeforCancer.com
For Ellagic Insurance Formula   (866) 294-1119
(Also can order from www.GreenwoodHealth.com)

Section Three

Key Cancer Recovery Issues

18

To Alkalize or Not to Alkalize

If you have cancer, you will probably hear from many sources that you should try to alkalize your body. This is because it is known that cancer cells thrive best in acidic environments. It is also known that, in general, cancer patients are much more acidic than non-cancer patients—even to the point of being 1,000 times more acidic.

Do cancer patients start out with more acidic bodies in the first place? Often they do—especially when cancer develops in adults. When cancer develops in children, however, this is often not the case. I have come across cases of brain tumors, for instance, that occurred in children with perfectly optimal pH and I suspect that many other pediatric cancers, as well as many adult cancers, also occur under perfect pH conditions. Thus, acidic bodies are not the *only* cause of cancer, but simply one of many possible triggers (as in the forest fire analogy.)

In general, though, it is widely thought that overly acidic body tissues are prone to developing cancer. Then, once a person *has* cancer, the body may become even *more* skewed toward the acidic end of the scale due to the cancer cells themselves producing lactic acid—and this allows the cancer cells to thrive in their own little acidic environment which they have created.

Of course, the reason that overly acidic bodies are good environments for cancer is because acidic tissues carry less oxygen than optimally alkaline tissues (the extracellular and intracellular fluids of tissues, to be more exact), and cancer prefers to be in low oxygen environments. In this chapter, we'll look at what the acid/alkaline balance is, talk about how to alkalize the body, and clarify some common misconceptions about alkalizing and cancer.

Cells and Homeostasis

Most of us could go our whole lives without wondering how our extracellular and intracellular fluids are doing. Normally, we shouldn't *have* to worry about them because these fluids are usually well-maintained by the body through a process called "homeostasis." But if we want to understand cancer, we have to get down to the cellular level and understand what our cells need and want from their immediate environment. To do this, it helps to look at how multicellular organisms developed in the first place and I'd like to present the scientific evolutionary viewpoint on this. (If this does not agree with your own belief system about how life developed on earth, remember that this is just a theory. It does, however, give us one way of understanding cells that seems to make sense.)

From a scientific evolutionary viewpoint, life on Earth first evolved in the primordial waters of our planet, which became our oceans. This ocean environment was perfect for fragile, single-celled organisms to develop in because it was constant in temperature, pressure, and nutrient availability. Living in the ocean was like being in a womb for these early single cells. Chaotic characteristics of the dry land environment, such as weather fluctuations, landslides, earthquakes, floods, and so forth, were not felt in the ocean womb. Thus, in this ideal environment, single-celled organisms thrived, and the entire surface area of each cell could happily interact with the outside watery environment to allow food in from the ocean as well as to expel waste back out into the ocean.

Being in such a good situation, these early single-celled forms of life evolved and progressed into more complex life forms. They eventually became "multicellular" organisms. But amassing more than a few cells together risked cutting some cells off from their watery environment which each cell desperately needed to survive. In essence, multicellular organisms solved this problem by developing an *inner* fluid environment for all the cells to interact with—an "inner ocean," so-to-speak, that they could carry around with them. In fact, this inner ocean probably mimicked the original pH, osmotic pressure, ionizing capabilities, mineral composition, and other features of the outside ocean of primordial days.

Since those primordial days, some of the characteristics of Earth's oceans have changed. Evaporation, erosion of land into the water, and climate changes causing large portions of water to be frozen into polar ice caps, have all contributed to the oceans of today being saltier than they used to be when single-celled organisms were evolving. But the original inner ocean that multicellular organisms developed is still a part of our physiology today and still allows each individual cell to gain its nourishment from and excrete its wastes into the fluid around it. It is called the "extracellular fluid" of our bodies. Our cells depend on it to survive. This fluid is maintained by the body at constant conditions through a process called "homeostasis." Homeostasis is carried out in *other* ways as well. Six overall examples of homeostasis in the body are:[1]

1. Keeping the body temperature constantly around 98.6°F

2. Keeping blood acidity/alkalinity levels constant

3. Keeping certain chemical concentrations in body fluids constant

4. Keeping the glucose level of the blood constant

5. Keeping the levels of oxygen and carbon dioxide constant

6. Keeping the volume of blood and body fluids constant

From the evolutionary viewpoint, all of the above processes of homeostasis could be said to be the body's way of mimicking the constant conditions of earth's primordial waters wherein life first developed.

The Body's Acid/Alkaline Balancing Act

Of course, *all* of the above constant conditions are important to the functioning of a healthy body. But many believe that the acid/alkaline balance of the extracellular fluids is of *particular* importance to whether or not normal cells turn into cancer cells, as well as to whether cancer cells, once established, rage out of control.

The body has a variety of ways that it maintains proper pH levels, but the primary way that it does this is through the use of minerals from the diet. Contrary to what some people might believe, it is *not* the acidity or alkalinity of the foods we eat that keeps us in balance. In fact, it is a common misconception that eating or drinking something acidic will make the body acidic—and that eating or drinking something alkaline will make the body alkaline.

In reality, whether a food is acidic or alkaline *before* it goes into our bodies is not necessarily an indication of whether it will make us more acidic or alkaline once that food (or drink) is digested. For example, citrus fruits such as limes and lemons are very acidic *outside* the body, but they promote alkalinity when they are broken down and digested *inside* the body. This is because certain minerals, such as calcium, magnesium, potassium and iron, among others, are very alkalizing to the body's inner environment and many fruits and vegetables (including limes and lemons) tend to be high in these alkalizing minerals. Thus, the digestion of fruits and vegetables tends to have an overall alkalizing effect on the body, even though some of them may be quite acidic before we ingest them. Another example is apple cider vinegar, which is extremely acidic in itself but aids in alkalizing the body once digested.

What a food breaks down into when digested, or how a food aids digestion or the assimilation of nutrients are key factors when it comes to influencing body pH. Therefore, it is best to forget about whether a food is acidic or alkaline itself, and instead, look at which foods are "acid-forming" or "alkaline-forming" in the body.

Unfortunately, typical dietary habits in the modern industrialized world generally include high quantities of refined and processed foods. These foods tend to be robbed of their natural minerals, vitamins, and enzymes. Very refined foods, such as white sugar and white flour, are so severely stripped of their mineral content, they are virtually all acid-forming in the body. In contrast to refined sugars, raw fruits (which are also very sweet due to their fructose content) contain such an abundance of alkalizing minerals that the total fruit is alkaline-forming in the body.

Also, when people no longer had to work hard to hunt down their meat and could buy it instead from a grocery store or fast-food restaurant, the consumption of meat became easier and more frequent. Animal foods such as meat, fish, poultry, and eggs are acid-forming in the body, primarily because of the extremely acidic byproducts that are produced during digestion. These byproducts, such as sulfuric acid, phosphoric acid, and uric acid, tend to overwhelm the alkalizing effects of the minerals contained in these foods.

A brief look at some common acid-forming and alkaline-forming foods and beverages can give us a quick understanding of how a person's acid/alkaline balance can get skewed to the acidic end of the scale over many years of modern eating habits. The current tendency toward acidity as a result of diet is then *compounded* by the fact that chronic stress *also* contributes to acidity in the body, as do many prescription medications.

Lists of acid-forming versus alkaline-forming foods may vary slightly from source to source, but most foods and beverages are commonly listed in the following way:

Acid-Forming Food

all meats	most nuts and seeds
fish	peanut butter
poultry	lentils
eggs	most legumes
margarine	soft drinks
most commercial cheese	coffee
pasteurized milk	commercial teas
most processed grains	most alcoholic beverages
pastas	ice cream
crackers	chocolate and cocoa
noodles	tobacco
refined sugar	NutraSweet, Equal, Sweet'N Low
pastries and candies	most prescription drugs

Alkaline-Forming Food

most raw vegetables	olive oil
most ripe, raw fruits	goat cheese
sprouts	raw milk
sprouted whole grains	honey
wheatgrass	molasses
sauerkraut	maple syrup
apple cider vinegar	stevia
algaes and sea vegetables	spices
miso	herbs and herbal teas
soy sauce	green tea

Almost Neutral (slightly alkaline-forming)

> soured dairy products (yogurt)
> butter
> almonds
> buckwheat
> millet

Optimally, people's diets should be made up of approximately three-quarters alkaline-forming foods, and approximately one-quarter acid-forming foods to maintain a healthy pH balance. Yet, looking at the above lists, it is clear that most Americans ingest way too many acid-forming foods and beverages, and not nearly enough alkaline-forming foods and beverages. Just think about how many people eat sugary cereal or refined wheat toast with coffee and maybe eggs for breakfast, a meat sandwich with refined wheat bread and a soda for lunch (maybe along with a little salad). Then, for dinner, there is often a main course of meat, fish, or pasta, possibly followed by a sugary dessert. Not to mention the common extra cup of coffee or soda in the afternoon with a candy bar as a pick-me-up!

In general, understanding which foods tend to be acid-forming and which tend to be alkaline-forming is important. But these types of lists can only give us a partial understanding of how the acid/alkaline balance in the body can become skewed. For instance, if a deficiency of certain key nutrients builds up over time, then some important alkalizing features in the body may not be able to do their job no matter how many alkalizing foods you ingest. A good example of this is illuminated by the research of Dr. Johanna Budwig and her flaxseed oil and cottage cheese approach (see Chapter 13). Her findings showed that people who become severely deficient in omega-3 and omega-6 essential fatty acids (EFAs) can develop low oxygen cellular environments because their cell membranes cannot attract as much oxygen when they don't have enough of these vital, electron-rich EFAs. In other words, fish for instance, is considered acid-forming in general, but prolonged dietary intake of certain kinds of fish that are high in essential fatty acids and vitamin D may *promote* alkalinity in the body over time.

Thus, another common misconception is that people should *only* eat alkaline-forming foods. There are important health benefits to some of the acid-forming foods, too. If not careful, those who eat *only* alkaline-forming foods and cut out all animal products may suffer from a deficiency of complete proteins, essential fatty acids, or iron. So, when it comes to diet, moderation and balance are often the key and optimum health may result from a diet made up of about 75 percent alkaline-forming foods and 25 percent acid-forming foods.

Of course, diet is not the only contributor to over-acidity in our bodies. Chronic stress, caffeine, and dehydration (which are all rampant in modern living) also contribute. Stress triggers the sympathetic nervous system, which increases cellular metabolism, which in turn increases acidity.[2] Also, chronic dehydration is an increasingly common problem of modern living where people are rushing around between work, taking the kids to school, talking on the cell phone, making dinner, etc., while keeping themselves going with caffeinated drinks that are diuretics. Chronic dehydration can promote acidity in the body in various ways and certain toxins in our bodies can too. One easy way to help maintain a good acid/alkaline balance is to drink plenty of good clean water every day. This reduces dehydration and flushes out toxins.

A Detailed Look at pH, Oxygen and the Heart

So why is it that an overly acid environment in the body is also a low oxygen environment? The answer to this question is somewhat detailed on a biochemistry level, but basically it is because all acidic conditions consist of excess hydrogen ions. In the absence of sufficient minerals to neutralize this acidity, the body must combine these excess hydrogen ions with any oxygen that is available, thereby creating water as a harmless byproduct. Thus, if a person is continually creating an acidic inner environment and they *don't* have enough alkalizing minerals in reserve from their diet, then their body is constantly having to neutralize their overly acidic state by depleting the body's oxygen. However, if there *are* enough alkalizing minerals available for the body to use first, such as calcium, magnesium, or potassium, then it is not necessary for the oxygen of the body to be used up in order to neutralize the excess hydrogen ions.

According to Robert Barefoot and Carl J. Reich, M.D., authors of *The Calcium Factor: The Scientific Secret of Health and Youth*, calcium is the most important of all the alkalizing minerals we assimilate from our diets. They claim that "calcium to acid is like water to a fire,"[3] and we'll be talking about calcium shortly.

A body pH of 7 is considered neutral on a scale of 0 to 14. The more you go down the scale from 7 (toward 0), the more *acidic* you are. The more you go up the scale from 7 (toward 14), the more *alkaline* you are. Our bodies "like" to be slightly alkaline to function optimally. All of our cells and enzymes function best in slightly alkaline environments.

The pH level of our blood, however, is the *most* important for our bodies to maintain and the blood is always kept at a constant level of about 7.4. This is partly because it is critical that the blood be able to maintain sufficient oxygen in order to circulate oxygen to all of our cells. If the blood becomes too acidic, the heart might relax to the point where it could cease to beat. If the blood becomes too alkaline, on the other hand, the heart might contract to the point where it could also cease to beat.[4] Thus, the blood pH *has* to be given priority over pH anywhere else in the body if the person is to survive.

There are numerous ways that our bodies maintain a virtually constant blood pH of about 7.4. (It literally must be maintained at the very narrow pH range of 7.35 to 7.45.) If necessary, the pH of the rest of the body will be "sacrificed" so that the pH of the blood can be maintained at this critical level. Our bodies do this by using up reserves of alkalizing minerals from other parts of the body. These alkalizing minerals may come from body tissues such as the bones, teeth, cartilage, muscles, kidneys, and liver, among other places. Thus, a person's tissues and extra-cellular fluids can become way too acidic for good health throughout many areas of the body, even though the blood remains at a constant optimum alkaline/acid balance.

The constant optimum pH level of the blood, along with the constant optimum oxygen level of the blood, may be why cancer of the heart is virtually unknown. This is helped by the fact that blood flowing into the heart comes directly from the lungs and has the highest pH and oxygen levels of any blood within the body.

But *all* of our bodies' cells are highly sensitive to proper pH levels of the fluid environment around them, and they will not function well if this environment becomes overly acidic. Robert Barefoot and Dr. Carl Reich explain the above concepts in the following passage from their book *The Calcium Factor*:

> In chemistry, alkali solutions (pH over 7.0) tend to absorb oxygen, while acids (pH under 7.0) tend to expel oxygen. For example, a mild alkali can absorb over 100 times as much oxygen as a mild acid. Therefore, when the body becomes acidic by dropping below pH 7.0 (*note:* all body fluids, except for stomach and urine, are supposed to be mildly alkaline at pH 7.4), oxygen is driven out of the body thereby, according

to Nobel Prize winner Otto Warburg, inducing cancer. Stomach fluids must remain acidic to digest food and urine must remain acidic to remove wastes from the body. Blood is the exception. Blood must always remain at an alkaline pH 7.4 so that it can retain its oxygen. When adequate mineral consumption is in the diet, the blood is supplied the crucial minerals required to maintain an alkaline pH of 7.4. However when insufficient mineral consumption is in the diet, the body is forced to rob Peter (other body fluids) to pay Paul (the blood). In doing so, it removes crucial minerals, such as calcium, from the saliva, spinal fluids, kidneys, liver, etc., in order to maintain the blood at pH 7.4. This causes the de-mineralized fluids and organs to become acidic and therefore anaerobic, thus inducing not only cancer, but a host of other degenerative diseases, such as heart disease, diabetes, arthritis, lupus, etc.[5]

As mentioned above, there are certain systems of the body that have different acid/alkaline ranges. Here is an overview of *all* the body's pH ranges:[6]

Common pH Ranges

Blood	7.35–7.45
Saliva	6.50–7.50
Urine	4.50–8.40
Liver bile	7.10–8.50
Stomach fluids	1.00–3.50

Over-Acidity and Cancer

The Nobel Prize winner, Dr. Otto Warburg, believed that cancer cells are normal cells which have been forced to adapt to a low oxygen environment in order to survive. Could it be that, by switching to anaerobic functioning, these normal cells are simply "remembering" how they once functioned in the primordial oceans when they were single-celled organisms? This might be the case since, according to current scientific theory, *all the cells that existed at that time were living in a largely anaerobic environment.*

We don't generally think about this, but oxygen did not become prevalent in the earth's atmosphere until after plants evolved. So, all single-celled life *before* plants had to function anaerobically. It may be that every cell in our body retains the ability (a memory, if you will) to function anaerobically if it needs to in order to survive. This concept is supported by the fact that normal healthy muscle cells frequently revert to anaerobic functioning under adverse conditions. In other words, when we exercise so strenuously that the supply of oxygen to our muscles is not sufficient for normal functioning, then our muscle cells switch to anaerobic functioning. This involves utilizing glucose for energy, instead of oxygen, and it results in the production of lactic acid—just as with cancer cells. It is largely this production of lactic acid in the muscles that causes muscle soreness after strenuous exercise. Luckily, muscle cells have the capacity to switch *back* to normal aerobic functioning once the strenuous exercize has stopped and oxygen delivery to the muscle cells has been restored. (Cancer cells, on the other hand, are generally damaged cells that no longer have the capacity to switch back to aerobic functioning.)

Another problem that over-acidity may cause is related to the fact that enzymes of the body do not function well in acidic environments. Thus, some of the body's best defenses against cancer are neutralized. And yet another problem may be related to micro-organisms. There are some researchers who believe that, when the pH balance of the body is skewed, certain harmless micro-organisms can then change form, become pathogenic and thrive. We saw in the chapters on Royal Rife and Gaston Naessens that some micro-organisms can change form and become cancer-causing micro-organisms when conditions are unhealthy in the body.

It is interesting to note that how fast-growing or slow-growing a tumor is may be directly related to the rate at which it uses anaerobic functioning. Some cancer cells rely more on anaerobic functioning than others. Decades ago, two researchers at the National Cancer Institute performed some experiments where they actually measured the fermentation rate of different cancers known to grow at different speeds. What they found was that the more aggressive (fast-growing) a cancer was, the higher its glucose fermentation rate was, and that the slower-growing a cancer was, the lower its fermentation rate was.[7]

Though over-acidity is not the only cause of cancer, it is generally accepted that a poor acid/alkaline balance can contribute to the development of the disease and that maintaining optimum alkalinity can go a long way toward helping a person avoid a cancer diagnosis. For people who already *have* cancer, alkalizing the body through diet and supplements may help slow down cancer growth and help the rest of the body function better as well, but it should not be relied upon as a curative measure.

Alkalizing Minerals

An understanding of the health benefits of alkalizing minerals, and in particular of calcium, was first developed by Carl Reich, M.D. Dr. Reich was a medical maverick who, in the early 1950s, suspected that most of the diseases of his patients could be related to overly acidic bodies and calcium deficiency. In fact, Reich worked together with the Nobel Prize winner, Otto Warburg, for many years to formulate an understanding of the role of ionic calcium and cancer.

Dr. Reich started his medical practice in 1950 in Calgary, Canada. When he suspected calcium deficiency in his patients, he began to experiment with prescribing several times the RDA of calcium to his patients along with magnesium and vitamin D which helped the assimilation of the calcium. Reich was immediately rewarded with a high percentage of his patients (who were suffering from a variety of chronic degenerative diseases) getting better. By the 1980s, Dr. Reich had cured thousands of suffering patients. He did not specialize in cancer, so most of his patients received treatment for conditions such as asthma, arthritis, colitis, dermatitis, rheumatism, migraine, fatigue, and depression. But his findings on calcium deficiency applied to cancer as well.

In the early 1970s, Dr. Reich discovered that the pH level of saliva is an outstanding indicator of ionic calcium levels in the body. And he was able to validate clinically that a simple three-second test of the saliva using litmus paper strips could indicate whether a person was functionally deficient in calcium or not. He found that the pH of saliva for healthy people is generally 7.0–7.5. On the other hand, when a person was deficient in ionic calcium, he found their saliva pH would be around 4.6–6.4 (much more acidic).[8] Reich was able to prove that a few weeks to a few months of supplementation, along with dietary changes, would produce a gradual increase in saliva alkalinity and a corresponding increase in wellness.

For anyone wanting to find out what their own pH level is and whether they are overly acidic or not, pH strip testing is easy to do. Saliva strips are inexpensive and generally available in health food stores as well as from a number of sites on the Internet. Strips usually come with a color-coded chart. According to Barefoot and Reich, a healthy person with sufficient alkalinity and ionic calcium levels will generally show a result of dark green to blue on the pH strip. (Remember to give at least 15 seconds for the color to develop.) Most children test blue. But over 50 percent of adults are green-yellow, indicating a pH of 6.5 or lower and calcium deficiency. Amazingly, according to Barefoot and Reich, "terminal cancer patients are usually a bright yellow, a pH of 4.5. This is more than 1,000 times the acidity level of a normal healthy individual at pH 7.5, causing the body to self-digest."[9]

The Importance of Vitamin D

Dr. Reich also reasoned that the minimum daily requirements of vitamins and minerals were way too low and he was the first doctor in North America to prescribe "mega doses" of vitamin and mineral supplements. He figured out that a big factor behind why so many people showed signs of calcium deficiency was not having enough vitamin D in their bodies. Even though calcium is one of the most important bioelements, it is also one of the more *difficult* elements for the body to assimilate. This is because, once calcium has been fully dissolved in the stomach, its absorption into the body is completely dependent on adequate levels of vitamin D in the intestinal tract. No matter how much dietary calcium a person ingests, without adequate vitamin D to aid in its absorption, most of this calcium will just pass through the body. Dr. Reich made the important discovery that many people who had enough calcium in their diets were actually not assimilating the calcium they were ingesting due to insufficient levels of vitamin D.

Unfortunately, vitamin D is quite rare in most foods. The only common food source with significant amounts of vitamin D is fish (and fish oils). Possibly one of the richest food sources of vitamin D is eel, a delicacy found in many sushi bars. A less common food source with significant amounts of vitamin D is Shiitake mushrooms, which may account for some of this type of mushroom's healing action. But, in general, food sources of vitamin D are rare. Luckily, Mother Nature has made up for this by providing our bodies with the ability to *manufacture* vitamin D at the surface of our skin when exposed to sunlight. This sunlight-induced vitamin D then gets relayed to our intestinal tracts. If the vitamin D receptors of the small intestine are saturated, a person's body can increase its absorption of calcium by a factor of 20.[10]

Vitamin D deficiency could be considered yet another nutritional deficiency of modern living because, before modern times, humans spent much more of their time outdoors exposed to sunlight. If they lived in cold climates, such as in the northern latitudes, and couldn't be exposed to a lot of sunlight, then they tended to subsist on large amounts of fish.

(Mainly because very cold climates do not support agriculture or even sufficient game hunting.) In the old days, when people lived in warm climates, they generally had minimal clothing covering their skin and spent many hours every day exposed to sunlight while they did their hunting, gathering, farming, preparing of tools, and so forth.

Nowadays, many people spend most of their time indoors in artificial lighting, which does *not* provide the spectrum of light needed to produce vitamin D. And when people today are outdoors, they often have clothing covering most of their skin. For people wearing loincloths and spending most of their time outdoors, their bodies could produce between 1 million and 3 million IUs of vitamin D every day. This is quite a contrast to the ridiculously low recommended daily allowance (RDA) of vitamin D which is 400 IUs. To put this RDA amount in perspective, 400 IUs can easily be produced on the average person's skin surface in less than 18 seconds if that person's body is in full exposure to sunlight![11] So, calcium is critical for maintaining optimum pH in the body, and vitamin D is critical for assimilating calcium.

In *The Calcium Factor*, Dr. Reich and Robert Barefoot make the following points:[12]

- No mineral is involved in as many biological functions in the body as calcium.

- Calcium is the key "biological workhorse" that brings nutrients into all of our cells (helping to nourish all the cells of the body).

- None of calcium's jobs is more important than its role in helping to maintain proper pH levels in the body.

- One problem that can occur if the intracellular and extracellular fluids are too acid is that cell walls can begin to disintegrate. When this happens, toxins and carcinogens are able to get inside the cell and possibly bind with the DNA's nucleotides. Some of these toxins and carcinogens can then cause the DNA to mutate with a result of cancer.

In a sense, Dr. Reich actually considered cancer to be *"'tailor made'* to survive and to thrive in an ionic calcium deficient environment."[13]

It is interesting to look at the diet and lifestyles of the longest-lived and healthiest people in the world, because doing so supports the importance of a high assimilation of ionic calcium. For instance, the Hunzas in Pakistan; the Armenians, Azerbaijanians, and Georgians in Russia; the Vilcabamba Indians in Ecuador; the Titicacas Indians in Peru; the Bamas in China; and the Tibetans are all mountain-residing people who drink highly mineralized water from glaciers. This water is so full of minerals, including high levels of calcium, that it is "milky" color and is called "milk of the mountains." According to Barefoot and Reich, these long-lived people may ingest on any given day 100,000 milligrams of calcium. The Okinawans are another group of people who are incredibly healthy and long-lived and though they live at sea level, they do just as well by drinking water full of coral calcium. This is a result of dissolved coral reefs and the water is also milky white in color and called "milk of the oceans."

All of the above groups of people are virtually disease-free and are not limited to our required daily amounts, or RDAs, of minerals. In fact, they consume about 70 times the RDA of calcium, 22 times the RDA of magnesium, and 18 times the RDA of potassium, to name just a few of their abundant dietary nutrients.[14] All of these minerals are highly alkalizing to the body and are therefore preventive to disease.

Barefoot and Reich suggest that a change in diet alone can, over time, bring a person's body back into correct pH balance. But if a person has cancer, they suggest that the person will want to bring about their pH re-balancing as quickly as possible—and that requires high doses of certain supplements. Calcium, magnesium, and vitamin D are very important for regaining pH balance, and in particular, many people find that supplementing with a coral calcium product helps immensely. Of the various coral calcium products on the market today, the "marine harvested" and "high-grade" versions are probably the best. Vitamin D is added to coral calcium products, but people who are starting out acidic should also either get a lot of skin exposure to sunshine every day or supplement with extra vitamin D.

Alkalizing Once You Have Cancer

Reich and Barefoot made it clear in their book that cancer cannot survive in an optimally alkaline environment. Though this is true, it has also sparked a common misunderstanding that can be dangerous to the cancer patient. What *has* been proven scientifically is that cancer cells in *artificial* environments, such as petri dishes, cannot survive if the environment is alkaline enough. This has caused many people to assume that if they are able to raise their body pH to the point where saliva testing shows it to be in the optimally alkaline range (a pH of 7.0–7.5), then all the cancer in their body will necessarily die off.

What people *don't* take into account is that active tumors within the body are very different from a small number of microscopic cells in a petri dish. Since a tumor is made up of millions of cancer cells, all thriving and producing energy for themselves through the anaerobic respiration process called glycolysis, the environment immediately around the tumor will generally become quite acidic as a result of glycolysis producing lactic acid as a byproduct. Thus, the area immediately surrounding the tumor may remain acidic even when the rest of the body is optimally alkaline! So, it is critical that people do *not* think that all they need to do is bring their alkalinity up to get rid of their cancer. (The exception to this rule is Cesium High pH Therapy as described in Chapter 16. Cesium is not an everyday supplement and not sold at most health food stores. It is also only a trace mineral in our foods. While normal alkalizing supplements like calcium, magnesium, potassium, and vitamin D alkalize the extracellular environment of the body, Cesium High pH Therapy is a specific treatment method that is capable of alkalizing the *intracellular* environment of cancer cells. In other words, cesium is readily absorbed into cancer cells, where it then alkalizes them to death *from the inside.*)

Having said that, it does appear that bringing one's general body pH up to a healthy slightly alkaline level should be able to help slow the growth of cancer and improve the body's functioning and overall health. To this end, many cancer patients take significant doses of calcium, magnesium and vitamin D. In general, it is best to consult with your physician, nutritionist, or alternative cancer specialist about how to alkalize your body when you have cancer. This is to ensure that the alkalizing supplements and/or diet changes you choose are compatible with your cancer treatment approach and support your optimum recovery.

Also, it is important to understand that many alternative treatments for cancer have historically worked *without* the person alkalizing his or her body at the same time. Two very powerful approaches that come to mind, for instance, which don't require alkalizing are Protocel® and Dr. Burzynski's Antineoplaston Therapy.

Resources:

Books

Robert R. Barefoot and Carl J. Reich, M.D. *The Calcium Factor: The Scientific Secret of Health and Youth.* Wickenburg, Arizona: Deonna Enterprises Publishing, 2001. (Can be ordered from Exxel Audio by calling: 800-443-9935.)

Herman Aihara. *Acid and Alkaline.* Oroville, California: George Ohsawa Macrobiotic Foundation, 1986.

Websites

www.superior-coral.com (also can call 877-287-3263)

www.healthtreasures.com

www.cureamerica.net

www.hopeforcancer.com/OxyPlus.htm (Also contains information about Warburg's Oxygen Boosting and alkalizing formula, "Oxy Plus.")

www.alkalizeforhealth.net

www.cocoonnutrition.org

www.gethealthyagain.com

19

What Women Must Know
About Hormones

There can be many contributing factors to the development of cancer. But one particularly important factor for women is hormone imbalance. Many important hormones in our bodies work together and, when in balance, contribute to our overall health and well-being. Some of these important hormones are thyroid, DHEA, testosterone and cortisol. However, for women with cancer, the most important hormones to monitor closely are estrogen and progesterone, and those are the hormones we will be focusing on in this chapter.

Estrogen, Progesterone, and Hormone Imbalance

Generally, hormone imbalance in women occurs when there is too much estrogen and too little progesterone in their bodies. In our discussion of women's hormones and cancer, two concepts need to be clarified up front. The first concept is that "estrogen" is really a *group* name because every woman actually makes three different estrogen hormones in her body. These three types of estrogen are called: estradiol, estrone, and estriol. Whenever hormones are discussed, these three versions of estrogen tend to be *collectively* referred to as "estrogen."

The second concept is that, in discussing hormone imbalance, it is the *natural* estrogen and *natural* progesterone to which I am referring. So, if you are a woman and thinking something like, "Well, I am getting my hormones balanced right now because I am on hormone replacement therapy," then you may need to think again. The hormones provided in conventional hormone replacement therapy, such as those in "Premarin" and "Provera," are *not* natural in the sense that they are not *bioidentical* to the hormones we produce in our bodies. Thus, they do not rectify hormone imbalance in the body. Actually, most hormone replacement therapies prescribed by conventional doctors involve *non-bioidentical* hormones and the hormones in birth control pills are also *non-bioidentical*. The functional differences between bioidentical and non-bioidentical hormones will be discussed soon, but remember, it is only the bioidentical forms of hormones that can bring about true hormone balance in a woman.

All hormones perform very important physiological functions. In doing so, hormones can be *so* powerful that nature has created checks and balances for them. The way that our bodies naturally keep the estrogen levels in check, for instance, is by producing the hormone progesterone to oppose the estrogens. The opposing effects of progesterone keep the effects of the estrogens in balance, and this balance is necessary if a woman's body is to function normally and stay healthy. If a healthy balance is not maintained, and a woman has too much estrogen and too little progesterone functioning in her body over a significant period of time, then she is prone to many serious health problems. These health problems can even be life-threatening, and include stroke, heart attack, osteoporosis (or brittle bones), and yes, even cancer. The types of cancer in women that are most frequently caused by an estrogen/progesterone imbalance are the cancers of the sex organs. Thus, these tend to be breast cancer, endometrial (uterine) cancer, and ovarian cancer. But other cancers can result, in part, from hormone imbalance as well.

Estrogen/progesterone imbalances can also play a role in the development of cancer for men. The type of cancer most frequently caused by this type of hormone imbalance in men is prostate cancer. But there are reasons why an imbalance between estrogen and progesterone *can often be a much bigger cancer factor* for women than for men. One reason is that a woman's natural life cycle includes big changes in her hormone levels during her mid-life years, before and during her transition into menopause, that can throw her into imbalance.

In general, a woman's progesterone production will begin to decrease 10 to 15 years before menopause begins, then will continue to drop even lower for several years afterward. Her estrogen levels, on the other hand, will not decrease much during her premenopausal years. Just before menopause her estrogen levels will, however, become more variable, with up and down surges. It is not until a woman is actually experiencing menopause and no longer having menstrual cycles that her estrogen levels have finally decreased a significant amount. Thus, hormone imbalance in women occurs partly because, during the pre-menopause phase, their estrogen and progesterone levels do not drop equally.

This gap between estrogen and progesterone is then widened even more by environmental and dietary factors that contribute to *increases* in a woman's estrogenic activity. (These other factors will be discussed in more detail when we look at the causes of estrogen dominance.) Women in the modern western world suffer from these added environmental and dietary factors the most. This is why they tend to suffer more from menopausal symptoms than many women in third world or Asian countries.

Another *major* reason women are much more likely than men to suffer serious hormone imbalance is that they are so often recipients of some form of prescribed, synthetic hormones. These synthetic hormones are most often in the form of: (1) birth control pills, or (2) hormone replacement therapy (HRT). HRT is usually prescribed for symptoms of menopause, including the frequently occurring "surgically induced" menopause that is a result of hysterectomy. These two sources of prescribed hormones can cause many women to actually spend decades of their lives on a hormone regimen that can cause a very unhealthy imbalance in their bodies. And many of them are not told, and are thus not aware, that this imbalance can significantly increase their chance of developing cancer and other life-threatening conditions.

Estrogen Dominance

When women develop an imbalance between estrogen and progesterone, it is almost always the estrogen levels that are too high and the progesterone levels that are too low. It very rarely happens the other way. John R. Lee, M.D., spent many years researching and writing books about the dangers of hormone imbalances in modern women. In discussing what causes these imbalances, Dr. Lee coined the term "estrogen dominance." Estrogen dominance refers to the *ratio* of estrogen to progesterone. In other words, before, during and after menopause, a woman may suffer from various menopause symptoms as a result of her estrogen levels being low. These symptoms of low estrogen might be hot flashes, depression, foggy thinking, dry skin, vaginal dryness, low sex drive, and insomnia. But even with low estrogen levels, she may *still* be estrogen dominant. This is because her progesterone level most likely is even lower than her estrogen, and the ratio of estrogen to progesterone in her body is still imbalanced in the direction of too much estrogen.

Breast cancer, which is one of the second leading causes of cancer death among women, is linked to this type of hormone imbalance. Luckily, the good news is that the *correction* of hormone imbalance can not only help to *prevent* cancer in women, especially breast cancer, but may also improve a woman's chances of recovery from cancer.

To understand how estrogen dominance contributes to cancer, we must first understand estrogen and progesterone a little better. The estrogens perform many functions in our bodies. But for women, one of the most important functions of the estrogens could be described in this simplified way: The estrogens prepare a woman for reproduction. (The word "estrogen" was coined originally when researchers first discovered its "estrus-producing" capabilities.) In other words, the estrogens bring on menses in teenage girls (or stimulate the proliferation of endometrial cells in preparation for pregnancy), and they stimulate the development of breast tissue in young women to prepare them for breast-feeding. Both of these important functions involve the stimulation of new cell growth.

On the other hand, one of the most important functions of progesterone in women could be described in this simplified way: Progesterone protects pregnancy once pregnancy has been initiated. (The word "progesterone" was coined originally to mean "pro-gestation.") In other words, there are many health benefits to the body that progesterone provides throughout the life of every woman, but it has a *particularly* important job during pregnancy. During pregnancy, a woman's progesterone production shoots sky high. This high level of progesterone in her body then protects the developing fetus by preventing ovulation and the ensuing sloughing off of the endometrial lining. In fact, women who have low levels of progesterone will sometimes experience repeated miscarriages because their bodies are not producing enough natural progesterone to safeguard the normal process of gestation.

Another thing to keep in mind is that estrogen is dominant in a woman's body throughout the first week of her menstruation, and progesterone is the dominant hormone in a woman's body right after ovulation and for the two weeks preceding her menstrual period. When a woman does not produce enough progesterone she will often experience symptoms of PMS. This is because the progesterone hormone is supposed to be dominant the two weeks before menstruation, and if there is insufficient progesterone at this time, a woman will feel noticeable symptoms. Thus, many women have reported great relief from their PMS symptoms after they started supplementing their bodies with natural progesterone.

So, it is a direct result of women being the child-bearing sex that initially sets them up for a roller-coaster ride with their hormones. Women's bodies must be able to switch between two drastically different modes—gestation and non-gestation—and these different modes require different hormones being dominant at different times. Men don't have to switch between these different modes, and so their hormone balance is easier for their bodies to maintain. But normally, this roller-coaster ride should not be too difficult. Women's bodies have evolved to handle the changes in their hormones. It is largely because of modern living that these changes have resulted in far more out-of-balance states in women than ever before.

Estrogen Dominance and Cancer

The cancer risk from estrogen dominance results from the fact that the estrogens tend to stimulate cell growth. Because of this simple factor, estrogen dominance puts a woman at serious risk for developing cancer. And if a woman *already* has cancer, the state of estrogen dominance can make it more difficult for her to achieve recovery. This cancer-promoting factor of estrogen is widely accepted by the medical community and is the reason most doctors will refuse to prescribe estrogen for menopausal symptoms to a woman who has cancer.

Exactly how does estrogen promote cancerous cell growth? It does this by activating an oncogene, or cancer-stimulating gene, in cells. The cancer-stimulating gene that responds to estrogen is called "Bcl-2." Progesterone, on the other hand, *down-regulates* this very same Bcl-2 gene, and up-regulates a tumor-suppressor gene in the same cells. This tumor-suppressor gene is called "p53." When p53 is activated, it slows cell reproduction and restores proper programmed cell death. This programmed cell death is called "apoptosis" (pronounced with the second p silent), and is an integral function of all normal, healthy cells. Thus, estrogen tends to stimulate uncontrolled cell growth by activating the Bcl-2 gene, and progesterone tends to stop uncontrolled cell growth by activating the p53 gene, which slows cellular reproduction and restores proper programmed cell death.

As we have seen so many times before, nature tends to provide checks and balances for all physiological processes. As long as a woman's estrogen and progesterone levels are balanced, she will not experience out-of-control cell growth. But once her estrogen level is "dominant," then the many different effects of her estrogen can go unchecked.

So far, we have been discussing the type of estrogen dominance that can occur in a woman's body with her own natural hormones. But even more of a cancer risk is when a woman is prescribed estrogen for menopause symptoms and is *not* prescribed natural progesterone along with it. This is referred to as prescribing "unopposed estrogen," and it rarely happens anymore because doctors are now very aware that they should not prescribe unopposed estrogen. The dangers of doing this became all too clear after mainstream medical doctors had been prescribing unopposed estrogen for about 20 years to menopausal women and then found out that a high number of these women were developing endometrial cancer.

But what conventional doctors have not yet fully admitted is that this practice of prescribing unopposed estrogen for two decades not only caused uterine cancer, but it also caused many women to develop and die of breast cancer. In his book, *What Your Doctor May Not Tell You About Breast Cancer*, Dr. Lee comments on the rapid rise in breast cancer during the middle of the twentieth century:

> The probable cause of the rise in breast cancer deaths was the prescription of unopposed estrogen (not balanced with progesterone) to menopausal women, a common practice from the early 1950s to the mid-1970s. While the medical community acknowledged that this practice caused endometrial (uterine) cancer, it never admitted that it also caused breast cancer.[1]

Thus, using prescribed estrogen *without* also supplementing with natural progesterone is a *huge* cancer risk to women. As Dr. Lee stated, this practice not only can cause fatal breast cancer and uterine cancer, but as we shall see later on, it can also cause fatal ovarian cancer.

Natural Progesterone and Breast Cancer

Over the last decade, the mainstream medical community has focused a lot on genetic predisposition factors for breast cancer. Some conventional doctors are pushing the genetic origins of breast cancer so much that some women who do not even have cancer are actually deciding to get "preemptive" mastectomies just because there is a history of breast cancer in their family. But according to Dr. Lee and his colleagues, only about 10 percent of all breast cancer cases in this country can be attributed to "inherited" genetic causes. And these genetic causes only *predispose* some women to breast cancer—they don't guarantee that cancer will develop. On the other hand, Dr. Lee believes that something as controllable as estrogen dominance can be a powerful contributing factor to cancer in women.

Support for the link between estrogen dominance and breast cancer comes from a study that was done back in the early 1980s by L. D. Cowan and colleagues at Johns Hopkins University. These researchers discovered that women who had low levels of progesterone in their bodies ended up having a 540 percent higher incidence of cancer than women who had good progesterone levels.[2]

An even more interesting study was carried out from 1975 to the mid-1990s (over an 18-year period) in England. This study was conducted by P. E. Mohr, M.D., a British physician, and the results were published in a 1996 issue of the *British Journal of Cancer*. Dr. Mohr and his colleagues went to the top three surgical hospitals in London and asked them to measure a variety of hormone levels in women at the time of breast surgery for all breast cancer patients in those hospitals. This was done, and the results were fascinating. (Incidentally, all of the women in this study were node-positive cases, meaning their breast cancer had already metastasized.) What Dr. Mohr's study showed was that those women whose breast cancer surgery was performed in the *second half* of their menstrual cycle (which is when their own production of progesterone was at its highest) were *much less likely* to have their breast cancer recur later on.

This study showed that, of the women who had higher levels of progesterone in their bodies at the time of surgery, about 65 percent were still alive 18 years later. But of those women who had low levels of progesterone on the day of their surgery, only about 35 percent were still alive 18 years later.[3] In other words, if you are a woman preparing to undergo breast cancer surgery, Dr. Lee says, "You *double* your survival rate just by having your progesterone level satisfactory on the day of your surgery!"

Dr. Mohr's study looked at women whose progesterone levels were high or low on the day of surgery simply due to the part of their menstrual cycle they were in. Dr. Lee believes that if these women had been *supplementing* with natural progesterone at ages when their own levels began to drop, it is possible that they would have done even better. One of the reasons he believes this is that, since 1978, Dr. Lee has put many of his own female patients on natural progesterone for osteoporosis. In cases where the woman had a history of cancer, no estrogen was prescribed along with the progesterone because of the cancer stimulating effects of estrogen. Over the next 20 years, Dr. Lee made a point of following these women who had a history of cancer that he had put on natural progesterone. Amazingly, he found that *not one* of them died of cancer in those 20 years.

Thus, both the 18-year study done by Dr. Mohr and Dr. Lee's own experience with his female patients showed that supplementing with therapeutic levels of natural progesterone can *significantly decrease the likelihood that a woman will have a recurrence of her breast cancer.*

Natural Versus Synthetic Hormones

Unfortunately, when the medical community was finally forced to accept that they could not safely prescribe unopposed estrogen to women, rather than add *natural* (bioidentical) progesterone to their prescriptions, they chose to add *synthetic* (non-bioidentical) progesterone. There are various forms of synthetic progesterone, and they are all technically referred to as "progestins." (The most commonly prescribed progestin today is Provera.) Most likely, this practice came about because pharmaceutical companies could not patent and make high profits from selling natural progesterone, but they *could* make high profits from selling synthetic progesterone. Many hormones are "synthesized" in laboratories, and natural progesterone is synthesized from various plant sources. However, the end result is bioidentical to what we make in our bodies, thus the end result is natural progesterone. Progestins, on the other hand, like Provera, are called "synthetic" because they never become bioidentical to what we make in our bodies.

Because they are not bioidentical, synthetic progestins do *not* protect against cancer as natural progesterone does. After years of prescribing synthetic progestins along with estrogen, the medical community finally began to see evidence that progestins did not control the cancer risk of unopposed estrogen. In fact, it made it worse.

The problem is that doctors do not tend to be aware of the very important differences between "synthetic" progestins and "natural" progesterone.

Since they know that estrogen and progestins can contribute to cancer, doctors often wrongly assume that natural progesterone will contribute to cancer as well. If you have cancer, and your doctor is leery of supplementing you with natural progesterone, keep this in mind: Synthetic progestins contribute to cancer. Natural progesterone protects against cancer. It is terribly unfortunate for women that many doctors still do not understand this functional difference.

Understanding the structural difference between natural hormones and synthetic hormones is simple. In a nutshell, *natural* hormones are those hormones that occur naturally in our bodies, or are produced in a laboratory to have *exactly* the same biochemical structure as those in our bodies. Each hormone in our bodies has a specific chemical structure that is unique to that hormone. For example, there is only one specific molecule that is estradiol, one specific molecule that is estrone, one specific molecule that is estriol and one specific molecule that is progesterone. Because pharmaceutical companies cannot patent and thereby cannot make exorbitant profits on any natural substance, they prefer to modify the hormones they sell. They do this by changing the natural hormone molecule in some way so that it is no longer the exact same molecule (or hormone) that occurs naturally. Then, they have a substance they can patent. Whenever a hormone molecule is even one atom different from the natural hormone found in nature, it is referred to as "synthetic."

However, natural hormones can also be "synthesized" in laboratories. For example, natural progesterone is produced by our bodies, but it can also be synthesized in a laboratory from plant sources to be completely "bioidentical" to the progesterone we make in our bodies. These plant sources tend to be either wild yam extract or soy, and contain "diosgenin," which is similar to our own natural progesterone. In laboratories, diosgenin can easily be altered just a little bit to become exactly bioidentical to the progesterone found in our bodies. Thus, in the field of hormone research and prescription, the synthesized result is called "natural progesterone." It is synthesized from something that is natural to plants, and it only requires a minimal change to turn it into something that is natural to humans.

One way to look at this terminology is the following: to "synthesize" something just means putting something together from parts. But "synthetic" refers to any substance *not found in nature*.

As long as the natural progesterone, which is synthesized in laboratories to put into natural progesterone creams and pills, is exactly bioidentical to the progesterone in our bodies, then it is completely safe and will carry out all the same functions in our bodies as the progesterone we naturally produce. Synthetic hormones, on the other hand, are produced to have almost the same, *but not exactly the same*, chemical structure as those hormones that occur naturally in our bodies. Thus, they carry out some of the same functions in our bodies as our own natural hormones, but not all of them. This is not a good thing for women because *all* of the functions of our natural hormones are there for a reason. Also, synthetic hormones can bind to receptor sites for much longer periods of time than their corresponding natural hormones would, which means they can *block* the action of a woman's own natural hormones that her body may still be producing.

In the case of progesterone, the synthetic forms (called progestins) definitely do not have many of the protective and beneficial effects on the body as the natural, bioidentical form of progesterone. Progestins do *not* provide the protective effects against stroke, heart disease, osteoporosis, and cancer that natural progesterone does. And because they block a woman's own natural progesterone from binding to cell receptor sites, they actually make estrogen dominance *worse*. Plus, one of the key ways that natural progesterone helps to prevent cancer is by activating the p53 gene in cells—the tumor-suppressor gene that slows cell proliferation and stimulates normal cell death. However, according to Dr. Lee, most synthetic progestins do *not* activate the p53 gene. In fact, because progestins are so dangerous and promote so many serious health risks, Dr. Lee states, "Prescribing a progestin to a menopausal woman should be considered medical malpractice." Yet, synthetic progestins are the progesterone-like hormones in all birth control pills as well as in conventional hormone replacement therapy for menopause!

The fact that synthetic hormones are not exactly the same in molecular structure as those hormones naturally found in our bodies turns out to be a *huge* distinction. In the world of chemical molecules, changing just one atom can sometimes turn a molecule into a completely different thing—such as a completely different hormone. Nowhere is the difference between natural and synthetic hormones so clear as in diagrams of their chemical structures. For example, here is a graphic representation of three different molecules. The first shows the chemical structure of the hormone "testosterone," the second shows the chemical structure of the hormone "progesterone," and the third shows the chemical structure of the synthetic progestin "Provera."

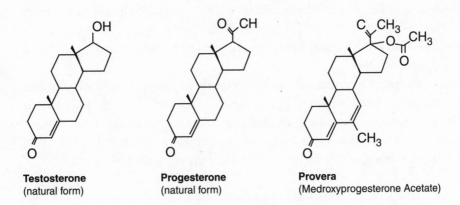

Testosterone
(natural form)

Progesterone
(natural form)

Provera
(Medroxyprogesterone Acetate)

As you can see, the two hormones, testosterone and progesterone, are extremely similar in chemical structure. Yet, virtually everybody knows there is a big difference in how these two hormones function in the body. Thus, a very small change in chemical structure can produce a large change in how the molecule functions in the body. Look at the drug Provera. It is obvious this molecule has quite a few differences in its chemical structure from that of natural progesterone. In fact, natural progesterone is actually *more* similar in structure to testosterone, a completely different hormone, than it is to Provera, its synthetic counterpart.

The most common hormone replacement therapy regimen being prescribed to menopausal women today is a combination of the two drugs Provera and Premarin. This is the regimen that is supposed to "replace" their insufficient levels of progesterone and estrogen. We have already seen how different Provera is from the natural progesterone women need. Now, let's look at Premarin to see how similar it is to the natural estrogen women need.

Plain and simple, Premarin is a strange form of estrogen for women because it is made up of *horse* hormones. Yes, that's right. Premarin is synthesized from horse urine taken from pregnant mares. Because horses are a different species and their hormones are thus different from ours, this drug puts estrogen hormones into women that may be natural to horses but are not natural to humans. Premarin, therefore, is considered a prescription drug that provides "synthetic" estrogen for women because the estrogen is not bioidentical to what human women produce in their bodies. Moreover, the process of creating the Premarin drug is very cruel to the horses that are used. Pregnant horses are kept in inhumane conditions so their urine can be used to create this very profitable drug. If you have any doubt as to whether this is where the drug Premarin comes from, just look at the name: "Premarin" is short for *pregnant mare's urine*. In technical publications, Premarin is sometimes referred to as "conjugated equine estrogen."

The point to remember is that *all* synthetic estrogens and *all* synthetic progestins are *un*-natural hormones. And they *all* create an imbalanced situation in a woman's body that can contribute to stroke, heart disease, brittle bones, and cancer. Yet, how many reasons are there for women to be prescribed synthetic hormones? Here are six common ones:

1. To alleviate menopause symptoms.

2. To supply hormones depleted by hysterectomy.

3. To avoid pregnancy through use of "the pill."

4. To treat osteoporosis.

5. To alleviate painful or irregular menstruation.

6. To reduce acne.

The cruel reality is that, ever since the development of synthetic hormones, modern women have been turning into stroke, heart disease, and cancer casualties in alarming numbers.

In its January 26, 2000, issue, the *Journal of the American Medical Association* published a study that was done on a whopping 46,000 women. This huge study concluded that the most commonly prescribed form of HRT (Premarin and Provera) produced a 40 percent higher risk of breast cancer in women who used it for five years as compared to women not using conventional HRT. This breast cancer risk factor was deemed to increase by 8 percent for each year of use. So, women on Premarin and Provera for 10 years could be assumed to have an 80 percent higher risk of developing breast cancer, women on Premarin and Provera for 20 years could be assumed to have a 160 percent higher risk, and so forth. Yet, a combination of Premarin and Provera is *still* the most common form of hormone replacement therapy prescribed to women today.

Unfortunately, the truth of the above study has still not completely reached the public. This is partly because, when the above study results came out, newspapers and other media around the country (such as medical writers and TV commentators) reported the study inaccurately.

They mistakenly used the term "progesterone" when they were referring to the synthetic "progestins" used in the study.[4]

The same thing happened with an even more recent study that captured a lot of media attention—the now famous Women's Health Initiative (WHI) Study. This study followed over 16,000 women and was originally scheduled to run from 1997 to 2005. But it was halted prematurely in 2002 because of the high rate of life-threatening side effects women receiving the HRT were experiencing. This study caused countless women to give up their hormone replacement therapy. It is important to understand that bioidentical hormones were not used anywhere in the above studies. They both focused only on the use of Premarin and Provera. Provera appears to have been the *most* damaging of the two drugs, probably because it replaced the use of natural progesterone which has so many protective effects that progestins don't have.

Thus, it is critical that the public and doctors distinguish between progesterone and progestins. And it is critical that people realize there are *many* results from studies and statistics showing that progesterone in its natural form carries a protective effect against cancer and other health problems. For instance, its cancer-protective effect is evidenced by the fact that the most common age for women to start showing the beginning stages of breast cancer is about five years before menopause.[5] This is exactly when a woman's own progesterone level has dropped dramatically, yet well before her estrogen levels have fallen.

The cancer-protective effects of natural progesterone are also evidenced by the statistic that going through a full-term pregnancy by age 24 can *reduce* the risk of breast cancer for a woman by more than half.[6] During pregnancy, a woman goes through many months where her progesterone level is extremely high as compared to those times when she is not pregnant. This high level of progesterone contributes to normal differentiation of breast tissue and can have a long-term protective effect against cancer developing later on in the breasts.

Since birth control pills are made with synthetic progestins, the use of birth control pills at young ages can contribute to breast cancer as well as synthetic HRT. Dr. Lee states,

> It has been well established that when girls between the ages of 13 and 18—and to a lesser but still significant effect, women up to the age of 21—use birth control pills, their risk of breast cancer can increase by as much as 60 percent. The younger a girl begins to use contraceptive hormones, the greater her risk of breast cancer.[7]

Dr. Lee and his colleagues believe that this predisposition to breast cancer caused by birth control pill usage happens in two ways: (1) the synthetic progestins in the birth control pills block the beneficial and cancer-protecting activity of a woman's natural progesterone; and (2) because the pill blocks ovulation, it thereby blocks a certain amount of a woman's own supply of natural progesterone from being produced in the first place.

It is extremely unfortunate that the medical community has resorted to using Big Pharma studies such as those mentioned above to warn women against *any* use of hormones—even bioidentical ones. In fact, the misunderstanding has gone so far as to terrify women if their breast cancer cells are not only estrogen receptor positive, but *also* progesterone receptor positive. Once again, conventional medicine has now adopted the erroneous idea that natural progesterone is bad, when the studies that have been scaring them have only been done on non-bioidentical progestins. Given that natural progesterone promotes apoptosis and down-regulates the Bcl-2 gene, it would appear to be a *good* thing if a woman's cancer cells are progesterone receptor positive. If your doctor tells you there is no difference between progesterone and progestins, just show him or her a picture of how different the two molecules look.

Other Causes of Estrogen Dominance

If hormone imbalance *only* occurred as a result of conventional HRT or birth control pills, then many women who had never taken either of these would be able to rest easy. However, this is not the case. There are other causes of hormone imbalance and estrogen dominance in modern women as well that do *not* involve prescribed hormones. For those women who have never undergone prescribed synthetic hormone use, the main factors contributing to estrogen dominance are: environmental xenoestrogens, diets high in refined carbohydrates and low in phytochemicals, and excess body fat.

Xenoestrogens

Xenoestrogens are petrochemically derived compounds that are "estrogen-like," which most people are exposed to on a regular basis. (The *x* in xenoestrogens is pronounced like a *z*, as in "xylophone.") The prefix "xeno" means "foreign" and indicates that xenoestrogens are not normally found in nature. These unnatural compounds are considered "estrogenic" because they produce estrogen activity in our bodies.

We are exposed to xenoestrogens in a variety of ways:

- We ingest xenoestrogens from pesticides used on crops whenever we eat nonorganic supermarket fruits and vegetables.

- We absorb xenoestrogens into our bodies through our skin whenever we come in contact with common lawn and garden sprays, as well as indoor insect sprays.

- We breathe in xenoestrogens from car exhaust and smog.

- We drink in xenoestrogens in areas where industrial waste dumps have contaminated the ground water supply.

- We eat xenoestrogens when we ingest eat meat or dairy products from livestock fed estrogenic drugs to fatten them up.

- We are exposed to xenoestrogens through the use of common solvents, soaps, and plastics.

Xenoestrogens are everywhere. They are nonbiodegradable and accumulate in our bodies over time. Because they build up in our bodies and mimic our own estrogen, they dangerously contribute to the condition of estrogen dominance. According to Dr. Lee, all xenoestrogens (as well as other xenohormones) should be considered toxic.

There are two main ways that environmental xenoestrogens contribute to estrogen dominance. The first way is that they bind to estrogen receptors in our bodies and produce an increase in estrogenic activity. The second way that xenoestrogens contribute to estrogen dominance in women is that they can damage a woman's egg follicles and cause ovarian dysfunction.[8] Ovarian dysfunction can then result in the decrease of a woman's own progesterone production. Chronic xenohormone exposure to adult women can bring about this ovarian dysfunction and result in reduced progesterone production, but it can happen much earlier, too. It is now known that exposure to xenohormones as early as during embryo development can cause this functional loss of ovarian follicles.[9] This means that estrogen dominance for many of us women may be partly caused by the environmental xenohormones *our mothers were exposed to when they were pregnant with us.*

It is imperative that the public at large become more aware of the dangers of xenoestrogens in our environment. These dangerous, nonbiodegradable chemicals are already reducing the populations of many other species on our planet, and are seriously contributing to reduced fertility in women and men as well. In general, men in industrialized countries are already showing greatly reduced sperm counts (compared to their grandfathers) as a result of these xenohormones. Some researchers believe that humans may, at some point, become an endangered species because of the multitude of xenohormones in our environment.

Diet

It is well known that eating lots of fresh fruits and vegetables on a regular basis can protect against all kinds of cancer. This is in large part due to the cancer-fighting vitamins and minerals, as well as the natural fiber that these healthful foods provide. However, few people know that diets high in fresh fruits and vegetables also protect against the cancer-prone condition of estrogen dominance. One of the ways they do this is by providing our bodies with what are called "phytoestrogens."

Phytoestrogens, or plant estrogens, are natural compounds found in plants that have weak estrogen-like activity in humans. They are part of the larger family of compounds known as "phytochemicals," and are a natural and important part of any healthy diet. There are presently 18 different phytochemicals known to be estrogenic in humans. These phytoestrogens bind to estrogen receptors in the body and convey many of the health benefits of human estrogen to men and women alike. And because they bind to estrogen receptors, they compete with our own estrogen hormones for the same receptors.

This is particularly helpful for women battling estrogen dominance because the weaker plant estrogens block some of the activity of the excess, stronger human estrogens. They do not cling to the receptors for long and are easily processed out of the body.

The seven subgroups of phytoestrogens are: isoflavones, coumestans, flavanones, flavones, flavanols, lignans, and chalcones. The isoflavones and coumestans are the most powerful of the phytoestrogens, with about a 10-fold stronger estrogenic effect than the others. Virtually all plants, including vegetables, fruits, seeds, legumes, and grains, have some form of phytoestrogen in them. Flavanones are primarily concentrated in citrus fruits, lignans are found in all fruits, vegetables, and cereals, and the stronger isoflavones and coumestans are mostly found in legumes.

Because of so much processed food in our diets, Americans generally don't eat as many "whole" foods as people in other countries do. There are many other populations around the world where a higher percentage of the daily diet consists of various forms of whole vegetables, grains, seeds, legumes and fruits than in the United States. In those populations, women generally don't have to deal with as much estrogen dominance because they haven't spent a lifetime eating processed and refined foods virtually devoid of phytochemicals.

The isoflavones are some of the most potent phytoestrogens to humans, yet, ironically, they are the most lacking in the modern western diet. This is because when most westerners eat a phytochemical-containing plant, it is usually in the form of a piece of fruit or a salad vegetable. It is not usually in the form of some type of legume (or bean). Yet, in countries where women suffer the *least* from symptoms of PMS and menopause, legumes are part of their staple diet. In the orient, this staple legume tends to be the soybean, and in Central and South America, this staple tends to be made up of more than one legume, including chickpeas and lentils.

The important isoflavone category of phytoestrogens can be broken down into four *specific* isoflavones. These are: genistein, biochanin, daidzein, and formononetin. Every time we eat a legume, we are consuming at least one of these four beneficial isoflavones. A great deal of research has been done on the effects of isoflavones. Besides helping to alleviate the many uncomfortable symptoms of estrogen dominance, isoflavones have also been shown to have potent anti-cancer properties. They fight cancer in a variety of ways, including by inducing apoptosis (normal cell death) and inhibiting angiogenesis (new blood vessel growth to cancer cells). In addition to their direct anti-cancer properties, isoflavones are also known to be diuretics, have anti-inflammatory properties, are antioxidants, and can stimulate the immune system and improve cardiovascular health.

Thus, women who have diets low in fresh fruits, vegetables, and legumes, are deprived of many of the hormone-balancing nutrients these foods can supply. Soy products are becoming a more and more common way for women to naturally treat their health issues, but there is some controversy around soy as well. Unfermented soy products actually contain some anti-nutritive agents in them that are somewhat harmful to the body. Therefore, the healthiest way to get isoflavones is by eating fermented soy products, such as miso, tofu, and tempeh, as well as a variety of other legumes, such as various beans, chickpeas, and lentils.

In this discussion of diet, it is also important to note that the consumption of excess alcohol can contribute to estrogen dominance. This is because estrogen is processed out of our bodies through the liver. If a woman regularly consumes alcohol, she may be compromising the functioning of her liver and thereby not be as able to process out the excess estrogen from her body as well as she should.[10] Excess ingestion of prescription drugs can also have the same effect on the liver as alcohol. Over time, the continued excess intake of alcoholic drinks and/or prescription drugs can compromise the functioning of a person's liver, which compromises the processing out of excess estrogen and thereby contributes to excess buildup of estrogen in the body and to estrogen dominance.

Body Fat

Yet another reason women in the modern western world have more problems with hormone imbalance than others is that they tend to be more overweight. Easy access to highly processed and fast foods, overly generous restaurant meal proportions, abundant candy and snacks, and less than optimum exercise levels have all taken a toll on both men and women. Little do most women know, however, that fat cells produce estrogen. In general, the more fat a woman has, the more estrogen she is likely to be making in her body, even *after* menopause.[11] These extra fat cells, each making estrogen, complicate the problem by being storage cells for xenoestrogens as well. It is no wonder that a largely overweight country like the United States is also a largely estrogen-dominant country.

So, when it comes to estrogen dominance, there are four main causes:

1. Synthetic hormones from HRT and birth control pills

2. Xenoestrogens from pesticides and other environmental sources

3. Diets low in phytochemicals and high in refined carbohydrates

4. Excess body fat

For more information on estrogen dominance, and how to correct female hormone imbalance, I highly recommend *any* of Dr. John R. Lee's books, videos, and audiotapes. According to Dr. Lee, one of the quickest and easiest ways to start correcting this imbalance, if you have it, is by using natural progesterone.

Pesticides and Breast Cancer

In examining direct causes of breast cancer, xenoestrogens and other toxins from pesticides also need to be looked at closely. These dangerous chemicals may promote a high risk of breast cancer in women for two main reasons. One reason is that toxins from pesticides and industrial waste tend to be stored in the body in fatty tissues and women's breast tissue is made up of about one-third fat. As long as these toxins sit in the fatty tissue, they pose a risk of genetic damage to cells. Another reason is that these and other toxins can *accumulate* in breast tissue over time, posing a greater and greater threat to each woman as she grows older. Corporations that cause pollution often refer to the small amount of toxins that people are exposed to at any given time as being safe, without ever addressing the fact that these toxins can accumulate and concentrate in the body and have a cumulative effect over time.[12] This is an example of how science can be misused and facts can be presented in a misleading way.

If you think that pesticides are safely controlled by laws, you may not know that many of the pesticide chemicals used today are exempt from current laws. For instance, in 1970 the EPA set certain safe pesticide limits. But within this legislation, congress allowed "the continued use of all pesticides approved before 1970." (This is a curious way to enforce environmental protection regulations.) Similarly, in 1978, more accurate measures of testing pesticides for safety were enacted, but this legislation once again exempted *all pesticides that had been approved prior to 1978.*[13]

One of the most telling studies about the relationship between pesticides and breast cancer involved the entire country of Israel. After breast cancer deaths had been rising in Israel for about 25 years, they dropped sharply between the years of 1976 and 1986. The only apparent reason was a strict ban of three organochlorine pesticides that had been enacted in the early 1970s. (These pesticides were DDT, BHC, and lindane).[14] Organochlorines are considered to be "complete" carcinogens, which means that they both *initiate cancer as well as promote cancer once it has gotten started.*[15] Moreover, along with the decrease in breast cancer cases in women after this ban, it was noted that there was also a corresponding decrease of these pesticides in cow's milk and in *Israeli women's breast milk. Breast milk, therefore, is one way that infants can receive concentrated doses of pesticide xenohormones.*

It is important that we, the public, exercise more control over what pesticides we are exposed to. And it is not just those pesticides that are used on crops that we must think about, but also those used in public buildings, on lawns, gardens, and in our own homes.

Breast Cancer Statistics

The number of women getting breast cancer has been steadily increasing over the past century, and this increase appears to be accelerating. According to the National Cancer Institute, the incidence of breast cancer rose by a whopping 40 percent between 1973 and 1988. Breast cancer is now the most common cause of death from cancer in women between the ages of 18 and 54, and the *leading* cause of death for *any* reason in women aged 45 to 50.

It is not easy to come across accurate figures of what the "cure rates" for breast cancer through conventional medicine really are. This is because all official statistics are based on the definition of "cure" as being "alive five years after diagnosis." Keeping a woman with breast cancer alive for five years is often achievable through surgery, radiation, and chemotherapy. But it also often involves the woman going in and out of remission, feeling frequently ill, being surgically mutilated, and never becoming cancer-free.

This bogus way of defining "cure" is one of the biggest ways that official statistics are misleading and directly give women false hope.

There is another way organized medicine has made official breast cancer cure rates misleading. It is by including something called DCIS in their breast cancer statistics. DCIS stands for "ductal carcinoma in situ," and is classified as a form of breast cancer within the duct. But many experts debate whether DCIS should even be classified as a cancer at all. When a woman is diagnosed with DCIS, it means she has abnormal cells scattered here and there, *not* clustered together into a tumor, which are *contained within* the duct and are *not* penetrating or infiltrating the deeper layer of cells in the breast.[16] The bottom line is that DCIS is essentially known to be a *benign* condition. If the abnormal cells begin to invade the deeper tissue, then it is no longer considered DCIS. The critical thing to understand is that only a very small fraction of DCIS cases go on to become actual malignant cancer, and therefore DCIS is really more of a pre-cancerous state.[17]

According to many experts, DCIS is 99 percent curable.[18] This makes it similar to many skin cancers in that it is not generally a life-threatening condition. But the cancer industry includes this easily curable, mostly benign condition in their official breast cancer cure-rate statistics, and thereby makes the overall cure rate for *all* breast cancers look considerably better. Over the past 20 years, DCIS diagnoses have comprised approximately 30 percent of all breast cancer diagnoses.

Conventional Breast Cancer Treatments

Surgery

For virtually all breast cancer cases, surgery is the primary treatment used. Following that, radiation, chemotherapy and hormone-blocking drugs are the treatments of choice. Whether a lumpectomy (removal of the lump and surrounding tissue) or a mastectomy (removal of the entire breast and surrounding tissue) is recommended, depends on the type and stage of the breast cancer. For women whose cancer has not yet metastasized, so that they only need surgery with *no* follow-up radiation or chemo, their chances of long-term recovery are the greatest in conventional medicine. In fact, Ralph Moss reports in his book *Questioning Chemotherapy* that for cases of non-metastasized breast cancer (lymph node-negative), surgery alone will cause about 90 percent of these cases to *not have a recurrence of the disease.*[19] Many women have survived their breast cancer under these conditions and gone on to live long, normal lives.

But surgery for breast cancer is generally only curative when the cancer has not yet metastasized. Once metastasis has occurred to *any* other location, including the lymph glands, the surgery may be considered only "palliative,"[20] or simply a procedure that is not expected to bring about long-term cure but merely to buy the patient time.

Unfortunately, when metastasis has occurred and follow-up treatments after surgery are required, long-term life expectancy drops dramatically for a woman with breast cancer using conventional approaches. Here are some comments on those follow-up treatments.

Radiation

The benefits of radiation treatment for breast cancer are questionable, yet radiation is still the most commonly used treatment for breast cancer after surgery. A recent article in the British medical journal, *The Lancet*, showed that, according to one study, the use of radiation on breast cancer patients *did* reduce deaths from breast cancer by 13.2 percent. However, these same radiation treatments *increased* deaths from other causes by 21.2 percent.[21] These "other cause" deaths were largely from heart disease as a result of the radiation administered right around the heart area. As Dr. Lee puts it, the only conclusion that can be made from this study on the use of radiation for breast cancer is that "the treatment was a success but the patient died."

Chemotherapy

After surgery and radiation, chemotherapy is the next most often pre-scribed treatment for breast cancer. However, it is *also* debatable as to how effective this type of treatment for breast cancer is. Ralph Moss reports that there is literally *no evidence* that chemotherapy can bring about long-term survival in cases of breast cancers that have already metastasized. Yet, over two dozen chemotherapy drugs have been approved for use in metastasized breast cancer. In these cases, it is apparently hoped that the chemotherapy treatments may be able to *extend* the life of the patient somewhat.[22] Once again, we are looking at a *palliative* treatment, with the doctor hoping to buy the patient time but not necessarily expecting a cure.

As mentioned earlier, surgery alone can prevent recurrence for about 90 percent of the women surgically treated for non-metastasized breast cancer. Of those 10 percent who do have a recurrence, it has been esti-mated that only about 3 percent could benefit in any long-term way from chemotherapy.[23] If Ralph Moss's research and the above statistics are accurate, we must conclude that *no* patient with metastasized breast can-cer will benefit in a long-term way by the use of chemotherapy, and only about 3 percent of those patients with very early stage, non-metastasized breast cancer will benefit in a long-term way from chemotherapy.

By the early 1980s, the medical community was so discouraged with their lack of long-term success in treating breast cancer, that they tried something radical. For a period of about 10 years, from the mid-1980s to the mid-1990s, a new regimen of extremely high doses of chemotherapy (about 10 times the normal amount) followed by a bone marrow transplant was tried. For a while, this highly risky combination treatment was thought by many doctors to be a woman's best chance of surviving advanced breast cancer. The high-dose chemotherapy was the cancer treatment. The bone marrow transplant was the follow-up treatment used to save the woman's life after the chemo had destroyed her bone marrow and her body's ability to produce new red blood cells.

Before the mid-1980s, about a hundred of these treatments each year were performed for breast cancer. By 1994, this number had grown considerably with about 4,000 high-dose chemotherapy/bone marrow transplant procedures being performed each year in the United States for breast cancer. This type of combination treatment is truly barbaric. It might not be out of line to say that it is the most horrendous type of treatment for any patient to undergo. The high-dose chemotherapy seriously damages the intestinal lining from mouth to anus, causing patients to endure great pain whenever they swallow or defecate. Making this unbearable are the alternating bouts of nausea, vomiting, and diarrhea the chemo causes. On top of this, the patient has to undergo extreme loneliness by being kept in an isolation room for weeks while their bone marrow recovers. This isolation is necessary because their immune system has been so damaged that they are highly susceptible to infection at this time. Thus, it is too risky for even their family members to approach them.

In the early years, one out of every five women died directly from this treatment. In later years, after the procedure had been perfected considerably, the death rate directly caused by this treatment "improved" to one out of every 10 women it was used on. Those who survived the treatment often sustained *permanent* damage to their heart, kidneys, lungs, liver, and nerves.

Finally, after many years, the medical community realized that the long-term survival gain for patients who received this type of treatment for breast cancer was debatable. One revealing article in the August 2002 issue of *Discover* magazine summed it up as follows:

> Most oncologists now agree that high-dose chemotherapy is simply the wrong treatment for breast cancer. Chemotherapy works by killing cells when they're dividing, so the faster cancer cells divide, the harder they're hit. Blood cancers—some leukemias and lymphomas—grow rapidly and so are acutely vulnerable. But breast cancer cells reproduce more slowly and tend to be far more resistant to cancer drugs. No matter

how many breast cancer cells are killed, at least a few survive, and they keep dividing after the chemotherapy ends.

The slow pace of most breast cancers also helps explain why transplanters were so optimistic. Breast tumors can take years to reappear after treatment, but the transplanters were used to leukemia, which tends to come roaring back in a matter of months. If they found no evidence of breast cancer after a year and a half—the usual waiting period for blood cancers—they assumed a patient was cured, or at least in long-term remission. Yet the cancer was often lurking in the background, gathering its forces for another, more devastating appearance.

From the moment [Dr.] Peters first administered high-dose chemotherapy until the first clinical trials were concluded, nearly 20 years passed. During that time, hundreds of physicians practiced the unproven treatment. An estimated 30,000 breast cancer patients suffered through high-dose chemotherapy, only a fraction of them as part of a clinical trial. All told, the nation spent around $3 billion paying for it, while an estimated 4,000 to 9,000 women died not from their cancer but from the treatment.[24]

According to the above article, doctors initially talked about high-dose chemotherapy/bone marrow transplant procedures as the "long-sought cure" for breast cancer they had been waiting for. Even many insurance companies were finally persuaded to pay for this expensive treatment.

But after longer-term studies were concluded, the medical community was forced to realize that any survival advantage the treatment may have provided for patients was actually wiped out by the fact that so many patients *died from the treatment itself.* One of these long-term studies was performed by the National Cancer Institute over almost 10 years and the results were presented to the public in 1999. This randomized NCI study only included patients whose breast cancer had not yet metastasized, but even in these cases of early breast cancer the survival benefits of high-dose chemotherapy followed by bone marrow transplant were negated by the number of women who died from the treatment. Thus, even for breast cancer that had been caught early, the high-dose chemotherapy/bone marrow transplant procedure was deemed ineffective.

It seems that if normal doses of chemotherapy had been saving the lives of women with breast cancer and having worthwhile long-term results, then the medical community would never have spent so much time and money on such a risky procedure—one where the treatment itself killed from 10 to 20 percent of the patients it was used on.

Tamoxifen

Tamoxifen is a nonsteroidal, estrogen-blocking drug that has become the most common conventional treatment for breast cancer after surgery, radiation, and chemotherapy. The reasoning behind the use of this drug is that Tamoxifen is actually a synthetic form of estrogen, but it is a *weaker* estrogen than estradiol (every woman's *strongest* natural estrogen in her body). By binding to the estrogen receptors of the breast, Tamoxifen blocks a woman's own more powerful estrogen from binding to those same sites and doing their work. Thus, in breast tissue, Tamoxifen is considered an "anti-estrogen."

However, what doctors don't generally tell their female patients is that Tamoxifen acts as a *stronger* estrogen in the uterus and is actually classified as a "cancer-causing" drug because it can *cause* endometrial cancer.[25] Moreover, according to Dr. Lee, the endometrial cancer caused by Tamoxifen is far more aggressive and more lethal than endometrial cancer caused by unopposed estradiol.

The following are five major downsides to using Tamoxifen:

1. About 20 to 30 percent of all breast cancers are not estrogen-driven, and therefore are not affected by Tamoxifen at all.

2. Even for estrogen-driven breast cancers, there is evidence that Tamoxifen is *not* effective once the cancer has metastasized to the lymph nodes.[26]

3. Research has now shown that Tamoxifen does not *permanently* stop cancer cells from growing, but rather puts them into a sort of "deep sleep." Once the Tamoxifen is removed from the body and a woman's own estrogen is again allowed access to those receptors, the cancer cells, if still there, will begin to grow again. For this reason, Tamoxifen is called a "cytostatic" drug rather than a "cytotoxic" one.[27]

4. There are many serious side effects that may accompany the use of Tamoxifen, some of which can be life-threatening. For instance, a woman's risk of developing a potentially fatal blood clot in the lung is *tripled* on Tamoxifen, and her risks of suffering a stroke, blindness, and liver dysfunction are also significantly increased.[28] Less serious side effects that this drug can induce are hot flashes, night sweats, depression, nausea, and vomiting.

5. As already mentioned, Tamoxifen can actually cause aggressive endometrial cancer in the very women who are taking it to recover from
their breast cancer.

Short-term studies on the use of Tamoxifen for breast cancer in the
United States have made the drug look a lot more successful than the
long-term studies that have been performed in Europe on the same drug.
For instance, Dr. Lee comments,

> The only large U.S. study was cut short, supposedly because the inci-
> dence of breast cancer dropped so much in the Tamoxifen group that
> they couldn't justify withholding this treatment from the placebo group.
> It's worth noting, however, that the trial was stopped at about the same
> time that breast cancer began to reappear, despite the Tamoxifen, in the
> two European studies.[29]

Thus, it appears that a number of European studies have concluded
there is no long-term life extension gain for women with breast cancer
who use Tamoxifen. One article in the *Lancet* suggested that the different conclusions from the American versus the European studies may
have resulted from the fact that Tamoxifen only *temporarily suppresses*
tumors, and that if the American studies had followed the women for a
longer period of time, their conclusions would have been more like the
European conclusions.[30]

Yet, despite the fact that European studies showed no long-term life
extension through the use of Tamoxifen, despite the fact that Tamoxifen is not effective for lymph-node positive cases of breast cancer, and
despite the life-threatening side effects that may be caused by this drug,
approximately 60 percent of the women with breast cancer in the United
States are being treated with Tamoxifen right now.[31] Surely, if women
were made fully aware of all Tamoxifen's drawbacks, there would be a
lot fewer women willing to use it.

Another estrogen-blocking drug currently being considered by the FDA
for use on breast cancer is "Raloxifene." It apparently does not tend to
cause uterine cancer the way Tamoxifen does; however, it *does* also carry
with it some very dangerous side effects. Like Tamoxifen, Raloxifene tends
to cause blood clots in the veins, and if one of these blood clots travels to
the lungs, it can threaten the life of the patient.[32]

It seems odd that most conventional doctors are so willing to prescribe very expensive, very dangerous, and not very effective estrogen-blocking drugs to women with breast cancer, yet they so rarely consider prescribing low-cost, entirely safe natural progesterone. Natural progesterone safely opposes the effects of estrogen in the body, including normalizing cell growth, while at the same time providing other great health benefits to the body as well.

Estrogen Dominance and Other Cancers

Earlier, I referred to a study done at Johns Hopkins that showed women with low progesterone levels (estrogen dominance) to have a 540 percent *greater* risk of developing breast cancer. But that same study also showed that women with low progesterone levels had a *10-fold higher incidence of all types of cancer* compared to women with good progesterone levels.[33] In other words, women with insufficient progesterone carry a 1,000 percent higher risk of developing cancer *of any type* when compared to women with good progesterone levels. This study clearly indicated that breast cancer is not the only type of cancer that can result from estrogen dominance.

Evidence has been available for many years that proves the prescription of unopposed estrogen can cause uterine cancer. There is also evidence that the prescription of unopposed estrogen can cause ovarian cancer. One large study, done at Emory University, looked at 249,000 women over a period of seven years to find out more about which factors might be linked to fatal ovarian cancer. (The researchers had to study such a large group of women in order to be able to have a significant number of cases of fatal ovarian cancer naturally occur.) A computer was then used to analyze and compare common characteristics of those women who developed fatal ovarian cancer. What it came up with was this: *every one of the women in this very large group who developed fatal ovarian cancer was on prescribed, unopposed estrogen.*[34]

Also, Dr. Lee believes that estrogen dominance may be a contributing factor to prostate cancer in men. As we have discussed, estrogen dominance is not usually as serious a problem for men as it is for women, but men's progesterone levels do decline as they get older, and men are also subjected to many xenoestrogens from the environment which can make them estrogen dominant. Dr. Lee claims he has also had very good results supplementing his prostate cancer patients with natural progesterone.

Testing for Hormones—Blood or Saliva Test?

Let's say you are a woman who wants to know whether or not you are balanced or imbalanced in your estrogen and progesterone. Most *conventional* doctors will have you do a blood test to find out, and most *alternative* doctors will recommend a saliva test. What is the difference and which type of test is more accurate?

The answer to this question is somewhat controversial, but Dr. Lee makes a very good case for why the saliva test for these particular hormones is much more accurate and reliable than the blood test. His reasoning is that saliva testing is much more useful because it measures the amounts of bioavailable (or "free") hormones in the blood, whereas blood testing measures a lot of "bound up" hormones that will never be available to the cells in the body. According to Dr. Lee:

> Saliva tests are more useful than blood tests because they measure the bioavailable (free) hormone in the blood. After steroid hormones (progesterone, cortisols, estrogens, DHEA, testosterone) are manufactured by the ovaries, adrenal glands, or testes, they're released into the bloodstream, where they attach or bind to very specific hormone carrier proteins and, to a lesser extent, to red blood cells. Progesterone and cortisol bind to cortisol binding globulin (CBG). The estrogens (estradiol, estrone, estriol) and testosterone bind to sex hormone binding globulin (SHBG). All of the steroids also bind to albumin, which is a protein present in very high concentrations in the blood. For every 100 steroid molecules bound to these carrier proteins, only about 1 to 5 percent escape the binding proteins and make it into the cells during circulation through the blood. The small 1 to 5 percent of steroids that escape the binding proteins are considered the free or bioavailable hormones, and these are what you want to measure, because they represent the amount of hormone that the tissue actually receives and responds to.
>
> Some of the steroids also bind to red blood cells. The more fat-loving a steroid hormone is, the more likely it is to hitch a ride on a red blood cell. Steroids hang on less tightly to red blood cells than they do to carrier proteins. This means that steroids bound to red blood cells will dissociate more easily and therefore are more bioavailable for use by your cells. Studies have shown that when red blood cells pass through the capillaries of tissues, the steroids bound to them can dissociate and enter tissues within milliseconds.[35]

The two problems associated with using blood tests to measure estrogen and progesterone levels are: (1) blood tests measure hormones that are bound to carrier proteins, only a small percentage of which will be available for use by the body; and (2) because blood tests generally measure the serum or plasma of the blood (meaning the blood cells have been removed), these tests are not able to measure those hormones bound to the fatty membranes of red blood cells which are largely available to the body because they tend to dissociate from the blood cells when they pass through the capillaries.

Progesterone is more likely to bind to red blood cells than other hormones. Dr. Lee refers to the research of one of his colleagues when he explains:

> According to hormone researcher David Zava, Ph.D., progesterone is by far the most lipophilic, or fat loving, of the steroid hormones. It circulates in the blood, carried by fat-soluble substances such as red blood cell membranes. Some 70 to 80 percent of ovary-made progesterone is carried on red blood cells and thus is not measured by serum or plasma blood tests. This progesterone is available to the body for use and readily filters through the saliva glands into saliva where it can be measured accurately. The remaining 20 to 30 percent of progesterone in the body is protein bound and is found in the watery blood plasma where it can be measured by serum or plasma blood tests. However, only 1 to 9 percent of this progesterone is available to the body for use. That is why saliva testing is a far more accurate and relevant test than blood tests in measuring bioavailable progesterone.[36]

If you consult with a naturopathic or holistic physician who uses saliva testing, they will generally have a laboratory with which they work. However, you can order your own saliva tests *without* a doctor's prescription if you'd like to assess your hormone balance yourself. One very competent laboratory you can contact to do this is:

ZRT Lab, (503) 466-2445, www.salivatest.com

If you live in any state of the United States *other than* California or New York, you can order your own saliva test from ZRT Lab without a doctor's prescription. If you live in California, however, you will need a doctor's prescription, and if you live in New York, you will not be able to order from this lab even *with* a prescription. You can also access more detailed information about saliva tests and hormone balancing on ZRT's website (www.salivatest.com).

Cream Versus Oral Progesterone

Once a woman has determined through testing that she needs to supplement her body with natural progesterone, there are two main ways she can do this. One way is by using a non-prescription natural progesterone cream that is rubbed onto various areas of the body. Another way is by getting a doctor's prescription for pharmaceutically compounded natural progesterone in pill form and taking it orally.

Both ways can be successful, but evidence indicates that the cream, or transdermal route, is the most efficient way. Since natural progesterone is so lipophilic (fat-loving), it is easily absorbed through the skin. When taken in pill form, on the other hand, as much as 90 percent of the natural progesterone is destroyed in the gastrointestinal track within 15 minutes, and thus no longer available to the body.[37] This means that a much higher dose of progesterone must be taken when used orally as opposed to transdermally.

The important thing to remember if you decide to use a cream, however, is that not all natural progesterone creams are alike. It is critical to choose a cream with the correct amount of progesterone in it. Dr. Lee states that women should always use a cream that has at least 400 milligrams of progesterone per ounce. Most of the good progesterone creams provide about 480 milligrams of progesterone per ounce. Since the levels of progesterone in creams are not regulated, some progesterone creams on the market have carried as little as 10 mg of progesterone per ounce. (What a difference!) So looking into which creams have the right amount of natural hormone in them and are best to use is very important.

Also, some creams are sold as hormone-balancing creams when they only have wild yam extract in them. It is true that progesterone is often synthesized from wild yam extract, but that does *not* mean that the wild-yam extract itself is going to be the same as progesterone. If a cream boasts its wild yam extract content, but does not claim to have progesterone in it, then it will not do a woman any good.

There are many good natural progesterone creams on the market today, and I do not wish to recommend any particular one. But as a general help, I will mention some of the progesterone creams that I have heard are good hormone balancing creams. These are just *some* of the creams that have been independently tested and assessed as having about 400 to 600 milligrams of progesterone per ounce.

Natural Progesterone Creams

ProGest	by Emerita www.progest.com	(800) 648-8211
Natural Prog. Cream	by Heartland Products www.heartlandnatural.com	(888) 772-2345
Awakening Woman	by Alt. Med. Network www.altmednetwork.com	(877) 753-5424
Balance Cream	by Vitality Lifechoice	(800) 423-8365
Gentle Changes	by Easy Way, Internat'l.	(800) 267-4522
Renewed Balance	by AIM Internat'l.	(208) 465-5116
FemGest	by Bio-Nutr. Formulas	(800) 950-8484
Woman	by Nature's Garden www.progesteronecreme.net	(909) 898-1466
Eternal Woman	by Mind/Body Solutions www.eternalwoman.com	(818) 879-1203
Natural Prog. Cream	by Young Again Nutr. www.youngagain.com	(877) 205-0040
Kokoro Balance	by Kokoro, LLC www.kokorohealth.com	(800) 599-9412
ProBalance	by Springboard www.springboard4health.com	(866) 882-6868
Natural Prog. Cream	by Source Naturals www.sourcenaturals.com	(800) 815-2333
Woman To Woman	by Woman To Woman www.womantowomanco.com	(888) 267-5032
ProgestaCare	by Life-flo www.life-flo.com	(888) 999-7440

There are many more good balancing creams on the market, and the creams listed here should not be seen as the *only* ones to choose from. There is a great deal of information on the Internet about natural progesterone creams, and visiting various sites can give you more information about each cream's specific number of milligrams of natural progesterone, as well as other ingredients that might be included.

For women who do not have cancer, or who are in remission from cancer, supplementing with natural progesterone is easy and safe. Instructions on how and when to apply the cream are provided with each product, as well as in Dr. Lee's and other books on natural progesterone. However, for women who are dealing with active cancer (especially those with large and aggressive tumors), seeking the guidance of a physician or holistic practitioner is recommended. This is because the first few weeks on natural progesterone *may* temporarily sensitize the estrogen receptors in a woman's body and initially cause mild symptoms of estrogen dominance. Thus, depending on your particular case, your practitioner may suggest you add natural progesterone supplementation very gradually, or may even suggest that you wait until the alternative approach you are using has your cancer growth under control first, before adding natural progesterone to your program.

Resources:

Books

John R. Lee, M.D., David Zava, Ph.D., and Virginia Hopkins. *What Your Doctor May Not Tell You About Breast Cancer.* New York: Warner Books, 2002.

John R. Lee, M.D., with Virginia Hopkins. *What Your Doctor May Not Tell You About Menopause.* New York: Warner Books, 1996.

John R. Lee, M.D., Jesse Hanley, M.D. and Virginia Hopkins. *What Your Doctor May Not Tell You About Premenopause.* New York: Warner Books, 1999.

Websites

www.johnleemd.com (All of Dr. Lee's books, videotapes, and audiotapes can be ordered from this site.)

www.salivatest.com (For saliva testing.)

20

What Men Must Know About Prostate Cancer, the PSA and Hormone-Blocking Drugs

W omen are not the only ones who have to worry about a hormone link to cancer—nor are they the only ones who must wonder whether hormone-blocking drugs are safe or effective. With prostate cancer being the second most common cause of cancer death in men (after lung cancer), and hormone-blocking drugs such as Lupron and Casodex being so commonly prescribed, this is a very big issue for men, too.

For women with cancer, the hormone that is blocked is estrogen. For men, the hormone that is blocked is testosterone. In Chapter 19, we saw that blocking estrogen in women is fraught with negative side effects and does nothing to help bring about a long-term cure. In fact, some women die as a *result* of the estrogen-blocking drug given to them. Is there any evidence that testosterone-blocking drugs are any more effective for men who have cancer? This is what we will be exploring in this chapter. In the process, we'll look at:

1. Diagnosing Prostate Cancer

2. Conventional Prostate Cancer Treatment

3. The PSA Test and It's Limitations

4. What the PSA *Really* Does and Why the Body Produces It

5. Hormone-Blocking Drugs

6. The Misunderstood Role of Testosterone

Diagnosing Prostate Cancer

Over the past century, prostate cancer occurred primarily in older men and was known for being slow-growing in most cases—so slow-growing, in fact, that men over 65 could often simply live with their cancer without getting any treatment at all. This was because they had a good chance of dying of old age before dying from their cancer. However, according to cancer treatment specialist Dr. Contreras of the Oasis of Hope Hospital, recent years are showing more and more cases of aggressive (fast-growing) prostate cancers being diagnosed. Plus, men of younger and younger ages are developing prostate cancer and the younger cases tend to have a higher incidence of aggressive forms.

Methods for diagnosing prostate cancer have improved over the years and include digital rectal examination (DRE), transrectal ultrasound, PSA testing, and needle biopsy. Digital rectal examination involves a physician using a lubricated gloved finger to manually feel the prostate gland through the rectum. This takes only a minute or less and is done to detect a lump or unusual hardness on the back side of the prostate. It is an easy, virtually painless procedure and a good diagnostic tool, but it cannot detect tumors that are on the front or embedded in the middle of the gland. Since approximately one-third of all men diagnosed with prostate cancer have normal DRE's, the digital exam is never conclusive by itself.

Transrectal ultrasound (TRUS) is a 5 to 15-minute outpatient procedure that involves an ultrasound wand inserted through the rectum up toward the prostate. Though not able to detect every mass 100 percent of the time, this procedure will detect most masses and is also a valuable tool for ascertaining the size and shape of the gland. Together, the DRE and TRUS are important diagnostic tools for detecting a mass or a change in size or shape of the prostate gland.

The PSA test is the easiest diagnostic tool, because it is a simple blood test. This test is not able to detect cancer definitively, but it can often detect the likelihood of cancer at an early stage, *before* a mass is noticeable. The PSA blood test looks for levels of a compound in the blood called "Prostate Specific Antigen." Though different clinics or doctors may vary in how they evaluate PSA scores, the following are how PSA levels are categorized in general:

0 to 2.5 is considered low

2.6 to 10 is considered slightly to moderately elevated

10 to 19.9 is considered moderately elevated

20 or more is considered significantly elevated

In the past, doctors considered any PSA count below 4.0 as "normal." Then it was found that a small percentage of men with prostate cancer had PSA counts below that, so 4.0 is no longer considered a definitive number that indicates no cancer. Now, the normal PSA level for most men is considered to be less than 4.0 and it is thought that men under the age of 40, in general, should have a PSA count under 2.7. For older men who have enlarged prostates or calcium deposits in their prostate glands, a count of 6 to 10 may be considered normal.

Thus, there is no "normal" or "abnormal" PSA level which can apply to everyone. This is because PSA levels are only an *indirect* measure of something happening in the prostate gland. As we will see in the next section, there are many reasons why a man's PSA count may be elevated, and *cancer is only one of those possible reasons.* The PSA level goes up in response to enlargement of the prostate gland or because of pressure in the prostate gland. This pressure may be caused by a tumor growing, but there can be other sources of pressure, too. Since most men experience enlargement of the prostate as a normal part of aging, the age of a man as well as other factors must *always* be considered in order to understand the meaning of a man's PSA count.

Keep in mind that PSA results alone do not confirm the existence of cancer and that this diagnostic blood test simply helps to narrow down the "likelihood" of cancer. For example, for a 40-year-old man with no obvious infection or inflammation in the prostate, an elevated PSA count above 4 indicates a 20–25 percent chance of prostate cancer and a PSA count higher than 10 indicates about a 50 percent chance of cancer. As the count goes up from there, the likelihood of prostate cancer increases.

PSA testing is an important early detection tool, but it is not a definitive cancer marker test.

The needle biopsy procedure, on the other hand, *does* give the definitive answer as to whether a man has prostate cancer or not. It can also indicate how fast-growing or slow-growing the cancer is. This rate of growth is assigned a number between 1 and 10 and is referred to as the "Gleason score" or the "Gleason scale rating." 2 on the Gleason scale indicates the slowest growing type of prostate cancer and 10 indicates the fastest-growing type. Typical prostate cancer Gleason ratings might be 3, 4, or 5. Ratings of 7, 8, 9 or 10 indicate aggressive (fast-growing) forms of prostate cancer.

This way of determining the aggressiveness of prostate cancer was developed in 1966 by a pathologist named Dr. Donald Gleason. Actually, the Gleason score is really the sum of two preliminary scores from two sites—a primary site and a secondary site. Each score is obtained by needle biopsy and assigned a number from 1 to 5. Then these two preliminary scores are added together. For example, a score of "4" from the primary site may be added to a score of "3" from the secondary site to produce an overall Gleason score of "7."

It is not uncommon for between 12 and 24 needle biopsy sticks to be required in order to get an accurate sampling of cancerous tissue. The down sides to this procedure are: It can be extremely painful; there is a risk of secondary infection as a result of moving bacteria from the rectum into other tissue or the bloodstream; and, worse, there is a serious risk of spreading a man's cancer by promoting metastasis down the needle tracks into the rectum. Some clinics are using Doppler transrectal ultrasound to pinpoint the tumor more accurately and thereby require fewer than the usual number of needle sticks in their efforts to obtain adequate prostate tissue sampling. So, anyone planning to get a needle biopsy might want to search for a clinic that uses TRUS to guide their needle biopsy procedure.

Conventional Prostate Cancer Treatment

Since men are being diagnosed with prostate cancer at younger and younger ages and often face more aggressive forms of it today, they don't have the luxury of being able to "live with it" as commonly as they did in years past. Thus, there are many more men today who must receive effective treatment or their prostate cancer *will* kill them. Unfortunately, the types of treatment offered by conventional medicine are problematic. The four most commonly used treatment methods for prostate cancer are:

1. Surgery

2. Radiation

3. Chemotherapy

4. Hormonal Therapy

Surgery

This is the most effective treatment that conventional medicine has to offer for prostate cancer that is caught very early and involves the complete surgical removal of the prostate gland (radical prostatectomy). When the cancer has not yet metastasized, prostatectomy may result in a long-term cure. However, "getting all the cancer" is not guaranteed, and this type of surgery is something most men would like to avoid if possible since it is often an emasculating procedure with a high likelihood of some degree of impotence and other dysfunction occurring as a result. (For instance, besides impotence, some men experience incontinence for years after this type of surgery.) If the cancer does recur at some point post-surgery, it will then be considered metastasized prostate cancer and surgery will no longer be a curative option.

Radiation

Once the cancer has metastasized to other areas of the body, such as to the lymph system, liver or bones, surgery is no longer a curative option. At that point, radiation and/or chemotherapy must be relied upon. Radiation treatments can either be done through external beam radiation, or through radioactive seed implants (called brachytherapy). Either form of radiation can cause sexual dysfunction and damage to sensitive tissues in nearby areas such as the bladder, urethra, and rectum that may cause a man serious physical difficulties for the rest of his life. Urinary and rectal irritation can involve pain, burning, and bleeding, and increased urinary frequency and urgency may occur. Sometimes these symptoms dissipate over time, but according to a recent study published in the *Journal of Clinical Oncology*, a significant number of men report new symptoms developing up to 6 years after radiation treatment. Men who receive radioactive seed implants appear to suffer the worst outcomes for sexual dysfunction and incontinence. Moreover, radiation has also been proven to sometimes cause prostate cancer cells to mutate into more aggressive forms that may then be even *more* difficult to treat than the original cancer was.

Chemotherapy

Chemotherapy comes with many possible negative side effects: hair loss, nausea, exhaustion, liver, kidney, heart and nerve damage, to name just the most common ones. And, like radiation, it rarely has any long-term curative effect. Don't let official "cure" rates fool you. They do not reflect real long-term cures. They simply reflect 5-year survival rates. Whether a man continues to suffer from cancer or even dies from his cancer *after* the 5-year point is of no consequence to these statistics. Doctors will refer to these statistics when they talk about your chances of being "cured" because mainstream medicine has defined "cured" as being alive five years after diagnosis. But the truth is that toxic treatments (any form of chemo or radiation) may be able to "knock down" the cancer for a while and sometimes put a patient into "remission", but they can rarely get rid of *all* the cancer cells in a person's body. Therefore, chemo and radiation are rarely able to make a person cancer-free.

Hormonal Therapy

To try to improve the efficacy of conventional treatment for prostate cancer, mainstream medicine added "Hormonal Therapy" to their list of recommended treatments. With this form of therapy, a hormone-blocking drug is prescribed to block the man's production or use of testosterone. Two of the most common hormone-blocking drugs for men are Lupron and Casodex, however there are others as well. The use of these drugs is based on the conventionally-accepted idea that testosterone feeds cancer growth. Hormonal therapy is generally listed as "palliative" because it is not even considered by mainstream medicine as a possible curative treatment for a man with prostate cancer. In other words, hormonal therapy is simply used in an effort to *prolong* a man's life. But whether it actually does prolong men's lives, or shortens them, is in question. At the core of this question lies the controversy around the testosterone-cancer link.

According to Dr. John R. Lee, the current commonly accepted medical concept that testosterone feeds cancer growth is a fallacy that should have been corrected decades ago. (We'll go into more detail about this issue very soon and look at why the concept that testosterone feeds cancer does not hold up to scientific scrutiny.)

Other less common conventional treatment methods for prostate cancer are orchiectomy and estrogen therapy. Orchiectomy involves surgical castration through the removal of the testicles. About ninety-five percent of a man's testosterone is produced by the testicles, with the remainder being produced by the adrenal glands. Orchiectomy is performed as an attempt to stop as much testosterone production as possible which, of course, is due to the widely-held belief that testosterone feeds cancer. Since testosterone-blocking drugs were developed, however, the use of drugs to block testosterone tends to be chosen as a more favorable approach over surgical castration—especially since it was found that the adrenal glands in men who underwent orchiectomy would often step up and produce more testosterone after the surgery to compensate for the loss of production by the testicles. Thus, men who undergo orchiectomy often have to take hormone-blocking drugs post-surgery, anyway, to block the testosterone their adrenal glands are making. This is no longer a preferred approach because it is irreversible and also since men still need to take testosterone-blocking drugs afterward anyway.

Side effects of all hormone therapy methods used to block or reduce a man's testosterone include impotence, hot flashes, weight gain, loss of muscle mass, fatigue, loss of sexual drive, nausea, vomiting, and breast swelling and tenderness.

Estrogen therapy is another hormone therapy that is sometimes used in an attempt to block testosterone. Though not one of the more common protocols, administration of estrogen not only suppresses the production of a man's testosterone, but it is thought to also have a negative effect on prostate cancer cells. Historically, this type of treatment has been used primarily in late-stage cases in patients who have developed hormone-resistant prostate cancer and a synthetic estrogen called diethylstilbestrol (DES) has been the estrogen of choice. However, this approach is only used occasionally today and may carry with it some risk of developing a blood clot, heart attack or stroke.

Even with all of the above treatment options to choose from, conventional medicine has not had significant success curing prostate cancer other than through complete surgical removal of the prostate gland when the cancer is caught early. Many alternative cancer treatments, on the other hand, *have* shown excellent track records for curing prostate cancer—even after it has metastasized. Some of the most effective alternative methods for bringing about long-term prostate cancer cures are: (1) Protocel® Formula 23, (2) the Flaxseed Oil and Cottage Cheese diet, (3) Essiac Tea and (4) Low-Dose Naltrexone. Other alternative methods have been known to work for prostate cancer as well. Thus, it is no surprise that more and more men are turning to alternatives that don't involve surgical mutilation or damage to the body through toxic treatments.

However, because drugs such as Lupron and Casodex can very quickly lower a man's PSA count, men with prostate cancer are convinced they should *still* take a hormone-blocking drug even though they choose to rely primarily on an alternative non-toxic method to treat their cancer. The medical establishment seems to have everyone convinced that less testosterone in the body is best for a man with prostate cancer and that a lower PSA count means less cancer. But, as we will see, lowering the PSA count through the use of testosterone-blocking drugs is simply an *artificial* way of reducing the PSA and does *not* correlate with a decrease in cancer. Moreover, there is reason to believe that less testosterone in the body may actually cause a hormone imbalance that can *promote* the growth and spread of cancer! Therefore, the issue of whether a man with prostate cancer should use a hormone-blocking drug or not is of utmost importance. But, in order to fully understand this issue, we must first understand more about the PSA.

The PSA Test and Its Limitations

Men choosing either conventional or alternative treatment will generally want to follow their progress by getting regular scans as well as by checking their PSA levels. The good news is that the PSA test can be used as a valuable tool in the diagnostic process. The bad news is that the PSA test is *not* as accurate at measuring cancer as many doctors lead patients to believe, and anyone using this test should be aware of its limitations.

As already mentioned, PSA stands for "Prostate Specific Antigen," which refers to a protein produced primarily within the prostate gland. However, as Dr. Lee points out, calling this substance *prostate specific antigen* is not completely accurate since it is *not* specific only to the prostate gland—in fact, PSA is also produced within breast tissue in both men and women. That issue aside, it is normal for healthy men to have a small amount of PSA always leaking out into the bloodstream. The amount of PSA that is leaked, so-to-speak, is what the PSA test is designed to detect.

When the prostate gland is enlarged, infected, or diseased, greater than normal amounts of PSA are released. Because high elevations in PSA tend to correlate with the growth of cancer in the prostate gland, the PSA test was approved by the FDA in 1986 for helping to monitor and care for patients who had already been diagnosed with cancer. Then, in 1994, the test was approved for the general public as an early detection blood test for cancer. Since then, the PSA test has become more often relied upon as a cancer diagnostic, and its limitations have become more often ignored.

What surprises many men is that there are conditions *besides* prostate cancer that can cause a man's PSA count to rise. For instance, prostatitis and lower urinary tract problems can cause the PSA to rise and remain elevated. BPH (benign prostate hypertrophy), which is simply enlargement of the prostate gland, can also cause the PSA to rise and remain high. Temporary increases in PSA levels may be caused by ejaculation within 24 hours before the test, digital rectal examination before the test, or prostate biopsy. (In fact, prostate biopsy can cause such a dramatic rise in the PSA that it can take up to a month for the PSA count to return to normal after this procedure.)

In other words, a man with a high PSA count might have cancer, or he might just have inflammation in the prostate gland or some other reason for an elevated PSA. The truth is that *a whopping two-thirds of men with elevated PSA levels do not have prostate cancer!*

Thus, the poorly-named "Prostate Specific Antigen" is not only *not* specific to the prostate gland, it is also not specific to prostate cancer. Too many men are being scared into thinking that a certain PSA level means they must have cancer. And other men who are dealing with prostate cancer are being scared into thinking that even a one-point rise in their PSA count is an indication that their cancer is growing, when there could be many reasons why their PSA count might go up one or more points at any given time.

On the other hand, one might at least hope that if a man *does* have prostate cancer, the PSA test will definitely flag it. Not necessarily. *In about 20 percent of the cases where men are known to have early prostate cancer, the PSA level is normal!* For example, this will generally be the case when a malignant tumor is "occult"—meaning it occurs on the *outside* of the prostate gland rather than inside it. Doctors even classify some prostate cancers as "low-PSA producing cancers." Frank Critz, M.D. is founder and medical director of Radiotherapy Clinics of Georgia (RCOG) and has treated 8,000 men with prostate cancer over 25 years. In a question and answer posting on his website, Dr. Critz made some very illuminating statements. He wrote:

> Some prostate cancers will not make very much PSA and are called *low-PSA producing cancers*. Low-PSA producing cancers can be very advanced and fool doctors. For example, the worst cancer we have treated at RCOG in the past 10 years was in a man whose highest PSA was only 0.5 ng/ml. However, he had a Gleason score of 10 and the cancer had already spread (metastasized) into his bones and he was incurable. The PSA is usually a good indication of the amount of cancer you have, but it is far from foolproof.[1]

So what is this all about? Haven't men been led to believe that a PSA test can tell them whether they have prostate cancer or not? For the next level of understanding, we must look at what the PSA does in the body and why it is produced in the first place.

What the PSA *Really* Does and Why the Body Produces It

The clearest explanation of the real functioning of the PSA comes from a 28-page booklet called *Hormone Balance for Men*, by Dr. John R. Lee. Dr. Lee produced this booklet in 2003, and in it he challenges common misconceptions about the PSA and the role of testosterone and cancer. Throughout the rest of this chapter, I'll refer to the main points Dr. Lee makes, but readers should get his booklet for a more in-depth technical understanding. It can be ordered online for just $14.95 at www.johnlee md.com/store/books_booklets.html, or by calling (877) 375-3363.

In *Hormone Balance for Men*, Dr. Lee explains that the PSA has only recently begun to be understood in medicine. First of all, the PSA is not something that *only* cancerous cells produce. In fact, PSA is produced in large part by normal healthy cells of the prostate gland. The most important concept that Dr. Lee explains is that *normal healthy cells of the prostate gland produce PSA simply in response to crowding (or pressure).* This is why an infection or any type of inflammation in the prostate gland will generally cause a rise in a man's PSA production—the inflammation causes swelling, and the swelling causes pressure against the surrounding normal cells. It is also why benign calcium deposits in the prostate gland can cause general irritation and result in a rise in the PSA as well. Even manually applying pressure by massaging the prostate gland will often cause an elevation in PSA production. Basically any significant or sustained pressure against normal healthy cells of the prostate gland will tend to cause those cells to produce more PSA, and this will show up as a rise in a man's PSA count.

In the same way, when a man's PSA count rises due to prostate cancer it is because a tumor developing inside the gland presses on the surrounding healthy cells as it grows—thereby crowding them. The crowded healthy cells of the prostate then respond by producing higher amounts of PSA. This is why there is a *general* correlation between higher PSA levels and prostate cancer.

The concept that increased PSA production is caused by cells being crowded is not generally accepted throughout mainstream medicine, but it elegantly explains why so many different types of situations can cause a rise in a man's PSA—and it is also supported by the fact that an occult tumor on the *outside* of the prostate gland will *not* cause a rise in PSA. (Since a tumor on the outside grows outward and away from the prostate, it does not crowd the healthy cells of the gland.) In his booklet *Hormone Balance for Men*, Dr. Lee has, in essence, explained a *new* way of undrstanding what causes the PSA production in a man's body to rise. And he points out that there is ample scientific support for this new way of looking at the PSA.

So, if we accept that a man's body responds to increased pressure against normal healthy prostate cells by having those cells that are being crowded produce more PSA, then the obvious question to follow is, "*Why* do those cells produce more PSA when they are crowded?" Nature generally has a very good reason for any physiological action that repeatedly takes place—and this is no exception. According to Dr. Lee, the answer is that *the healthy prostate cells produce more PSA when they are crowded because the PSA has "anti-angiogenic" properties.* Voila! This is the key bit of information that allows everything else to make sense!

Anti-angiogenesis is a very interesting process. It is well-known that malignant tumors of virtually all types are able to stimulate the growth of new blood vessels to themselves. This is called "angiogenesis," and it occurs when a tumor is quickly outgrowing its food source and needs new blood vessels to feed itself. In other words, the tumor feeds its own abnormal growth by triggering the growth of new blood vessels to itself through angiogenesis. *Anti*-angiogenesis, therefore, refers to the process of *inhibiting* new blood vessel growth to a tumor and there are a number of different substances in nature that are known to be naturally anti-angiogenic. For instance, the use of shark cartilage by cancer patients was introduced decades ago because shark cartilage has anti-angiogenic properties. A number of different herbs also have anti-angiogenic properties and have successfully been used to help control cancer growth in many cases. (One such herb is called "Bindweed.") Since anti-angiogenesis slows down a malignant tumor's ability to feed itself and thereby slows the tumor's growth, it is *always* a good thing for a person with cancer to have this occurring.

So, now our understanding of the functioning of the PSA is complete, and it is really quite simple. Normal healthy prostate cells are crowded when a tumor *inside* the prostate gland starts growing. The crowded healthy cells produce higher amounts of PSA than they normally would and that PSA has angiogenesis inhibiting (or anti-angiogenesis) properties. Thus, the crowded surrounding healthy tissue is simply responding to the pressure from a tumor by producing more PSA to *slow* the growth of the tumor. This is the common sense that nature so often exhibits and is the body's way of allowing the prostate gland to protect itself against the spread of cancer. Apparently, a man's prostate is quite a smart gland!

At this point, it would be perfectly reasonable for a person to ask, "Are there any *other* sources of medical research that back up this concept that the PSA has anti-angiogenic properties? Or is Dr. Lee the only one saying this?" As it happens, various scientific studies have already supported this concept. For instance, the American Cancer Society summarized some groundbreaking research in November of 1999 in an article they posted on one of their online news sites. The title of the article was "Does PSA Fight Prostate Cancer?" In it, the American Cancer Society stated:

> When PSA levels rise above normal, it indicates prostate cancer may be present or returning. For this reason, men have generally thought of PSA itself as something undesirable. But this study from the *Journal of the National Cancer Institute* (Vol. 91, No 19) suggests PSA may not be the enemy but only a messenger.
>
> PSA may be fighting prostate cancer. It may be an angiogenesis inhibitor, meaning it may work to slow or stop the growth of tumors by shutting off the blood vessels that feed them.[2]

This ACS news article then went on to report some of the research findings from a Maryland biotech company called EntreMed that was trying to develop some anti-angiogenic drugs. It appears that, as background research, the EntreMed scientists had performed some interesting studies using human PSA. This is what the American Cancer Society reported about EntreMed's research:

> The researchers were aware that PSA had been found in cancers other than prostate cancer. For example, a study showed breast cancer patients with high PSA levels had a better prognosis. They theorized higher PSA levels in men with prostate cancer might reflect PSA being produced to fight growth of the tumors' new blood vessels and decided to test their theory with a series of experiments.
>
> The group first introduced PSA into lab dishes containing endothelial cells, the kind of cells that form blood vessels, and found that it did slow their reproduction. PSA also reduced the cells' ability to migrate, or to come together in preparation for forming new blood vessels.
>
> . . . The researchers then injected PSA into mice with cancer and found it reduced the number of new tumors in distant locations (metastases) by 40 percent. They concluded PSA does, in fact, reduce tumors' ability to grow new blood vessels and suggested other researchers might want to re-think the concepts behind 'anti-PSA prostate cancer vaccines' and other anti-PSA strategies now being developed. [3]

If Dr. Lee and the EntreMed scientists are correct, then an increased production of PSA in a man with prostate cancer is simply his own body's way of trying to stop or slow down the cancer growth. Clearly, no man would want to artificially *reduce* his body's production of PSA with this understanding. Unfortunately, this is exactly what hormone-blocking drugs do.

Hormone-Blocking Drugs

There are a number of hormone-blocking drugs that are prescribed to men with prostate cancer—Lupron and Casodex being two of the most common. Though various drugs have different mechanisms of action, the overall result of these types of drugs is that they either block the production of testosterone or they block the use of testosterone in a man's body by blocking the testosterone receptors. When testosterone is blocked either way, the PSA count goes down. Why? *Because the body needs testosterone to produce PSA.* Thus, using a testosterone-blocking drug is simply an *artificial way* of lowering of a man's PSA count that has nothing to do with reducing the amount of cancer in his body. In effect, blocking testosterone and seeing a reduction in PSA is simply like blocking the delivery of flour to a bakery and seeing that the baker can't make as many cakes as before!

So why do doctors love to prescribe testosterone-blocking drugs? One reason is because they like to see a man's PSA count go down. They know that higher PSA scores *tend* to correlate with more cancer and lower PSA scores *tend* to correlate with less cancer. But they don't understand the crowding issue or the anti-angiogenic property of the PSA, because those things have not gotten any attention in the mainstream medical world. *So they tend to categorically think of any elevated PSA level as a bad thing.*

But, "Wait a minute," you might ask, "When I use a testosterone-blocking drug for my prostate cancer, my PSA count goes down dramatically and stays down. Doesn't that mean the drug is reducing my cancer?" The answer is "No, it doesn't mean that." Hormone-blocking drugs for men artificially reduce the PSA count simply because they block testosterone and testosterone is needed by the cells of the prostate gland in order to efficiently produce PSA. This way of reducing the PSA count *has no correlation to a reduction in a man's cancer.* In reality, artificially lowering a man's PSA count with a testosterone-blocking drug, then thinking his cancer is going away, is like artificially tampering with the digital display on a weight scale so that it displays a significantly lower weight than it should—then standing on that scale and thinking you've actually gotten thinner!

Thus, the only way for a man on a hormone-blocking drug to really know if his cancer is receding or not is through some form of scan that can actually detect tumors in the prostate and/or metastatic lesions in distant locations. The PSA test should definitely *not* be used as a diagnostic tool when testosterone is being artificially blocked. At that point, a man's digital display has been tampered with, so-to-speak.

Another reason that physicians like to prescribe testosterone-blocking drugs is because there is a basic misunderstanding in the medical world about the role of testosterone and prostate cancer. This misunderstanding has been telling physicians that testosterone *feeds* cancer—a medical fallacy that began more than six decades ago. Unfortunately, as we know from women's hormone issues, medical misunderstandings are difficult to turn around and can take many, many years before they are finally corrected.

The Misunderstood Role of Testosterone

According to Dr. Lee, the misunderstanding about testosterone's role in prostate cancer began back in 1941, when a well-known physician named Dr. Charles Huggins carried out some ground-breaking medical research on men with prostate cancer. In *Hormone Balance for Men*, Dr. Lee describes this historical event which he calls "The Testosterone Fiasco" in the following way:

> In 1941, Dr. Charles Huggins showed that castration (orchiectomy) slowed the progression of prostate cancer. Castration removes much of one's testosterone production. He unfortunately assumed that the reduction of testosterone levels was the operative agent for his beneficial results. He failed to consider that castration also removes one's estrogen production. Thus, it is likely that the estrogen reduction was the real operative agent. Despite these faulty assumptions, Dr. Huggins was given the Nobel Prize for his research. As a result, conventional medicine came to believe that testosterone was the culprit in causing prostate cancer. The prevention and treatment of prostate cancer focused on either removing the prostate gland or reducing testosterone, or both. Techniques were found to castrate men surgically or chemically, as in Lupron, for example. Other doctors opted for radiation. In all of these treatments, all sex hormone production by the testes is stopped or arrested, and undesirable side effects are common. The sad fact is that survival of men with prostate cancer has not improved with these treatments. Further drugs (e.g., Flutamide) were developed to block all testosterone receptors (called total androgen blockade), thus eliminating the testosterone effect completely. It is now conceded that survival time is not affected; the men so treated instead developed depression, dementia, and diarrhea before dying right on time. [4]

The fallacy that testosterone feeds cancer was probably then kept alive by researchers who saw that blocking testosterone made men's PSA levels go down and who drew the conclusion that the cancer was going away because they did not have the understanding that testosterone is simply needed to produce PSA.

A very eye-opening point that Dr. Lee makes is that the erroneous "testosterone feeds cancer" concept still exists today *despite* the fact that (1) it has always been known that prostate cancer occurs most frequently in older men after their testosterone production has declined and that, until recently, prostate cancer was virtually *unheard* of in young men when testosterone production is highest, and *despite* the fact that (2) as far back as the 1950s, the University of Chicago was reporting on studies that showed pre-treating mice with testosterone *prevented* successful implantation of prostate cancer in those mice. Moreover, when cancer cells were implanted *without* testosterone and the cancer was allowed to develop—then testosterone was added at that point—the prostate cancer implants in the mice promptly stopped growing.[5] The University of Chicago studies are an example of how good science can be ignored if the results don't fit with the currently accepted medical paradigm.

So, if the PSA can slow down the growth and spread of prostate cancer by inhibiting angiogenesis, and testosterone is needed by a man's body to produce PSA, and if testosterone by itself has *also* been found to inhibit prostate cancer growth in laboratory animals, then it is clear that men should *not* be blocking their testosterone production if they have prostate cancer. If that's not convincing enough, Dr. Lee makes two more important points about testosterone which indicate that the more testosterone a man with prostate cancer has, the better.

The first important point is that testosterone has the ability to "oppose" estrogen. Men's bodies make estrogen, too, though not as much as women's bodies, and estrogen can fuel not only women's cancers of the breast, uterus or ovaries, but it can also fuel men's cancer in the prostate gland. Numerous studies have clearly shown that raised estrogen levels *promote* prostate cancer. Thus, the more testosterone a man has, the less likely he will be estrogen-dominant. Unfortunately, when a man's testosterone level is artificially reduced through the use of a testosterone-blocking drug, that allows a dangerous shift in hormone balance to occur—a shift, according to Dr. Lee, that *always* results in estrogen dominance. In fact, there is no doubt that estrogen dominance occurs when testosterone-blocking drugs are administered, because men can feel and see this shift happening. When men take Lupron, Casodex, or other testosterone-blocking drugs, they often experience enlarged or tender breasts and other symptoms that indicate the estrogen in their body is having a more pronounced effect than it was having before.

The second important point that Dr. Lee makes about testosterone and cancer is that, like progesterone, testosterone activates the p53 gene in cancer cells. As we discovered in the last chapter, it is the p53 gene that induces normal cell death, or apoptosis. In fact, Dr. Lee was so convinced that testosterone is actually *beneficial* to men with prostate cancer, that he prescribed both testosterone and progesterone to his own prostate cancer patients. Over a decade and a half, the results he had with those patients were excellent.

One of the reasons testosterone supplementation originally got labeled as dangerous was because, back in the mid-1900s, some drug companies produced and sold a synthetic and chemically altered testosterone called "methyltestosterone." They promoted it as if it were real testosterone even though it was a form not naturally found in the human body. After several years, some men using methyltestosterone developed liver cancer.

It is never a good idea to use a chemically altered hormone that is not naturally found in the body, and even supplementing with bioidentical hormones must be done carefully and *in balance* with other hormones. Thus, when men supplement with testosterone for body-building or for reduced libido due to normal aging, if they don't supplement in a balanced way, they may put themselves at risk for various health problems. Dr. Lee always looked at progesterone levels in men as well and prescribed bioidentical progesterone when needed along with bioidentical testosterone.

When it comes to the role of testosterone and cancer, one of the problems we face today is that conflicting studies keep coming out. Anyone doing a quick online search today can find recent scientific reports with titles such as "High Blood Testosterone Levels Associated With Increased Prostate Cancer Risk," and "Study Links High Testosterone and Prostate Cancer Risk." In the same search, however, one can find equally prestigious medical institutions putting out scientific reports that say just the opposite. Report title examples are "Testosterone Doesn't Affect Prostate Cancer Risk," and "Testosterone Seen Unrelated to Prostate Cancer Risk." Thus, if your doctor claims that scientific studies have *proven* that testosterone promotes cancer, you can assert that there are equally prestigious scientific studies that prove it doesn't. Obviously, the testosterone-cancer link is a complicated issue that medical science has not yet figured out.

In fact, more and more holistically-oriented doctors are prescribing bioidentical testosterone to men who are going through normal aging changes as a way to improve their health and functioning. According to a recent *Life Extension Magazine* article, "A recent study found that men with lower testosterone levels were more likely to die from cardiovascular disease and all causes compared with men who had higher levels. . . . Another review from the Baylor College of Medicine reported that there is a higher prevalence of depression, coronary heart disease, osteoporosis, fracture rates, frailty, and even dementia with low testosterone states."[6]

It is well-known that testosterone helps maintain strong muscles and bones, and the risk of osteoporosis and increased fracture rates in men with low testosterone is no small matter. In other words, suppressing one's testosterone while dealing with prostate cancer could cause other serious health threats that most men are not hearing about from their doctors. In fact, one MSNBC news release posted in 2005 stated, "Hormone-suppressing drugs increasingly used to suppress prostate cancer make men so prone to broken bones that the risks of the treatment may outweigh the benefits in those whose cancer was caught early."[7] The release goes on to explain that, for the elderly, broken bones can be lethal due to complications and that *"One-third of elderly men who break their hips die of complications within a year."*[8]

All of the above brings us to the unhappy conclusion that, when a man is given a testosterone-blocking drug for prostate cancer:

1. He is having his testosterone level artificially reduced . . . *even though testosterone helps to control prostate cancer by opposing estrogen and by activating the p53 gene to induce normal cell death,*

2. He is having his PSA production artificially reduced . . . *even though the PSA is his body's own defense against prostate cancer through its ability to inhibit angiogenesis and thereby slow a tumor's ability to feed itself,*

3. He is having his body thrown into an artificially-induced estrogen dominant state . . . *even though estrogen dominance is known to promote prostate cancer,* and

4. He is having his body thrown into an extremely low-testosterone state . . . *even though low testosterone is known to cause depression, dementia, and an increased likelihood of death from cardiovascular disease as well as from bone fracture complications in the elderly.*

These four situations are at a best, undesirable, and at worst, deadly. Yet a majority of men with prostate cancer will be faced with their doctor prescribing them a hormone-blocking drug. This is why it is so important for men to understand the *real* testosterone connection to PSA and prostate cancer and what PSA and testosterone really do in the body. As mentioned earlier, there are a number of alternative non-toxic methods that have excellent track records for prostate cancer. Specific approaches in *this* book to refer to would be Essiac Tea, Protocel®, Flaxseed Oil and Cottage Cheese, Cesium High pH Therapy, Low Dose Naltrexone, Pau D'Arco, and Ellagic Acid. (Remember, however, that when using Protocel® the PSA count may rise dramatically for a while as the cancer is breaking down.)

For those men who are still not convinced of the dangers of testosterone-blocking drugs and wish to use one while they pursue an alternative treatment approach, virtually no scientific study has been done on the associated impact that blocking testosterone may have on success with alternative therapies. One medical expert, Dr. Bernard Bihari, found this to be a serious issue with his own patients. In his work with non-toxic Low Dose Naltrexone (LDN), Dr. Bihari had a high rate of success putting prostate cancer patients into remission. (See Chapter 17.) However, he discovered that this success only applied to men who were not currently taking, *or who had not previously used* some form of hormone manipulation treatment. According to Bihari, the prostate cancer patients who had used a hormone manipulation treatment for their cancer did not respond as well as other patients did to the Low Dose Naltrexone therapy. This included men who had taken Lupron, Casodex, Eulexin, DES, or other drugs designed to reduce testosterone.

It may not be clear at this point as to what all the ways are that a testosterone-blocking drug could interfere with an alternative approach, other than making a man estrogen-dominant and speeding up the spread of his cancer. But it is particularly alarming that even men who were *no longer on a hormone-blocking drug*, but had taken one before, still did not respond well to Dr. Bihari's treatment.

Hopefully, more and more men will decide to decline hormonal therapy for their prostate cancer. If this is something you are considering, it may not be easy. Your oncologist may not be sympathetic to your decision to turn down what is considered an established medical approach. You may even find that your doctor will refuse to treat you or monitor your progress if you do *not* take a hormone-blocking drug. In that case, you may want to refer him or her to Dr. Lee's booklet *Hormone Balance for Men* for the scientific evidence that blocking testosterone in men with prostate cancer is not a good idea and indeed may cause harm. You may even need to find a different doctor to work with. The bottom line is that men have a right to refuse any treatment they don't want, and it may be time for men with prostate cancer to "just say no" to hormone-blocking drugs.

Resources:

Booklet

John R. Lee, M.D. *Hormone Balance for Men.* $14.95, 28 pages. To order, call (877) 375-3363 or go to www.johnleemd.com and select "Books" then "Booklets and Reports."

Websites

www.johnleemd.com (All of Dr. Lee's books, videotapes, and audiotapes can be ordered from this site.)

www.zrtlabs.com (For hormone testing.)

21

Toxic Teeth

Some of the most disturbing information about aspects of modern living that can contribute to cancer involves common dental practices. However, on the bright side, dealing with some of these dental issues can be a very powerful step to overcoming cancer in certain cases. Although not everyone with cancer has toxic teeth, the information in this chapter may provide some people with an important key that could influence whether or not the treatment they use for "outsmarting" their cancer is successful or not.

There are three main sources of toxic teeth in dental practice today that can contribute to cancer. They are: (1) silver fillings, (2) nickel-alloyed porcelain crowns, and (3) root canals. People who have any of these in their mouths may be carrying around an extra load of carcinogenic substances. Many people are healthy enough to be able to handle this extra load without obvious problems. But others, especially those people who are fighting serious illnesses, may not be.

Silver Fillings

First, let's look at the most common of these three practices—that of installing silver fillings. This type of cavity-filling material is not quite as prevalent today as it used to be, but is still being administered widely. For those of us in our mid-life years, this was the *only* type of dental filling that was ever offered to us as children or young adults. The truth we were not told, however, is that silver fillings are only half silver. Technically, they are silver "amalgams" because they are always combined with another material to make them more pliable. That pliable material, which comprises the other half of the silver filling, is mercury.

Mercury is one of the most deadly substances found on earth, if ingested. Even the *vapor* from mercury is extremely toxic. Most of us have heard the term "mad as a hatter," which was popularized with the mad hatter character in Lewis Carroll's tale of *Alice in Wonderland*. The mad hatter syndrome was prevalent in the 1800s and may have continued into the early 1900s because mercury was used extensively in the hat-making process. A mercury compound called mercury nitrate was commonly used to remove fur from pelts and to produce felt for hats more easily. (Abraham Lincoln's big stovepipe hat was made this way.) The hat-makers themselves were exposed to large amounts of vaporized mercury and began to display symptoms of brain damage. Doctors who did autopsies on hatters sometimes reported seeing large holes inside their brains. Although the use of mercury in hat-making has been banned, the use of mercury in dental fillings has not. Mercury still comprises about 50 percent of all silver (amalgam) fillings.

In some European countries, mercury amalgam fillings have been banned for decades. However, in the United States, they continue to be standard practice, and many dentists are still telling their patients they are completely safe. The true toxic nature of silver-mercury amalgams has been played down by the American Dental Association and most dentists believe the standard line of the ADA. However, other American dentists started wondering years ago how safe amalgams really could be when the instructions they receive with the filling material include some alarming directives. These instructions on how to handle mercury amalgam fillings are still given with the material, and include warnings to dentists such as:

- Don't ever touch it with your fingers.

- Don't leave it lying around uncovered.

- Leftover amalgam material, or an extracted tooth with an amalgam filling still in it, *must* be disposed of under strict toxic waste protocols.

In other words, dentists are warned that the mercury for silver amalgams is too toxic to touch, breathe, or to just throw into the waste basket. (Yet, it's okay to put it into someone's mouth and leave it there for many years.) As a result of instructions such as these, many clear-thinking dentists quietly stopped using amalgam fillings about 20 years ago and started using other materials whenever possible. This had to be done quietly, because dentists who were outspoken about the hazards of silver-mercury fillings often lost their license to practice.

One famous dentist who became probably the most outspoken against amalgam fillings was Dr. Hal Huggins. He wrote a controversial book about this issue and reported many illnesses such as multiple sclerosis, Parkinson's disease, and crippling arthritis that either cleared up or greatly improved when his patients' silver amalgam fillings were safely removed. Since so many of the side effects caused by silver amalgam fillings have been dismissed as "psychosomatic" complaints by doctors, Huggins aptly named his book *It's All in Your Head.*

Although the ADA still seems to hang onto the idea that the mercury in amalgams does not leak out once it is put into someone's mouth, there have been many scientific studies proving that it does indeed leak out into the body. Included in these studies is proof that a significant amount of mercury can get into the brain and stay there. Some researchers believe this is a contributing factor to Alzheimer's disease, since it is known that mercury in the brain can cause the sort of damage that is seen in the brains of Alzheimer's patients.

There are many ways that toxic mercury poisoning from dental work can bring about a gamut of illnesses. One of the ways this can happen is by weakening the immune system in general. Dr. David Eggleston of the University of Southern California measured T-lymphocyte levels in patients with mercury amalgam fillings. As an important contributor to health, T-lymphocytes normally comprise from 70 to 80 percent of the lymphocyte population in a healthy person's immune system. In one case, Eggleston found that a 21-year-old woman with amalgam fillings in her mouth had a T-lymphocyte level at only 47 percent of her total lymphocyte population. He removed her amalgams and replaced them with a plastic type of temporary filling. At that point, her T-lymphocyte levels rose from 47 percent to 73 percent. Next, he removed the plastic fillings and filled the teeth again with amalgam, and her T-lymphocytes fell back down to 55 percent. Finally, Eggleston removed this second set of amalgam fillings and filled the patient's teeth with safe gold inlays. At this point, her T-lymphocyte level went back up to a healthy 72 percent.[1]

It is very likely that a depressed immune system from mercury poisoning can predispose a person to cancer, not to mention the fact that mercury is, itself, a carcinogenic substance. This means that it can also directly *cause* cancer. One cancer story involving mercury amalgams was reported by the son of a dentist named Dr. Pinto. Dr. Pinto first learned about the dangers of amalgams at a conference in the 1920s. According to the story, Dr. Pinto was asked to treat a child who was complaining that her gums hurt. The child was also dying of leukemia. To try to save the child, Dr. Pinto quietly removed all of her amalgam fillings. This child's condition dramatically responded in just of few days and her doctors actually pronounced her leukemia as a case of "spontaneous remission."

Dr. Pinto then told the physician that he had removed her amalgams, but the physician and others in the medical profession wouldn't believe that had anything to do with the remission. To try to get through to them, Dr. Pinto re-inserted one amalgam filling in the little girl's mouth and told the doctor to look for a recurrence of the leukemia. There *was* a recurrence of symptoms, and Dr. Pinto then removed the amalgam filling, which was followed again by the child's recovery.[2]

Dr. Pinto did further research into the historical occurrences of certain types of diseases and found that Hodgkin's disease, another type of cancer, was virtually unheard of until 1832, shortly after amalgam fillings had been introduced into the very region where the first case of Hodgkin's disease was discovered. Unfortunately, no one in the dental profession would listen to Dr. Pinto.

However, recent research on amalgam fillings has been conclusive enough to cause some serious changes around the world. For instance, the government of Sweden performed its own research and concluded that 250,000 Swedes had immune system and other health disorders related to their amalgams. The Swedish government then put amalgam use on a schedule for complete phase-out. In 1994, a German company called Degussa, the world's largest producer of metals for use in dentistry, shut down its production of amalgam completely. Degussa apparently took the stance that it would reinstate the production of amalgam after mercury had been proved safe for the body. There are at least four European countries that currently have either banned the use of amalgam fillings for children and women of child-bearing age, or have put amalgam use on a schedule toward complete phase-out.

Even though the United States has not banned amalgam use, one survey published in the December 1989 issue of *Dentist* magazine reported that over one-third of the dentists polled *did* believe that all silver amalgam fillings should be removed and replaced with composite fillings. Yet, dentists who feel this way in the United States are up against very powerful opposing forces that appear to control the policies of the ADA. As of 1994, the ADA "Code of Professional Conduct" stated:

> . . . the ADA has determined through the adoption of Resolution 42H-1986 that the removal of amalgam restoration from the non-allergic patient for the alleged purpose of removing toxic substances from the body, when such treatment is performed solely at the recommendation or suggestion of the dentist, is improper and unethical.[3]

A CBS *60 Minutes* program aired a segment on the amalgam controversy in December 1990. Although it received one of the highest viewer responses ever, this segment was *not* repeated. Moreover, the Washington State Dental Association's response to this program was to immediately inform its dentist members that their patients "did not have a right to know that their 'silver fillings' contained mercury."[4]

The difficulty with this controversial issue is that not everybody with amalgam fillings has cancer or some other obvious illness. This is because many people's immune systems are strong enough to withstand the damage that the mercury does to the body. However, if you *are already* dealing with a serious illness, you may want to consider having your amalgam fillings safely replaced with another material.

What is *critical* to understand, however, is that there are safe ways to do this and unsafe ways. If you rush out and have your amalgams removed quickly by a dentist who does not understand the safety precautions required, you may be risking *even more damage to your health*. Sloppy removal of silver amalgam fillings can release even more mercury into your system than was leaking out before. You should definitely understand this issue if you are fighting a terminal illness and you opt for amalgam replacement. In fact, you may want to seek out the services of a "biological dentist." (This is a more and more common description of dentists who specialize in understanding and working with toxic teeth issues.)

When planning to get your silver amalgams replaced, two safety precautions to discuss with your dentist are the following:

1. Request a rubber dam. This is a piece of rubber designed to stretch between the lower right and left teeth with only the tooth being worked on uncovered. Its purpose is to keep any small pieces of

amalgam filling from falling onto your tongue or down your throat.

2. Request oxygen during the procedure. When amalgam fillings are removed, they must be drilled out. This can release mercury vapor into the air. The patient's nose, being closest to this vapor, can readily breathe it in. Your dentist should be able to provide an oxygen tube directly to your nose so that you breathe in clean oxygen rather than toxic vapor.

Once your amalgams are removed and replaced with a safe material, you may also want to opt for chelation. This is not always necessary, but is a way to get rid of any remaining mercury that may have gotten into your body. The most important thing to remember, however, is that the amalgams need to be removed *safely* in the first place.

If you are someone who is already dealing with cancer, unsafe removal of amalgam fillings may cause a worsening of your disease. In fact, if you are currently using an alternative treatment that you believe is effectively working on your cancer, you may not want to have your amalgams removed until *after* you are cancer-free. But if you are finding that your alternative cancer treatment is not working as effectively as you think it should, or if you are a healthy person and just want to avoid a cancer diagnosis, then seeking out a qualified dentist who knows how to safely remove silver amalgam fillings can be a great help to your health.

Nickel-Alloyed Porcelain Crowns

Although the toxicity of mercury in silver amalgam fillings is becoming more and more accepted, the toxicity of certain types of porcelain crowns and their possible link to cancer is not so widely accepted. Yet, about 75 percent of *all* crowns, including porcelain crowns, contain nickel, which is known to be an incredibly toxic substance and a powerful carcinogen. The way that porcelain crowns contain nickel is not in the white porcelain covering itself, but in the stainless steel inner metal band that the porcelain is bonded to for strength. What we aren't generally told is that this stainless steel is usually alloyed with nickel. The old-fashioned metal braces (used for straightening teeth) were also generally a stainless steel nickel alloy, and partial dentures often employ this form of alloy as well.

According to Dr. Eggleston, "Nickel is not nearly as active as mercury, however it corrodes and is far more carcinogenic."[5] In fact, Dr. Eggleston states that the nickel alloys being used in dental practices today are actually quite similar to a form of nickel that is commonly used by cancer research centers around the country to induce cancer in lab animals.

Two reported human cases involving nickel-alloyed porcelain crowns are particularly disturbing. The first one involves kidney disease, and the other involves breast cancer. The first story was a case of Dr. Eggleston's and is described by him. It involved a female patient who was admitted to Long Beach Memorial Hospital with kidney disease. However, the doctors attempting to treat her could not find the cause of her kidney problem. Her family physician then suggested special tests, which ended up showing she was highly reactive to nickel. The patient's doctor then asked her if she'd had any dental work done in the past seven years. She replied that she did have three porcelain crowns put in by her dentist. The doctor, knowing that porcelain crowns often have nickel-alloyed metal jackets underneath, suggested she get the crowns removed right away. The patient did this, and all of her kidney failure symptoms went away.

The other story involved breast cancer and was presented on one Internet site as told by Dr. Hal Huggins. According to Dr. Huggins, he came across a woman who had undergone a lumpectomy for breast cancer. While attending a support group for cancer in her area, she brought up the subject of the possible link between nickel crowns and breast cancer, since her husband had heard something about this from another source. One of the other women in the group replied that she had gone to a particular dentist down the street who had put nickel crowns in her mouth, and a couple of years later she developed the same type of breast tumor the first woman had undergone a lumpectomy for. It turned out that they both had gone to the same dentist, and both had gotten crowns put in. Then, these women found a third woman who had gone to the same dentist, gotten a crown, and *also* developed the same type of breast tumor. Amazingly, with a little more investigation, these women found a fourth woman, a fifth, and then a sixth—all who had gone to the same dentist, had one or more crowns put in, and who later came down with the same type of breast tumor.[6]

Coincidence? Possibly. It could also be that toxins or pesticides in that geographical region were contributing to this type of breast cancer. But the fact that there are thousands of articles that refer to nickel as a carcinogen make this sort of situation definitely worth investigating. How many other women, or men, have *paid dentists or orthodontists big money to unknowingly promote cancer in their bodies?*

As already pointed out, approximately 75 percent of the crowns placed currently in peoples' mouths in America contain nickel, which means that about 25 percent of them don't contain nickel. This is partly because gold alloys not containing nickel are also used sometimes as a metal base for crowns. It is also partly because, in recent years, the hardening process for porcelain used in dental applications has gotten better so that some crowns now do not use any metal at all and, instead, are 100 percent porcelain.

So there *is* a chance that, if you have a porcelain crown in your mouth, it might not contain nickel. But this could be worth calling your dental office about since, when nickel based crowns are used, the patient is generally not told this. And when asked directly, a common response from your dentist or orthodontist might be that what you're getting is "stainless steel." This certainly sounds good, but if you want to be sure, you must make it clear that you know stainless steel for dental work is generally alloyed with some other metal and that you want to know *specifically* if the stainless steel in your mouth is alloyed with nickel.

If you are told that the crown in your mouth is gold-based, then you are most likely better off. Gold in itself is not toxic or carcinogenic. However, gold is way too soft to be used by itself in dental procedures and is always alloyed with a stiffer metal for dental work. Therefore, you must also be sure that you know what the gold in your mouth has been alloyed with if you want to know whether it may be causing you illness or not. As far as I know, gold alloyed with platinum is a common and safe metal combination.

If you are unsure about the materials in your dental crown or crowns, you might look into being tested for levels of nickel in your body as an indicator. One way this can be done is through a hair analysis procedure.

Root Canals

So far, we have discussed silver-mercury amalgam fillings and nickel-alloyed crowns. Now, we come to the dental practice of administering "root canal" procedures. The very common practice of administering root canals may unfortunately be one of the biggest dental problems today because so many current dentists don't even know about the dangers of this type of treatment. In other words, many intelligent dentists will refuse to put mercury or nickel in people's mouths, but they will go right ahead and happily perform any number of root canals on their patients without any idea of the damage these procedures can cause.

Basically, a root canal is a procedure that is done when tooth decay or infection has advanced so far that the nerve in the root area of the tooth has become infected. The root canal is a narrow canal that runs from about the middle of the tooth down to the tips, or roots, of the tooth which are firmly buried in the jawbone. Front teeth have a single root into the jawbone and back teeth have two.

A healthy tooth contains a root canal that is lined with pink living tissue filled with tiny blood vessels, all of which surround a main nerve running down the center of the root and eventually connecting to other nerves in the surrounding jaw. Once this nerve is infected, the patient generally comes into the dentist's office in some degree of pain. This is in contrast to the more common dental decay that is confined to the hard shell of the tooth and is usually not painful because it does not involve nerves. When the nerve area in the tooth is infected, the most common procedure for the dentist to perform is called a "root canal." In doing this, the dentist removes the nerve and cleans out the entire root canal area, which is usually infected as well to some degree. Then, the inside of the tooth is disinfected, filled with some form of filling material, and sealed up again, usually with a crown on top.

The positive side of the root canal procedure is that the tooth remains in your mouth and does not have to be extracted. This allows the tooth to remain functional for chewing purposes, as well as to look good when you smile. On the negative side, the root canal-filled tooth is now a "dead" tooth because the inside living tissue and the tiny blood vessels that would normally bring nourishment to the tooth have been removed. Almost all root canal procedures appear, on the surface, to be wonderful solutions because rarely does the patient have any *noticeable* problem with the tooth itself after the procedure is done. Most dentists enjoy the fact that they rarely have a patient come back with complaints about a root canal-filled tooth.

The big problem, however, lies in the fact that the damage done by the root canal procedure is almost *never* noticeable at the location of the tooth. This of course is similar to the toxic effects of mercury from amalgams and nickel from crowns. But at least we know that mercury and nickel are extremely toxic substances, and we can test for those substances in the body with hair analyses and other procedures. Side effects from a root canal-filled tooth are much more difficult to pinpoint. The irony of the situation is that there may actually be more definitive research on the dangers of the root canal procedure than there is on any other type of toxic dental practice! But there is far less awareness of this research because it has been largely ignored by the dental profession for over 75 years.

The bulk of the research on root canal procedures was done between about 1900 to 1925 by a respected dentist named Dr. Weston A. Price. Dr. Price was a dedicated and thorough researcher who conducted meticulous laboratory research with a 60-man team. Over a 25-year period he conducted experiments on 5,000 lab animals after which he recorded and published his results in a two-volume report totaling 1,174 pages. Dr. Price also published 220 articles and two additional books, which can be found in the dental and medical literature.

It is extremely unfortunate for all of us that few dentists today have even heard of Dr. Weston Price and his research. In an effort to remedy this lack of awareness a noted dentist, Dr. George E. Meinig, recently undertook the mission of carefully reading all 1,174 pages of Dr. Price's two-volume report. Dr. Meinig then condensed Price's findings about the dangers of root canals into a much smaller and easy-to-read contemporary book called, *The Root Canal Cover-Up*. Dr. Meinig had the perfect background and experience to do this because he, himself, had practiced and taught root canal therapy, and was one of the founding members of the American Association of Endodontists (root canal practitioners).

According to Dr. Meinig, what Price and other researchers have been able to prove is that there is an unavoidable problem with the root canal procedure. The problem is that, no matter how much a dentist tries to disinfect the inside of the tooth after the root area has been cleaned out, there is really no way that all of the infection can be reached. This is because teeth contain microscopically small tubules that run through the dentin like a huge lattice of caverns in a mountain. The purpose of these tubules when the tooth is alive is to transport nourishment-carrying fluid and oxygen throughout the tooth. Thus, a healthy tooth is very much alive. To give you an idea of just how extensive this lattice of tubules is, it is estimated that if you were able to string all the tubules from just one average front tooth together, end-to-end, they would reach about 3 miles long. And since back teeth are much larger than front teeth, their tubules placed end-to-end would reach considerably farther.

Once infection has progressed into the depths of these microscopically small tubules in any tooth, there will inevitably be a certain number of bacteria that have roamed so deep that no disinfectant can reach them. So there will invariably be some number of bacteria that are still left alive in the tubules of the dentin after the root canal procedure is done and the tooth is filled and closed back up again.

But the root canal-filled tooth is now dead. There is no longer a supply of nourishment going in and out of the tooth, and there is no longer any fluid flowing into and out of the tubules. Without fluid flowing through the tubules, there is no mechanism for transporting antibiotics to the trapped bacteria. More importantly, there is no longer any transport of oxygen throughout the intricate maze of tubules. So the bacteria, which started out as normal "aerobic" bacteria, may now mutate to survive and become "anaerobic" bacteria. Unfortunately, the *anaerobic forms* of these bacteria can be much more dangerous than the aerobic form originally was and Dr. Price discovered that the entombed anaerobic bacteria are capable of creating powerful toxins that can then leak into the tissue surrounding the tooth. Once these toxins leak out of the tooth, they can get into a person's bloodstream and travel throughout the entire body.

Back in the early 1900s, after suspecting that some of the chronic illnesses of his patients were linked to root canal-filled teeth, Dr. Price started extracting those teeth. Then, by simply taking a piece of the extracted root canal-filled tooth and embedding this piece of tooth under the skin of a rabbit, he found that the rabbit would develop the same type of illness the person had!

For instance, Dr. Price found if he took a small piece of a root canal-filled tooth that had been extracted from a person who'd had a heart attack and placed it under the skin of a rabbit, that rabbit would die of a heart attack in about 10 days. He could then take that same piece of tooth *out* of the dead rabbit and put it under the skin of another rabbit, and in about 10 days, *that* rabbit would also die of a heart attack. Price found he could do this over and over with the same piece of tooth and get the same result for up to about 30 rabbits.

Moreover, heart disease only occurred in Price's lab animals when the person the root canal-filled tooth had come from had suffered from heart disease. If the person had suffered from another illness, *that* would be the illness that would show up in the rabbit. For instance, if the patient from whom the tooth was taken was suffering from kidney disease, then the rabbit with the piece of that person's tooth embedded in it would also develop kidney disease.

Dr. Price's first clinical case involved arthritis. In that case, he removed a root canal-filled tooth from a woman with severe arthritis and implanted the extracted tooth under the skin of a rabbit. Within 48 hours, the rabbit had developed crippling arthritis. Furthermore, after extraction of this tooth, the woman's arthritis improved dramatically. Dr. Price performed these types of experiments over and over, and kept getting the same results. Very rarely, did the rabbit *not* come down with the very illness the human patient was suffering from.

Price was a thorough researcher and he, of course, tested the possibility that just putting part of a human tooth into an animal was the problem. But he found that if he did the same procedure using a perfectly healthy, non-root-canal-filled tooth, then the rabbit would suffer no ill effects whatsoever. He also found that if he sterilized the piece of root canal-filled tooth first by using a powerful procedure involving steam heat, then the rabbit would suffer no ill effects, either.

Dr. Price found a high number of chronic degenerative diseases to be linked to root canal-filled teeth. The most common appeared to be various forms of heart and circulatory diseases, presumably because the toxins from anaerobic bacteria in the teeth leaked into and circulated throughout the bloodstream. Other chronic conditions that his research linked to root canal-filled teeth were various forms of arthritis, nervous system disorders, and even digestive disorders. For more detailed information about Price's discoveries regarding the toxic nature of root canal-filled teeth, I highly recommend Meinig's book, *Root Canal Cover-Up*.

A poignant description of the root canal procedure was given by Dr. Hal Huggins in a lecture he gave to the Cancer Control Society in 1993. Huggins stated, in his usual colorful way,

> . . . Then we get into the root canal business, and that is the most tragic of all. Isn't there something you can put in the center of the canal that is safe? Yeah, there probably is, but that is not where the problem is. The problem with a root canal is that it is dead. Let's equate that. Let's say you have got a ruptured appendix, so you go to the phone book, and who do you look up? Let's see, we have a surgeon and a taxidermist, who do you call? You going to get it bronzed? That is all we do to a dead tooth. We put a gold crown on it, looks like it has been bronzed. It doesn't really matter what you embalm the dead tooth with, it is still dead, and within that dead tooth we have bacteria, and these bacteria are in the absence of oxygen. In the absence of oxygen most things die except bacteria. They undergo something called a pleomorphic change—like a mutation. They learn to live in the absence of oxygen (and) now produce thioethers, some of the strongest poisons on the planet that are not radioactive.[7]

Huggins went on to say in this lecture that the thioethers do escape into the body's bloodstream and he points out a correlation between the increase in the rate of heart attacks in the United States since the early 1900s, and the corresponding increase in the practice of performing root canals. This would be consistent with what Dr. Price found in his research, which was that the predominant damage caused by root canals was to the cardiovascular system of the body since the mode of travel for the toxins is through the bloodstream.

The main problem in accepting the dangers of root canals over the years has been expressed in a debate over the "focal infection" theory. This is the theoretical idea that an infection focused in one part of the body can have a detrimental effect on a distant part of the body. Even though this debate continues, there are some transplant surgeons today who require root canal-filled teeth to be extracted before they will perform an organ transplant in a patient. This is because these surgeons believe there is a risk that focal infections in teeth might affect the new organ.

Josef Issels, M.D., of Germany, a world-famous cancer specialist, took the dangers of root-filled teeth very seriously. Dr. Issels was probably the first physician to require all of his cancer patients to have their dead teeth extracted as a part of his normal cancer treatment protocol. Over a 40-year period of working with more than 16,000 cancer patients, Issels had one of the highest total remission rates with late stage terminal cancer patients of any cancer practitioner. He also found that a survey of his cancer patients showed over 90 percent of them to have between two and 10 dead teeth in their mouths when they first arrived at his clinic for treatment.

In his well-written, in-depth book, *Cancer—A Second Opinion*, Dr. Issels talks about his research with root canals. In Chapter 8, titled "Focus on Foci," Issels found that dead teeth left in the mouth can become *toxin factories* and do, in fact, produce thioethers. Moreover, he presents very convincing evidence that thioethers have all of the qualifications of a substance capable of causing spontaneous cancer in humans.

Dr. Issels's writing is highly technical, and he uses medical terminology that is often difficult for the layperson to understand. But one simple experiment he reports is quite clear and impressive. Issels found that he could use an infrared-sensitive instrument to measure the level of infrared emission anywhere in a person's body. In doing so, he found that the infrared emission on the outer skin next to a root canal-filled tooth was elevated slightly higher than the area around healthy teeth. He could also monitor the infrared emission around a cancerous tumor area.

What Dr. Issels found was that, when a dead tooth in a cancer patient was treated (presumably by extraction), the corresponding infrared emission of that area of the mouth decreased, *and the infrared emission of the person's tumor area also decreased at the same time.*[8] Thus, he proved a definite interrelationship between the dead tooth and the cancer.

Yet another possible relationship between root canal-filled teeth and cancer may have to do with a different mechanism than toxins. This mechanism involves acupuncture meridians. Although little research has been done on this subject, one alternative cancer practitioner, Dr. John Diamond of Reno, Nevada, has said, "I have a number of patients with breast cancer, all of whom had root canals on the tooth related to the breast area on the associated energy meridian."[9] This is certainly something to think about for anyone with any type of cancer.

Of course, we all know people who have root canal-filled teeth in their mouths and appear to be perfectly healthy. This seems to confuse the issue. One alternative doctor clarified this issue in the following way. He said, "Root canals are like mortgages. As long as you can make enough money to pay the payment every month, everything is fine. But once you *can't* make the payment, then you're in big trouble!"[10] In other words, it is the strength of the immune system and the body in general that determines whether or not a root canal-filled tooth is going to bring about obvious health problems in any individual. This could be applied to the effects of mercury amalgam fillings and nickel-alloyed crowns as well. With diet, stress levels, and other factors varying greatly from person to person, the effects of these dental practices are necessarily going to vary from person to person also.

As with amalgam removal, having your root canal-filled teeth removed *safely* is of utmost importance. If your dentist or oral surgeon does not fully understand the issues of toxicity, there could be a danger that after the dead tooth is removed, toxic infection still remains in the surrounding bone socket. Once more, seeking out a competent biological dentist who knows how to safely extract root canal-filled teeth is a good idea. On pages 193–194 of his book, *Root Canal Cover-Up*, Dr. Meinig details how a root canal-filled tooth should be removed to ensure that none of the infection is left behind, and it might be a good idea to make sure your dentist or oral surgeon is familiar with those instructions in Meinig's book.

Although it is common practice for endodontists to leave behind the periodontal ligament when a tooth is extracted, Dr. Meinig and Dr. Hal Huggins both believe it is likely for root canal infections to have infected this ligament as well. They both recommend total removal of this ligament along with approximately 1 millimeter of surrounding jawbone following extractions. This procedure usually causes any residual infection from the root canal-filled tooth to be removed.

One last word of caution is warranted. Some alternative cancer specialists recommend that people who are in a weakened state from cancer may not be strong enough to have all of their toxic teeth dealt with at once. For some people, it might be best to have toxic teeth addressed slowly, over time. Again, consulting with a knowledgeable alternative cancer specialist, if possible, is a good idea.

Resources:

Books

Hal A. Huggins, D.D.S. *It's All in Your Head: The Link Between Mercury Amalgams and Illness.* Garden City Park, New York: Avery Publishing Group, 1993.

George E. Meinig, D.D.S, F.A.C.D. *Root-Canal Cover-Up.* Ojai, California: Bion Publishing, 1998.

Josef Issels, M.D. *Cancer—A Second Opinion.* Garden City Park, New York: Avery Publishing Group, 1999.

Websites

www.curezone.com/dental/root_canal.html

www.price-pottenger.org

www.whale.to/d/cancer.html

www.yourhealthbase.com/amalgams.html

22

Evaluating Conventional Methods

Are conventional cancer treatments ever warranted? Yes. For instance, surgery alone may sometimes be a curative approach when a tumor is localized and caught early. Other situations may warrant some amount of conventional treatment as well. For instance, if a person's tumor is so large that it is restricting a vital organ, or if the cancer is so advanced that there is not enough time left for an alternative treatment to have a chance to work, then immediate surgery, chemotherapy, or radiation, may be used to one's advantage. However, this is often simply short-term damage control. When it comes to long-term recovery, the efficacy of toxic conventional treatments is a different story.

The current medical establishment would like us to believe that *most* cancers, if caught early, are curable with standard medical techniques. Impressive-sounding conventional cure-rate statistics are advertised. But these statistics are achievable only after *gross* statistical manipulations have been done, and after key terms like "cure" have been re-defined. To review from Chapter 1, the following are six major ways that official cancer cure-rate statistics are often fudged so that conventional methods for treating cancer can look better than they really are:

1. By re-defining "cure" as *alive five years after diagnosis*, instead of using the word's real meaning, which is "cancer-free."

2. By simply omitting certain groups of people, such as African Americans, or by omitting certain types of cancer, such as all lung cancer patients, from the official statistical calculations.

3. By including types of cancer that are *not* life-threatening and are easily curable, such as skin cancers and DCIS.

4. By allowing earlier detection to erroneously imply longer survival.

5. By deleting patients from cancer treatment studies who die too soon, even if that is on day 89 of a 90-day chemotherapy protocol.

6. By using a questionable adjustment called "relative survival rate."

The problem is that if you are dealing with life-threatening cancer, the misleading official statistics are the numbers that will be offered to you as representative of your chances of survival, should you choose conventional treatment. It is critical that you understand how to *accurately* evaluate conventional cancer treatment methods because your life literally depends on the treatment decisions you make.

The Big Three—Surgery, Chemotherapy, and Radiation

What *are* the real statistics on conventional medicine's "big three" cancer treatments today? Unfortunately, nobody knows. Nobody *can* know when there are no data in mainstream medicine that reflect real cures. The only data we have to work with are figures that reflect the phony re-definition of the term "cure," that talk about short-term results, and that are recorded selectively in the first place in ways that defy correct statistical methodology. Thus, trying to figure out the *true* cure-rate statistics for conventional cancer treatments is a lot like trying to figure out which cup the magician's red ball is under.

Having said that, there are a number of things you *can* learn about conventional cancer treatment efficacy. For instance, out of all the conventional cancer treatments available today, it is probably safe to say that surgery alone has the best track record. Cancer researcher, Dr. Ralph Moss, claims that *most* of the conventional cancer cures today can be attributed to surgery alone.[1] However, the types of cases where surgery can be effective in a long-term way apply to only a small percentage of cancer patients. For instance, everyone agrees that surgery is virtually helpless as a curative procedure in any case where the cancer has already metastasized, and unfortunately, the *majority* of cancer patients are told they have metastasized cancer at the time they are first diagnosed.

Thus, for most people with cancer, surgery is no more than a "palliative" treatment (meaning it cannot save the patient, but is merely performed in the hope that it will buy the patient some time). For surgery to have a chance at actually being curative, it must be performed at a very early stage, before the cancer has spread past the primary site. Even for many of these cases, surgery cannot guarantee recovery. Some medical experts believe that there are early cancer situations where surgery may even cause the cancer to spread throughout the body by releasing free-floating cancer cells into the bloodstream or lymph system. But overall, the use of surgery alone probably still accounts for the largest number of long-term survival cases in conventional cancer treatment. And the best chance for long-term recovery through surgery may be when an entire organ can be removed (such as the thyroid gland, prostate gland, uterus, ovaries, etc.)

After surgery, we have radiation and chemotherapy. Unfortunately, the true long-term effectiveness of these methods can only be seen as *dismal*. Some studies have even produced evidence that cancer patients may be able to live longer *without* these treatments. For example, a *Science News* article, published August 1, 1998, presented a review of data about radiation treatment after surgery for lung cancer. The immense amount of data, which was collected from nine studies over a 30-year period, actually showed the two-year survival rate after lung cancer surgery to be 48 percent for patients who got post-surgical radiation treatments, and 55 percent for patients who underwent surgery alone. In other words, more patients who did *not* receive radiation treatments after surgery lived to the two-year mark than those who *did* receive radiation after surgery.

When it comes to chemotherapy, which is prescribed to about four out of five people with cancer in the United States today, Ralph Moss states in his book, *Questioning Chemotherapy:*

> A close look at chemotherapy yields some major surprises. Few would dispute its usefulness in acute lymphocytic leukemia, Hodgkin's disease, testicular and ovarian cancer, and a handful of rare tumors, mainly of childhood. But evidence for the life-prolonging effect in other common malignancies is weak, even for those cancers in which almost certainly it has some marginal success. And proof is simply non-existent for the majority of cancers, especially the advanced carcinomas.
>
> Even for the common cancers in which chemotherapy "works," such as small-cell lung cancer, the actual survival benefit is reckoned in weeks

or months, not in years. And during this time, the patient is likely to experience major, even life-threatening side effects from the treatment. Thus, the overall advantage to the patient is moot.[2]

Thus, the official claims of success for toxic treatments such as radiation and chemotherapy often refer to short-term effectiveness only. We will be going into more detail about radiation and chemotherapy in the next few pages, but first, let's look at the very important difference between "short-term" and "long-term" effectiveness.

Short-Term Versus Long-Term Effectiveness

Studying and quoting short-term effectiveness is just one tactic of a medical establishment that is *not* having success with long-term effectiveness. Since mainstream medicine is losing its war on cancer, it is very beneficial for those in charge to only study short-term effectiveness. This way, the actual long-term effectiveness (or *real* effectiveness) of conventional treatment does not have to be considered. Better yet, long-term side effects of treatment (which may kill the patient a few years down the line) do not have to be considered.

For example, in Chapter 19, we saw that many European studies showed the use of Tamoxifen for breast cancer to have no overall long-term survival benefit at all. According to Dr. Lee, Tamoxifen can temporarily suppress tumors, and that is why the short-term studies done in the United States made Tamoxifen look so good. However, the long-term studies done on Tamoxifen in Europe showed breast tumors *coming back* at just about the period of time when the studies in the United States were being cut short. The short-term U.S. studies did not show all the deaths caused by Tamoxifen's side effects later, such as from fatal blood clots in the lungs, stroke, liver dysfunction, or from uterine cancer, all of which can be directly caused by the Tamoxifen drug treatment.

But the most ludicrous aspect of short-term attention to conventional treatments is represented by how the term "cure" is re-defined. By re-defining the meaning of "cure" as *alive five years after diagnosis*, our current conventional cancer establishment is basically saying that the medical establishment considers five-year survival to be the best they can aspire to. Make no mistake—by labeling anyone with cancer who reaches the five-year mark as "cured," conventional medicine is proclaiming that once you have lived five years after diagnosis, they have done a great job—even if you still have cancer and have been miserably sick the whole five years. This official tactic of re-defining the word "cure" also frequently creates the ironic situation where a cancer patient can be listed as cured in the official statistics data base, yet *die from their cancer* a short while later!

Maybe for some people, living another five years is a great thing. For instance, it may be wonderful for those who are quite elderly when they are diagnosed with cancer, and they just want to live a few more years. But what if you are 25 or 40 years old, or 50 or 60? Living only five more years is not good at all! Or maybe you are one of many people raising small children when you are diagnosed with cancer. Most parents do not just want to see their children become teenagers—they also want to see them become adults, go to college, get married, have their own children, and so forth. And if it is your *child* who has been diagnosed with cancer, then to aspire to your child living just five more years is simply unacceptable.

One of the most important things to know when considering treatment for cancer is whether or not the statistics your oncologist presents to you reflect "long-term" or "short-term" effectiveness. After all, *you obviously want a long-term, not a short-term, recovery!*

Response Rates

One way that short-term results are used by mainstream medicine to imply long-term effectiveness is by the common conventional practice of studying and quoting cancer treatment "response rates." In mainstream medicine, the "response rate" of a particular treatment is often quoted as if it means *recovery rate*, or *cure rate*. But this is just another way that people seeking cancer treatment are misled by meaningless numbers. The phrase "response rate" is *not* synonymous to "recovery rate" or "cure rate." Quite the contrary. Common conventional cancer studies define a "response" as simply meaning a 50 percent reduction in tumor size over a particular period of time (usually about 28 days).

Because chemotherapy and radiation are "cytotoxic" (toxic to cells), it is easy to make malignant tumors shrink for a time when bombarded with these types of toxic treatments. However, that merely means that the tumor has died a little after being poisoned or burned. If there are any cancer cells left alive *after* the treatment, which there virtually always are, then the tumor will start growing again as soon as there is a break in the treatment. Since toxic treatments generally involve time breaks in their administration to let the patient's overall body recover, cancerous tumors often have a chance to grow back.

Thus, when tumor response rates are quoted, these rates do *not* indicate that patients regained their good health or their cancers were overcome. Response rates are just a convenient way for conventional cancer researchers to report the short-term *partial* effectiveness of a particular treatment. As Ralph Moss, Ph.D. states,

> It is one of the central fallacies of chemotherapy that shrinkages or 'response rates' have been proven to correlate with increased survival time. Yet, in answer to a patient's inevitable question, 'What are my chances?' the doctor may give impressive-sounding 'response rates' of, say, 60 percent.[3]

In other words, if your doctor tells you that the cancer treatment he or she is recommending to you has a response rate of 60 percent, you should know that what that *really* means is this: 60 percent of the time, that particular treatment protocol will cause tumors to "shrink" by at least half for at least a month. It does *not* mean that 60 percent of the cancer patients who get that treatment will become cancer-free.

Since toxic cancer treatments can often damage vital organs and suppress the immune system, the use of toxic treatments that are unable to effect a long-term cure must always beg the question as to whether or not the patient might have lived longer *without* the treatment. W. John Diamond, M.D., and W. Lee Cowden, M.D., report on this issue in their book, *An Alternative Medicine Definitive Guide to Cancer*. In it, they write:

> Virtually all the FDA-approved anticancer drugs are markedly *immunosuppressive*, because they ruin a person's natural resistance to disease, including cancer. Ulrich Abel, Ph.D., of the Heidelberg Tumor Center in Germany, conducted a comprehensive review of the world literature on survival among cancer patients receiving chemotherapy. He found that chemotherapy can help only 3 percent of the patients with epithelial cancers (e.g., cancers of the breast, lung, prostate, and colon). These cancers account for about 80 percent of all cancer deaths. In a study of chemotherapy-treated breast cancer patients, the researchers concluded, 'Survival may even have been shortened in some [breast cancer] patients given chemotherapy'.[4]

A few pages later, Dr. Diamond and Dr. Cowden follow with:

> German cancer researcher Ulrich Abel, Ph.D., observes that the

temporary shrinking of a tumor mass—defined as either a partial or complete remission—is not necessarily a good sign, because the remaining tumor cells often grow much faster and more virulently after the first series of chemotherapy treatments. Highly aggressive chemotherapy actually shortens survival times compared with patients in whom chemotherapy was delayed or administered less aggressively, says Dr. Abel. Paradoxically, patients whose tumors showed no response to chemotherapy actually survived longer than patients who did respond.[5]

Dr. Diamond and Dr. Cowden also report on evidence that some men with prostate cancer may survive longer without radiation treatments. They write:

> Radiation therapy—implanting radiation seeds in the prostate gland—routinely given for early signs of prostate cancer can actually hasten the development of that cancer. Prostate cells can double in as little as 1.2 months after radiation treatment while unradiated prostate cancer cells may take an average of 4 years to double.[6]

It is extremely misleading for doctors to allow cancer patients to believe that quoted "response rates" are the same as "recovery rates." It may be that many doctors who quote response rates don't know, themselves, the real meaning of what they are quoting. But for you, the person trying to get well, knowing the real meaning of response rate statistics will help you to more correctly evaluate treatment methods you may be considering.

Damage to the Heart

There are many ways that short-term effectiveness of conventional cancer treatments can look very good for a while, yet long-term effectiveness turns out to be *not* good at all. For instance, radiation to the chest area for either lung cancer or breast cancer can cause damage to the heart severe enough to cause a fatal heart attack at some point in the future. If the heart attack does not occur until the patient has been pronounced in remission, then the radiation treatment will look like it was successful. Deaths from subsequent heart attacks caused by cancer treatment do *not* have to be folded into the cancer treatment statistics. As mentioned in Chapter 19, one study on radiation treatment given to women with breast cancer showed that the use of radiation *did* reduce deaths from breast cancer by 13.2 percent, and this was most likely the figure that was publicly advertised. However, this same radiation *increased* deaths from *other* causes (mostly heart failure) by 21.2 percent!

Can Radiation or Chemotherapy *Cause* Cancer?

One fact that is often difficult for many people to believe is that many of the conventional treatments for cancer commonly used today are actually carcinogenic. This means they *can cause a secondary cancer to develop* a few years later, provided that the patient is lucky enough to survive their first cancer that long. This is just another way that short-term effectiveness of conventional cancer treatments may look good, while the long-term effectiveness may not look good at all.

Radiation-Induced Cancer

Evidence that radiation treatments can cause cancer goes back to the early days of X-ray technology. In *The Cancer Industry*, Ralph Moss reports:

> In 1902 a German doctor recorded the first case of human cancer caused by radiation: the tumor had appeared on the site of a chronic ulceration caused by X-ray exposure. Experimental studies performed in 1906 suggested that leukemia (cancer of the blood) could be caused by exposure to the radioactive element radium. By 1911, 94 cases of radiation-induced cancer had been reported, more than half of them (54) in doctors or technicians. By 1922, over 100 radiologists had died from X-ray-induced cancer, and many other research workers, laboratory assistants, and technicians had also succumbed. . . .[7]

More and more cases of people developing cancer due to X-ray technology were reported in the early to mid-1900s. Then, when radiation started being used as a treatment for cancer, secondary radiation-induced cancers began to be reported. Today, it is *well-known* that radiation treatments for cancer may also cause secondary cancers.

In her video, *Cancer Doesn't Scare Me Anymore*, Dr. Lorraine Day shows medical manuals that list the possibility of secondary cancers due to radiation treatment. She also talks about the many *other* serious and life-threatening side effects that can be caused by radiation treatments for cancer. Dr. Day makes the point that the ACS, AMA, and FDA refer to radiation treatments as "safe and effective" for cancer patients, yet radiation technicians, doctors, and nurses are all urged to protect themselves against much lower, indirect doses of the same radiation by wearing lead vests and carrying out other protective measures. In other words, it is quite ironic that extremely high exposure to directed radiation is considered safe for anyone with cancer, yet low indirect exposure is considered extremely dangerous for healthy radiation technicians!

All oncologists are well aware of radiation-induced secondary cancers in patients. An example is the real-life case of one woman who was able to successfully beat her breast cancer only to find herself facing another life-threatening cancer 10 years later. This time, she was facing inoperable metastasized lung cancer that her oncologist was convinced had been caused by the radiation treatments to her breast years before. Thus, while radiation treatments may be necessary in some cases where cancer is extremely advanced and needs to be reduced quickly, they are *never* without risk. Understanding this and only using radiation when absolutely necessary is important.

Chemotherapy-Induced Cancer

Many people are already aware that some sources of radiation can cause cancer because they have heard reports of cancer resulting from nuclear fallout, radiation accidents, and so forth. But it seems counter-intuitive that a carcinogenic drug would be intentionally given to someone trying to recover from cancer. A brief look at the history of chemotherapy will help to shed light on this.

The roots of modern chemotherapy go back to the early 1940s when poisonous mustard gas was being developed for chemical warfare. A potent form of mustard gas had already been used during World War I and, in 1942, the U.S. government contracted with various research centers to further investigate possible war-time chemical agents. Researchers at Yale University experimented with substituting a nitrogen atom for a sulfur atom in mustard gas, which, at the time, was called "nitrogen mustard."[8] A Yale anatomist then came up with the idea that it would be interesting to inject this nitrogen mustard into mice with cancer to see what would happen.

As luck would have it, the first such mouse experimented on showed impressive tumor regression. Although the mouse's cancer never completely went away, the mouse lived about four times longer than it was expected to live with no treatment at all and this got people's attention.

Researchers followed with more experiments and, though they could not achieve similarly good results on subsequent mice, it was eventually decided to try the nitrogen mustard treatment on a human cancer patient.

The first man experimented on had late-stage lymphosarcoma. Like the first mouse, he showed dramatic tumor regression after receiving nitrogen mustard. Researchers were ecstatic. But as with all the mice, the man's cancer was never cured. Within the first month of treatment, his white blood cell count fell dismally low. Then his cancer regenerated in his bone marrow and he died.[9] But because the man's tumor had regressed within the first few days, his case was considered to have been a "success." One-hundred-sixty more cancer patients were then administered experimental chemotherapy. The results showed that *not one* of these patients recovered from their cancer. In other words, all the evidence from early chemotherapy experiments indicated that the use of chemotherapy to treat cancer *was an unqualified failure!*

But in the early 1940s nitrogen mustard was the only synthesized chemical agent that had ever shown anti-tumor activity, and some people in positions of power were too excited about this to let it go. Chief of the U.S. Army Chemical Warfare Service, Cornelius "Dusty" Rhoads, was one of these people. Rhoads became a powerful advocate of chemotherapy when World War II ended and he became head of the Memorial Sloan-Kettering Institute for Cancer Research. He initiated tests on more than 1,500 different types of nitrogen mustard, and by 1955, about 20,000 of these types of chemicals were being looked at every year.[10]

Because chemotherapy was developed out of poisonous chemical warfare agents (and is still poisonous), there has always been a fine line between giving a therapeutic dose and killing the patient. In his outstanding book, *When Healing Becomes a Crime*, author Kenny Ausubel notes that in one clinical trial on the chemotherapy drug called "ICE," 8 percent of the patients died from the drug treatment directly, and in another trial on a chemotherapy drug studied for leukemia, 42 percent of the patients died from the drug treatment directly.[11]

From the days when chemotherapy was first used to the current day, this mode of treating cancer has *never* shown significant long-term effectiveness. Dr. Dean Burk was a chemist at the National Cancer Institute from 1939 to 1974. He also taught biochemistry at Cornell University Medical School from 1939 to 1941. When he retired in 1974, Dr. Burk left the position of chief chemist at the National Cancer Institute. The year before he retired, Dr. Burk wrote a letter to Dr. Frank Rauscher, a higher-up member in the NCI. In it, Burk wrote:

> Ironically, virtually all of the chemotherapeutic anti-cancer agents now approved by the Food and Drug Administration for use or testing in human cancer patients are (1) highly or variously *toxic* at applied dosages; (2) markedly *immunosuppressive*, that is, destructive of the patient's native resistance to a variety of diseases, including cancer; and (3) usually highly *carcinogenic* [cancer-causing]. . . . These now well established facts have been reported in numerous publications from the National Cancer Institute itself, as well as from throughout the United States and, indeed, the world. . . .
>
> In your answer to my discussion of March 19, you readily acknowledged that the FDA-approved anti-cancer drugs were indeed toxic, immunosuppressive, and carcinogenic, as indicated. But then, even in the face of the evidence, including your own White House statement of May 5, 1972, all pointing to the pitifully small effectiveness of such drugs, you went on to say quite paradoxically it seems to me, 'I think the Cancer Chemotherapy program is one of the best program components that the NCI has ever had.'. . . One may ask, parenthetically, surely this does not speak well of the 'other program areas?' [12]

Ralph Moss clarifies the subject of chemotherapy being carcinogenic even further in his book *Questioning Chemotherapy*, where he writes:

> Perhaps the strangest thing about chemotherapy is that many of these drugs themselves are carcinogenic. This may seem astonishing to the average reader—that cancer-fighting drugs themselves cause cancer. Yet this is an undeniable fact.
>
> It is sometimes said that only the alkylating agents, such as busulfan, carmustine, and melphalan, are carcinogenic. But this is not true. The authoritative International Agency for Research on Cancer (IARC) has identified 20 single agents or regimens which cause cancer in humans, and about 50 more in which such effects are suspected (236,248). Many, but not all, of these are alkylating agents. The offending drugs include doxorubicin and streptozocin (toxic antibiotics used as cytotoxic agents), BCNU (a nitrosourea), as well as the various hormone-like products. Perhaps the distinction between alkylating agents and other drugs in this regard is moot, since alkylating agents are predominantly included in most of the regimens commonly used in cancer.
>
> To give just one example of carcinogenicity, doctors looked at one-year survivors of ovarian cancer from five randomized trials. The incidence rates for acute nonlymphocytic leukemia and for pre-leukemia were about

100 times more common in women who got the drug melphalan than in those who received no chemotherapy.

'The magnitude of these risks suggests that the drugs are causally related to leukemia,' NCI epidemiologists cautiously concluded. However, they add, characteristically, that 'the identification of a carcinogenic effect does not preclude its use for treatment in patients.' In other words, the fact that these drugs cause cancer is immaterial in the doctor's decision to administer these cytotoxic agents.[13]

Using my home copy of *The PDR Family Guide to Prescription Drugs* (New Second Edition, copyright 1994), I looked up one commonly used chemotherapy drug called "Cyclophosphamide," which is also referred to as "Cytoxan." On page 167 of the Physician's Desk Reference, where side effects of Cytoxan are listed, I found this statement: "One possible Cytoxan side effect is the development of a secondary cancer, typically of the bladder, lymph nodes, or bone marrow. A secondary cancer may occur up to several years after the drug is given."

Cyclophosphamide, or Cytoxan, is an alkylating agent. It is also an integral part of the following commonly used chemotherapy protocols:

BACOP	CHOP	COMLA	MACC
CA	CHOP-B	COP	M-BACOD
CAMP	CISCA	COP-BLAM	Pro-MACE
CAP	CMF	CVP	Pro-MACE-cytaBOM
CAV	CMFP	CyVADIC	
CFPT	CMFVP	FAC	
COAP	Hexa-CAF	VAC	

Cyclophosphamide is also known as "Neosar" in the United States and "Endoxan" in Germany. According to Dr. W. John Diamond,

A study of over 10,000 patients shows clearly that chemo's supposedly strong track record with Hodgkin's disease (lymphoma) is actually a lie. Patients who underwent chemo were 14 times more likely to develop leukemia and 6 times more likely to develop cancers of the bones, joints, and soft tissues than those patients who did not undergo chemotherapy.[14]

And, the March 21, 1996, issue of the distinguished *New England Journal of Medicine*, reported:

Children who are successfully treated for Hodgkin's disease are 18 times more likely later to develop secondary malignant tumors. Girls face a 35 percent chance of developing breast cancer by the time they are 40—which is 75 times greater than the average. The risk of leukemia increased markedly four years after the ending of successful treatment, and reached a plateau after 14 years, but the risk of developing solid tumors remained high and approached 30 percent at 30 years.[15]

Some people may be willing to take the risk of developing a secondary cancer from the treatment they receive to rid themselves of their current cancer. But other people might not like the idea of seeing their cancer go into remission only to have to go once again into battle a few years later against a secondary treatment-induced cancer. (Especially when there are non-toxic, *non-carcinogenic* treatments they could choose from.) Do not assume your oncologist will tell you whether or not the chemo he or she wants to prescribe to you is carcinogenic or not. Generally, this subject is not addressed at all.

Also, the fact that so many chemotherapy drugs actually *cause* cancer is a very real threat to the public at large as well as to the environment. When cancer patients receive chemotherapy, much of their drug treatment gets passed into the public sewage systems through their urine. It thereby becomes an environmental poison that may eventually cause health problems or cancer to occur in other humans or animals. Remember, whenever we put poisons in ourselves, we are putting them in the environment, too.

False Hope?

How many times are doctors prescribing chemotherapy or radiation when there is very little evidence that this type of treatment will improve long-term life expectancy? About 80 percent of all cancer patients today are given chemotherapy, yet some researchers believe that chemotherapy may only show long-term effectiveness in as little as 2 to 3 percent of all cancer cases. And how often are radiation treatments prescribed to cancer patients when there is little evidence that doing so will help achieve long-term recovery for their particular type of cancer situation?

I know of a woman whose elderly father-in-law was prescribed radiation treatments for his late-stage, metastasized prostate cancer. When this woman called her father-in-law's oncologist directly to find out what his life-expectancy was, she was told by the oncologist that he had only about six months to live. The woman, being a clear thinker, then asked the oncologist if that prognosis for her father-in-law was "with" radiation treatments, or "without." The unbelievable answer she got was "either way." Yet her father-in-law had been prescribed radiation treatments and was *not* told that his survival chances were *exactly the same* whether he did the treatment or not. Both this elderly man and his wife thought the radiation treatments could cure him. These people were never told the truth, but instead were given "false hope" by their conventional oncologist.

I believe that the following statements are accurate: It is *false hope* when patients are prescribed a conventional cancer treatment and not told that the treatment is only considered to be palliative (not expected to cure the patient). It is *false hope* when response rates are quoted and presented in a way that implies long-term recovery. And it is *false hope* when any cancer cure-rate statistic that has been "fudged" is presented to a cancer patient as representative of his or her chances for real recovery and survival. Since all these things happen on a daily basis in conventional oncologists' offices, the logical conclusion is that conventional medicine is the biggest source of false hope given to cancer patients today.

Does Newer Mean Better?

It is wrong for the mainstream medical establishment to mislead patients about the actual long-term effectiveness of conventional cancer treatments. But one thing that plays into this problem is the readiness of the public to think that anything "newer" is "better." One of the most distressing patterns I have come across when talking to people who have recently been diagnosed with cancer, is their frequent willingness to overlook the proven long-term effectiveness of many alternative, non-toxic cancer treatments—and to eagerly look for the *most recent* conventional cancer drugs or procedures for their healing instead. I have heard people say things like, "There is a *new* cancer drug that is showing great results in clinical trials. I'm going to talk to my doctor about that."

Moreover, the media supports the newer is better fallacy, even when some of the new cancer drugs have not been tested for more than a few months. These drugs are often given great acclaim as possible "magic bullets" in newspaper or magazine articles. Ever since antibiotics were developed, and ever since strides in technology helped to make medical accomplishments soar, people in the modern world have come to think that anything new in medicine *must* be better. But cancer is not a simple bacterium that can be targeted by a simple antibiotic, nor is it a type of wound that can easily be closed up by modern technology and hardware.

Therefore, the "newer is better" stance does not necessarily apply to cancer, especially when cancer research continues to stick to the paradigm that cancer drugs must be toxic poisons in order to work and must be patentable.

Doctors play a role in the "newer is better" syndrome as well whenever they recommend that a cancer patient take part in a "Phase 1" clinical trial. You, yourself, may have been recommended this and are possibly considering it. But what all cancer patients should know about Phase 1 clinical trials is that they are little more than *toxicity* tests. They are clinical trials used to establish "safe" doses of new toxic drugs. In any Phase 1 trial, medical researchers have established acceptable response rates in laboratory animals, but they do not yet know the safe dose of that particular treatment for humans. So they put a bunch of patients through various doses of the new treatment in a Phase 1 trial and watch for side effects. Sometimes the doctors recommending Phase I trials don't even believe that the patient will be likely to benefit from the trial at all. But they hope that, in the long run, patients in the future may benefit from the trial. Basically, in Phase 1 clinical trials, you are little more than a guinea pig being used for determining human dosage levels. Phase 2 clinical trials are somewhat better because they have already done the Phase 1 for establishing toxic dosage levels, but they are still far from determining whether the new drug is truly effective for humans. Usually, Phase 2 trials show temporary shrinkage of tumors in some patients, but don't result in any long-term recoveries.

Of course, some new drugs may actually show promise. They might put a certain percentage of people into temporary remission. But, remember, remission simply means that all clinical evidence of the cancer is gone. It does not mean that all the cancer cells in the body are gone. Thus, remission often does not equate to long-term cure either. Basically, if a treatment has only been tested for a short time, then the *only* results available on it are short-term. In looking for *long-term* recovery, it makes more sense to go with a treatment that already has a good long-term track record.

When an oncologist says to a patient, "I'd like you to try this new treatment that clinical trials are just starting on," one has to wonder if this isn't just a little bit like a pilot saying, "Well, I don't have a plane available right now that I *know* can get you to where you want to go—but over here, on this other runway, is a brand-new type of plane we are just trying out. It's never been flown successfully before, but the pre-flight tests show it to be very promising." If it were me, looking for a plane to get me somewhere, I'd much rather walk a couple blocks down the road to another airport with a tried-and-true plane that has already successfully made the trip many times. This is what you do when you avoid the "newer is better" syndrome and look into which treatments (conventional or alternative) have actually worked in a long-term way for many people before you. Again, it all boils down to a simple question: Are you interested in surviving your cancer short-term or long-term?

A Deadly Double Standard

One of the things I have heard over and over from people looking into alternatives for cancer is, "What formal, large-scale studies have been done on this or that alternative cancer treatment?" When the person then hears that no large-scale studies have been done, they often figure the treatment approach must not be any good and no longer consider it.

The first thing to understand is that the developers of most of the alternative treatments mentioned in this book *did* try for many years to get formal, large-scale studies done on their innovative cancer treatments. If these approaches had been fairly evaluated by mainstream medicine, as they should have been, there *would* be large-scale formal studies to quote from. But only the richly funded mainstream research organizations (backed by pharmaceutical or government money) can afford to do these types of studies. So, if a treatment approach is not considered by pharmaceutical companies to be something that could be extremely profitable for them, large-scale formal studies will not be done. And, unfortunately, the government agencies involved in cancer treatment research, such as the National Cancer Institute and the FDA, simply act as watchdogs and protectors of Big Pharma's profits.

The second thing to understand is that, in many cases, small but significant studies *have* been done on alternative cancer treatments with great success. Some examples of these studies are:

- In 1946, a congressional committee looked into the Gerson therapy and officially concluded it was a sound and effective cancer treatment.

- In 1954, a team of 10 reputable doctors studied the clinical records of patients using the Hoxsey therapy and found it to be an effective cancer treatment. They strongly recommended it over other cancer treatments of that era.

- Between 1972 and 1977, Memorial Sloan-Kettering's head research scientist, Dr. Kanematsu Sugiura, studied Laetrile's effects on cancer in laboratory animals. He found Laetrile to be effective against cancers of all types, and pronounced it more effective than any substance he had ever tested for cancer.

- In the early 1980s, Dr. Nicholas Gonzales performed a detailed scientific analysis of 500 cases of cancer patients treated with Dr. Kelly's enzyme therapy with a focus on pancreatic cancer. He found it to be significantly more effective than anything conventional medicine had to offer.

- Several scientific studies done in the U.S. and Japan on Dr. Burzynski's antineoplaston therapy showed it to be significantly better than conventional methods for numerous types of cancer, and phenomenally so for brain cancers and lymphomas.

- In the early 1990s, in vitro studies done by the National Cancer Institute on Jim Sheridan's formula now called Protocel® showed results that were *much* better than chemotherapy results for a variety of different cancer cell lines. Yet they declined to study it further.

Generally, the public is not aware that any of these studies have been done, nor are they aware of their highly positive results. What most people want to see are modern large-scale clinical trials on alternatives for cancer. This is understandable considering that in most cases these people's lives are at stake. However, these types of expensive studies will not be done until the current medical climate changes.

But more importantly, people expect there to be unbiased, third-party, large-scale studies done on everything, without realizing that these types of studies have *not* even been done on *conventional* cancer treatments. In other words, cancer patients rarely say to their oncologist, "Doctor, I can't consider this particular type of chemotherapy or radiation treatment unless you are able to show me positive results from unbiased, large-scale studies showing that people who used this treatment got well—really got well, not just managed to live with their cancer for five years after their diagnosis." This is largely because patients assume that the studies for conventional treatments have already been done. They haven't.

What is so ludicrous about this double standard is that radiation and most chemotherapy agents are still officially listed as "unproven" cures by the FDA and are legally required in many cases to be classified as "experimental." The fact is that many doctors and most of the public mistakenly assume that anything approved by the FDA has been rigorously proven to be effective in scientific studies. In his June 6, 2003 newsletter, Dr. Moss shows us that this is not the case and gives an example of the process of officially approving a new cancer drug:

> The FDA has approved the drug Iressa (gefitinib) for the treatment of non-small cell lung cancer, despite evidence that it does not prolong the lives of patients. Approval came after an FDA panel heard testimony from patients, one of whom claimed to feel much better after taking the little brown pill. Her moving story helped convince members of the Oncologic Drug Advisory Committee to give final approval.
>
> . . . Some critics are beginning to wake up to the fact that the FDA is now approving drugs that emerge from "Big Pharma" without requiring the rigorous proof once considered necessary. In fact, when proof is offered that the drugs in question do *not* work it seems that the FDA is quite willing to throw out the studies and revert to anecdotal accounts.[16]

When extremely high standards of clinical results are required for under-funded alternative treatments but are *not* required for richly-funded conventional treatments, then we are dealing with a deadly double standard.

But it is not only Big Pharma that is biased toward their types of conventional treatments. There is also often a strong personal bias among conventional doctors against alternative treatments for cancer. Here is one story to illustrate some problems people face when they discuss treatment options with their oncologist. This was from a man whose wife was suffering from late-stage cancer, most of which was in her brain and growing fast. She didn't have much time. The man claimed he had looked into many alternative treatments for his wife, but said, "The problem with those is that so many of them turn out to be bogus." I found out later from him that the way he had decided they were bogus was by asking his wife's doctor what *he* thought of the alternative treatment every time he heard of one. Since the doctor looked at *all* alternative cancer treatments as bogus, that is what he replied in every case, without having any knowledge of the specifics of the therapy.

This man's wife died of her brain cancer a few months later. None of her doctors had anything effective to offer her, and yet they were all quite effective at keeping her from trying any alternative treatments— treatments they were totally uninformed about, but adamantly claimed were ineffective.

Unfortunately, most conventional doctors are completely uninformed or worse, *misinformed*, about any treatment that is not conventional. By this I mean that they usually know very little about anything not endorsed by pharmaceutical companies (or by medical organizations that are influenced by pharmaceutical companies). Thus, there is a very real problem in thinking that your doctor is going to know the truth about alternative cancer treatments. And doctors are not motivated to find out more about alternative cancer treatments because, in most U.S. states, it is illegal for them to prescribe any treatment for cancer *other* than what is specifically approved by the FDA.

We have been brought up to regard doctors and medical organizations as experts. We have been brought up to think that if we don't get our doctor's approval on some treatment approach we are interested in, then we are being irresponsible, maybe even "killing ourselves." We have not been brought up to believe that big industry, and not true science, is affecting which medical treatments are available to us.

New Cancer Drugs Are Big Business

It is difficult to accept that the most effective non-toxic approaches to treating cancer are *not* being used by oncologists and cancer clinics everywhere—and that toxic treatments that do not show significant effectiveness *are* being used. The only answer to this is that cancer treatments are "big business." In particular, new cancer *drugs* are big business. And the effectiveness of new drugs can easily be exaggerated and promoted in press releases by drug companies. Ralph Moss, Ph.D. shows how this can happen in his June 13, 2003, newsletter. Dr. Moss first states that,

> On July 30, 2001, Erbitux was hailed in a *Business Week* cover story, 'The Birth of a Cancer Drug.' The drug, then called IMC-225, was celebrated as a 'blockbuster' that 'halts the spread of cancer.' In an editorial entitled 'The Dawn of a New Era,' the magazine claimed that Erbitux 'seems effective against cancers of the colon, pancreas, head and neck and lungs.' It suggested that victory might be within sight in the war on cancer.[17]

Then, Moss goes on to explain that the Associated Press, CNN, and Wall Street all joined in with incredible excitement about this amazing new cancer drug. But what these news organizations *never* did was to look at the studies themselves. If they had, they would have found that, on average, the studies done on Erbitux showed the overall response rate to be only about 10 percent. (And we know that response rate is not equivalent to recovery—it just means that a 50 percent reduction in tumor size was achieved for a short while.) Plus, the studies on Erbitux showed an average of just 45 days to progression. This means that the common length of time that Erbitux could *slow* the cancer was only about one-and-one-half months before the cancer would progress and grow out of control again. Moreover, about 50 percent of the patients given Erbitux in the studies suffered what were considered *severe* side effects.

Yet, with so little effectiveness to boast, Erbitux went into clinical trials to get approval by the FDA as a cancer drug. If approved, Erbitux could be worth billions of dollars a year in sales to drug companies.

Apparently, FDA approval of cancer drugs like Erbitux does not require studies that show significant long-term effectiveness. For example, another highly touted cancer drug, "Iressa," has already achieved FDA approval. But according to Dr. Moss, "The approval came despite the fact that Iressa has been shown in rigorous studies not to prolong overall survival."[18]

The FDA itself appears to operate in ways that involve huge conflicts of interest. This organization is supposed to protect public safety where drugs are concerned, yet many of its personnel, including heads of departments, either have had or will move on to highly paid jobs in pharmaceutical companies. *The FDA personnel are not unbiased!* Not only are they not unbiased, they are practically autonomous and untouchable because much of what they do is *not* under direct control of Congress. Unbelievably, congressional hearings that uncover problems in the FDA are only allowed to "make suggestions" to the FDA where they think change is warranted. It appears that the FDA does not have to do anything Congress says!

Questions to Ask Your Oncologist

What can you do to protect yourself? At the very least, cancer patients have the right to know what the long-term efficacy of a treatment being offered them is, as well as what side effects they might experience. In other words, *they have a right to make a truly informed decision.* To make sure that you are able to make a truly informed decision for yourself, you can start by asking your doctor the right questions. Some questions I highly recommend that you ask your oncologist regarding the conventional treatment he or she is recommending to you are the following:

1. "What kind of *long-term* effectiveness does this type of treatment offer for my type of cancer? In other words, what are my chances of living longer than five years *and becoming cancer-free*?"

2. If your oncologist quotes "response rates" to you, you might want to say, "I am not interested in hearing about tumor response rates because I know that they only refer to short-term tumor shrinkage. What are the long-term, cancer-free statistics on this treatment?"

3. If you have a child who has been diagnosed with cancer, you might want to ask your pediatric oncologist, "What are the chances that my child will recover using this treatment and grow up to be a healthy adult? Have you seen any children fully recover from this type of cancer with this treatment and go on to live totally normal lives?"

4. "Is the treatment you suggest considered a *curative* treatment in this case, or just a *palliative* treatment?" (Remember, a palliative treatment is considered to be one that is *not* expected to save the patient's life, but is simply administered in the hope that it will prolong the patient's life. Sometimes this expectation for longer survival is only a few months.)

5. "What will this treatment do to my quality of life?"

6. "How long do you think I will live if I do *not* undergo any treatment at all? And how long do you think I will live if I follow your treatment suggestion?"

7. "Can you give me any phone numbers of other patients you have successfully treated with the type of treatment you are suggesting to me? Or, if you can't give out phone numbers, can you at least *describe* to me any cases of people who fully recovered from their cancer using the method you want to prescribe to me?"

8. "If I go through this treatment, what are all the serious, or even life-threatening, side effects I might experience? For example, is it possible this treatment could cause me to die from heart failure or a blood clot? Is it possible this treatment could cause me to develop a secondary life-threatening cancer within a few years?"

Do not be shy about asking these direct questions. This is information you have a right to know. You may be about to make a decision that your life depends on. Also, if your oncologist is not comfortable with these types of questions, then you should consider seeking out another oncologist who *will* answer them honestly. Remember, you are paying your doctor—he or she is working for *you*.

Hopefully, the information in this chapter will help you to evaluate conventional methods that may be recommended to you, and allow you to make a truly informed decision about the treatment method you want to go with. I suggest you be just as open and objective about considering the treatments your conventional oncologist recommends to you as you are when you consider any alternative treatment for your cancer. However, do not fall prey to a double standard. Do not let yourself be "rushed" into treatment before you have considered your options. Understand the terminology and statistics that are presented to you by your doctor. Be aware of short-term versus long-term effectiveness. Be aware of all possible side effects for any treatment you are considering, whether it is a conventional or alternative approach. And try to find out if other cancer patients have used that approach successfully to become cancer-free (not to just live 5 years after diagnosis). Never forget that your goal is to *recover* from your cancer and regain a normal cancer-free life!

Resources:

Books

Ralph W. Moss, Ph.D. *The Cancer Industry.* New York: Equinox Press, 1999.

Ralph W. Moss, Ph.D. *Questioning Chemotherapy.* New York: Equinox Press, 2000.

Video

Cancer Doesn't Scare Me Anymore, by Dr. Lorraine Day. To order, call (800) 574-2437, or visit Dr. Day's website: www.drday.com.

Newsletter

For the newsletter and special reports put out by Ralph W. Moss, Ph.D., go to www.cancerdecisions.com.

23

Choosing an Approach and Monitoring Your Progress

After reading the previous chapters of this book, I hope you have gained an understanding of some of the many options you can choose from to "outsmart" your cancer. However, if you make the decision for yourself to go with an alternative, non-toxic approach, you may also feel somewhat overwhelmed by all the possible options. This chapter will give you some important tips to help you choose an alternative treatment plan that is right for you. These tips address narrowing down your choices, contacting practitioners for more information, dealing with conventional doctors, prioritizing your overall treatment program, and monitoring your progress.

Narrowing Down Your Choices

How does one narrow down the choices? The best way to start is by evaluating four main treatment factors and how they apply to your particular situation. These are: (1) Efficacy of treatment; (2) Difficulty of treatment; (3) Cost of treatment; and (4) Level of supervision.

Keeping these factors in mind to see if there are some treatment options you may want to rule out may help you to more easily zero in on the approaches you want to consider. I would also recommend not just considering those approaches that have whole chapters devoted to them in this book. For instance, there might be an approach in Chapter 17 that is only briefly discussed, but after looking into it some more you decide it is the best option for you.

Efficacy of Treatment

Efficacy of treatment is, of course, going to be foremost in importance. But it is really impossible, without comprehensive comparative studies, to say that any particular alternative cancer approach is more effective than another in a general sense. And, with different people's physical conditions and medical issues varying so much, it is often very difficult to know which approach will be the most effective for any particular case. No cancer treatment, whether conventional or alternative, is 100 percent effective for 100 percent of the people that use it.

When trying to ascertain for yourself the overall effectiveness of any approach, there are some important issues to understand. For example, you may be concerned about some people you've heard about for whom that approach did *not* work. One thing to remember is that most of the people who use alternative approaches start them at a much later stage in their disease than is optimal. Because people are not usually aware of the benefits of alternative treatments when they are first diagnosed, they generally use conventional treatments first. It is only after these conventional treatments have failed that many people turn to alternative methods—and this tends to bring down the success rates of alternative approaches. (Because these people are often already seriously damaged by the chemotherapy and/or radiation they have been given, or possibly already damaged by the cancer that may have spread more extensively throughout their body.) The general rule is that, the sooner after diagnosis that you start *any* treatment, whether alternative or conventional, the better your chances for recovery will be. Another thing to remember is that, because alternative approaches are more often self-administered than conventional approaches, there will always be a certain number of people who do not use them as effectively as possible. I have heard more than once about someone who claimed that a particular approach did not work for them, but then I found out that they either did not give the treatment enough time, or there were things they were doing that interfered with the treatment. So, even though someone you know may not have had success with a particular approach, that does not mean it won't work for *you*. And you may be able to find others that it *did* work for.

One issue for some types of alternative approaches, such as the herbal therapies, is that it may be important to find sources that provide these treatments in as close to their original form as possible. Herbs are nature's medicine, but they must be grown, harvested, and used in optimal ways to be effective. The Hoxsey herbal formula, for instance, as well as Essiac, were both originally harvested from wild-crafted herbs grown in healthy, virgin soils. They were administered shortly after preparation and did not have to be prepared for mass marketing and long-term storage. Even though the Hoxsey therapy and Essiac are still achieving cancer recoveries for many people (especially in early stages of cancer), their overall effectiveness, particularly for late-stage cancer, may not be quite as good as when they were originally used.

Thus, if you are planning to use any herbal approach, I suggest you research that treatment as much as you can and try to find the best possible source to get the herbs from. If you decide to use the Hoxsey herbal approach, you may want to go *directly* to the clinic in Mexico that Mildred Nelson established to obtain good quality herbs and guidance on how to use them. For good quality Essiac, you may want to search out an independent herbal source that has high standards for the quality of herbs they sell rather than use a mass-produced herbal formula, or at least use a source that you know has brought about recovery for others.

In a similar way, diet-based approaches which focus primarily on high amounts of fresh vegetables and fruits, such as the Gerson therapy, may not be as effective as they were decades ago. This is partly because it is difficult in this modern world to find fruits and vegetables grown in truly balanced, healthy soils. Even organically grown fruits and vegetables are likely to come from soil that has been overused. Artificial fertilization techniques are helpful, but may not be able to produce crops that are as abundant in nutrients as virgin soils can. It is also partly because people are more toxic these days than they used to be. So the approaches that place a large focus on detoxification may have further to go in today's world than they did earlier in the 20th century.

However, we can learn from *all* of the successful non-toxic approaches and can often use parts of each in combination. For instance, pancreatic enzymes (Kelley), Laetrile (Krebs), herbs (Hoxsey or Essiac), diet (Gerson or Budwig), or coffee enemas (Gerson and Kelley) can often be combined with various other approaches to optimize one's chances for recovery.

Just make sure that the aspects you use from different approaches do not conflict with each other.

In general, alternative non-toxic cancer approaches tend to work well for *most* types of cancer, and they are *not* focused on treating specific cancers the way conventional treatments are. This is because they address the common characteristics of all cancer cells. Thus, the efficacy of any particular alternative approach will not be limited to one specific type of cancer the way conventional chemo drugs often are. Having said that, some alternative approaches may boast that they are *particularly* good at dealing with cancer in particular systems of the body. For example, Dr. Burzynski's antineoplaston therapy is particularly effective for primary brain cancer and lymphatic cancers, and Dr. Kelley's enzyme approach is particularly effective for pancreatic cancer. But both of these approaches have also achieved great results for cancers in other locations of the body, and there are other non-toxic approaches, such as Protocel® or flaxseed oil and cottage cheese that are effective for brain cancer and lymphomas as well.

The most important way to ensure effectiveness of any alternative, non-toxic approach is by acquainting yourself with it enough to make sure you are using it optimally, and by finding a qualified practitioner or support group to help guide you through it whenever possible. Taking care of yourself in other ways may also be important to your healing process. Some people may have to continue going to work while they are trying to recover from their cancer because of their financial needs. But if one can, it might be best to stay home and reduce stress while recovering. Some key aspects of taking care of yourself may involve getting the sleep you need, eating a nutritional and balanced diet, drinking lots of good water for hydration and detoxification, reducing unnecessary stress, and dealing with your emotions.

Difficulty of Treatment

In some cases, difficulty of treatment may be the biggest factor of all when considering which treatment approach to go with. This factor particularly comes into play when treating very young children or elderly people. In terms of sheer volume of work, the Gerson therapy presented in Chapter 5 is considered by many to be the most difficult alternative cancer treatment available. It requires the juicing of fresh, organic vegetables and fruits about 13 times every day, along with performing multiple coffee enemas every day and carrying out other specific daily requirements. Even some strong, young adults have found it necessary, when doing the Gerson therapy, to actually *hire* outside help in order to carry out the daily juicing requirement. And the daily coffee enemas may not be possible for young children, some older people, and even some middle-aged adults who do not have the energy or mobility to carry out the process. (However, for those people who want to use a strictly nutrition-based approach and *have* the energy or help required to do it, the Gerson therapy may be a great choice.)

Another issue to think about is the number of pills required by the approach you are considering. For example, the Gonzalez-Isaacs enzyme therapy presented in Chapter 7 requires an extremely high number of pills to be taken every day (up to about 150). This amount may be too difficult for young children to swallow or for the elderly to digest. There may be ways to work around this, such as opening the pills up and putting the powdered contents into a drink, but it is certainly a factor to consider when prioritizing one's treatment options.

Overall, some of the *easiest* approaches to administer to young children or elderly adults are the following: Protocel®, Poly-MVA, LifeOne, Burzynski's antineoplastons, flaxseed oil and cottage cheese, the Hoxsey therapy, Essiac Tea, low dose naltrexone, Lapacho/Pau D'Arco/Taheebo, and Ellagic Acid. (Remember, however, that Protocel® should *not* be done along with most other approaches unless compatibility is specifically listed, though most of the other approaches can be combined together without Protocel®.)

Thus, ruling out those approaches that may be too difficult to administer for your particular case can help narrow down your choices.

Cost of Treatment

Considering the cost of approaches is another way to narrow down your choices. The ideal situation would be for each person to have unlimited money and unlimited time, but this is not usually the case. Fortunately, most alternative treatments are much less expensive than conventional treatments for cancer. The down side is that health insurance policies rarely cover alternative methods, even if the doctor you are working with is a fully accredited M.D. Therefore, when it comes to using some of the more expensive alternative methods, it might be important to find out ahead of time if your insurance company will pay for any part of it or not or whether or not there is a way you can afford it.

The costs for different alternative treatment approaches vary considerably, so it is a good idea to consider the different prices listed at the back of each treatment chapter. These are only estimates, but they will give you a general idea of the expenses required. Besides the cost of treatment, one must also consider possible time away from work. If you start an effective treatment soon after diagnosis, you may have a very good chance of being able to carry on with your life normally while you recover. But many cancer patients may not feel well enough to work at all for at least some period of time. Or if you choose a very time-consuming method, then just carrying out the treatment may rule out time to go to work and bring home a paycheck. This means that when you consider treatment expenses, you may also need to factor in a reduction of income occurring at the same time.

The important thing to remember is that, when considering your treatment options, *more expensive* does not necessarily mean *more effective*. One of the more expensive approaches may turn out to be the best choice for one person, while one of the least expensive approaches may turn out to be the best choice for another. The good news is that, if you are particularly challenged financially, there are still excellent low-cost options available in the alternative cancer treatment world.

I believe that a good rule for anyone looking into alternative cancer treatments is to first try to decide which form of treatment you would choose if money were *not* an issue. In other words, put aside all of the money considerations you have, just at first, and try to evaluate what approach you think will give you the best chance for recovery. Once you have sorted out which treatment you would *like* to try, then see if you can come up with the money. Burzynski's antineoplaston therapy is the most expensive alternative approach and may be too expensive for most people. But it should always at least be considered whenever a person is dealing with brain cancer or lymphoma because of its high level of effectiveness for those types of cancer.

Think carefully before choosing a treatment approach that is not your first choice just because you can't afford your first choice approach. In some cases, it may be that there is no way around this. But whenever possible, it is a good idea to try to pursue the treatment approach you feel you can most fully commit to and have confidence in.

Level of Supervision

Another factor to consider is the type and amount of guidance or supervision you require to feel comfortable with your treatment approach. If you are the type of person who can feel comfortable primarily self-administering your own treatment after obtaining initial guidance, then there are certain approaches that can be considered. If you are the type of person who would be *most* comfortable with ongoing supervision and guidance from a medical practitioner, then there are *others* to consider. (E.g., Dr. Burzynski's Clinic in Houston, Dr. Gonzales's enzyme therapy in New York, Cesium therapy at the Reno Integrative Medical Center, the CAAT Protocol, Dr. Forsythe's clinic for Poly-MVA in Reno, or the Mexican or German cancer clinics.)

Preferably, geographical location will *not* be a deciding factor for most people, because airline flights are not that difficult to take. For instance, Americans who prefer treatment that is supervised by a doctor should not rule out clinics in Mexico. For about the equivalent of travelling to San Diego, California or San Antonio, Texas, these clinics can provide some of the very *best* doctor-supervised treatment and offer cancer patients the benefits of multiple alternative therapies combined.

Contacting Practitioners for More Information

If you decide to try an alternative cancer approach, you may want to quickly call each place of treatment you are considering. This could be to verify that they are still in operation as well as to ask some detailed questions about their treatment program. Feel free to ask what kind of success they have had dealing with your particular type of cancer, but don't expect formal statistics or studies. The best type of answer you will probably receive is a comment based on their own experience with their patients. This information is valuable, especially since they sometimes may be able to give you the phone number or email address of one or more of those patients. If they have not yet treated your particular type of cancer, this does *not* necessarily mean you should stop considering them for treatment. After all, there are many different manifestations of cancer, and yours may be one of the more rare types.

If your preliminary research looks promising, you may want to either start treatment immediately or consider making a consultation appointment first to discuss your particular case. This will use up some of your valuable time and money, but it can be an important step in choosing the treatment that will be best for you. Even if you have to go to several different treatment center consultations before you decide, it could be worth your efforts in the long run. Yes, it is important for you to start treatment as soon as possible—but it is also important to be able to make a *well-informed* decision as to which treatment you choose.

Most alternative doctors will want you to come in for a consultation with all of your diagnostic test results. These include biopsy reports, X-rays, CT scan results, blood tests, and whatever else you have been able to get from your conventional physicians so far. Ask first over the phone what types of records they want you to bring, and ask how much the consultation will cost. Often, an in-person consultation with an alternative practitioner or clinic can be of great help in determining which approach you want to follow. It not only will give you an idea as to whether you can feel comfortable with that practitioner or clinic, it also may give you a better idea as to the likelihood of that approach working well for you, and even possibly how long it may take. Another option is to ask for an informational packet to be mailed to you.

Time is *always* of the essence when dealing with cancer. But spending a little more time in the beginning can sometimes save time later on. It may be hard to take a few extra days for research or a consultation appointment in the beginning when your doctor and family members are urging you to rush into surgery, radiation or chemotherapy. But just remember that a well-spent number of days doing research in the very beginning can sometimes make the difference between life and death. Getting onto a cancer treatment plan as fast as possible is always the priority, but getting started on treatment that will give you your best chance for long-term recovery is also of utmost importance.

Dealing With Conventional Doctors

Every person who chooses to use an alternative approach to "outsmart" his or her cancer will be going against the grain of modern conventional medicine. One problem that can arise as a result of this is the difficulty involved with declining the treatment your conventional doctor thinks you should get. Most people with cancer are first diagnosed by a conventional doctor. If you are one of these people, you may have seen an oncologist who is very committed to the mainstream accepted approaches. It is not easy to turn down a medical specialist's recommendation—especially when you may be told that, in doing so, you will be killing yourself. One thing to remember in this situation is that, specialist or not, *your doctor works for you.* You are paying your doctor for his or her expertise and professional service. It is important to listen to and consider any recommendation for treatment your conventional doctor gives you. Doctors go through an immense amount of training and then experience a great deal clinically, so their input should be respected and sought. But when it comes to the final treatment decisions you make, that is up to you.

If you choose to use an alternative approach, you will most likely be in a situation where you still want to see your conventional doctor at certain intervals for diagnostic tests and monitoring of your progress. This is desirable whenever possible. Even people using alternative methods will want to have blood tests, CT scans, MRIs, or other tests done regularly to ascertain how well they are doing and make sure their cancer is responding to the approach they have chosen. Also, getting diagnostic tests performed by a conventional doctor will generally allow them to be covered by your health insurance policy. Another reason to seek help from a conventional doctor is in case there are any side complications arising from your cancer.

I recommend being as open as possible with your conventional doctor. I believe it is best to be honest and to give your doctor the opportunity of deciding to follow your progress while you use an alternative approach. You may be surprised to find that your doctor is more open-minded than you expected. If, however, your doctor takes a stance against alternative approaches and will *not* prescribe diagnostic tests to you unless you undergo conventional treatments, then you have the option of finding another doctor or oncologist who will. If you phone different doctors' offices, you may be able to find another doctor in your area who is willing to monitor your progress even though you are not using a conventional method. Though many people see their oncologist over and over and never tell him or her they are using an alternative approach, I recommend that you make an effort to find a doctor with whom you can work openly. In doing so, you are not only standing up for yourself and your right to openly choose your own treatment, you are also giving your doctor a chance to learn how effective alternative methods can be.

But if you do employ a conventional doctor to prescribe diagnostic tests for you, remember that, in some cases, your doctor may not know how to interpret the results of the tests. A good example is, when using Protocel®, cancer marker levels may rise as the cancer cells lyse and tumors break down. Conventional doctors may not interpret these results correctly, since they are trained to see any rise in cancer markers as indications that the cancer is growing or spreading. It is up to you to be informed about the particular approach you are using so that you can help your conventional doctor understand the process you are going through.

Prioritizing Your Overall Treatment Program

Once you have decided on the primary approach you wish to use, figure out your priorities. You may want to make a list to help you keep your overall recovery plan in mind. I would suggest that you list the primary treatment approach you have chosen as "priority number 1." Secondary to that, you can list any adjunctive treatments you would like to add to your program (as long as they are compatible with your primary treatment.) Then, lower on the priority list might be things like improving your diet, dealing with toxic teeth, working on emotional or psycho-spiritual issues, and anything else. Different people will list their priorities in a different order from other people.

Seeing the important issues prioritized and listed on paper can help to reduce some of the confusion that may arise when you think about what it is you need to do to "outsmart your cancer." As mentioned earlier, we can learn from *all* of the successful alternative approaches, and many of these can be combined effectively. Just be careful to not combine aspects of different treatments that might conflict. Most alternative cancer treatment approaches have very specific guidelines, and these guidelines are there for good reasons. Thus, an important rule to remember is to *always* thoroughly research any approach you are using and make sure you follow it or combine it with others correctly.

Monitoring Your Progress

Monitoring your progress is *critical*. One of the saddest things I have come across (and more than once) is when a person uses an alternative approach for a long time, maybe eight or ten months, and they just *assume* that it is working for them. Then they go in for a scan and find out their tumors have grown or their cancer has spread to new places, such as their liver. These people are devastated when they find out they are in a worse situation than when they started.

No matter how miraculous an approach may appear, and no matter how well it worked for your friend or your relative, you should *never* just assume that it will work as well for you at the same dosing schedule that was used for them. Every person's body is different and the success of the treatment may be affected by how toxic a person is (with heavy metals or other substances), how imbalanced hormonally a person is, whether one has toxic teeth issues, how much damage one's body has already undergone, etc.

Even though all of the alternative methods presented in this book have better track records than conventional cancer treatments in general, that does not mean they will cure 100 percent of the people who use them. Having success with an alternative cancer treatment might be easy for some people and the approach will definitely seem like a "magic bullet" for them. But for others, it may be more difficult. Also, when using a single product approach, such as Protocel®, Poly-MVA, 714X, or any others, you may not want to assume that the product is still being produced exactly the same as it was when this book was written. There is always the possibility that a company can be bought out by another company and a product may be produced slightly differently than it was before. There is no indication that this will happen to the products just mentioned, but it is yet another reason to be sure to always assess how well your cancer is responding to the treatment approach you are using.

Be sure to monitor your progress at reasonable intervals with whatever diagnostic tests you can get.

In most cases, scans (PET, MRI, CT or ultrasound) will be the best way to tell your cancer status and to ascertain whether the approach you are using is working effectively for you or not. How often one should get scans will vary from case to case. For instance, someone with a really fast-growing brain tumor may elect to get a scan every two months until the cancer is definitely regressing, then go to longer intervals. However, a person with a slow-growing prostate tumor may choose to wait four months after starting their alternative method to get a scan, and if things look good then, wait six months for the next one after that. But definitely monitor your progress at regular intervals if at all possible and *don't* just assume that the approach is working for you.

If your scans show that your cancer is still growing or that your cancer is stabilized but not going away, then you may simply need a higher dose of treatment. Thus, monitoring your progress isn't only for the purpose of deciding that the treatment is either working or not working at all—it may help you to find out whether the *way* you are using the treatment is optimal for your case or not. If not, you may be able to make adjustments.

One tricky situation that can arise for people using any self-administered type of approach is that there is a tendency to interpret every bit of discomfort, pain, or swelling as a sign that their cancer is getting worse. This is where an experienced alternative practitioner or support group for that particular approach can be invaluable. Often, some level of discomfort, pain, or swelling is normal on the path to recovery. But if you do not have an expert telling you that these symptoms are nothing to worry about, then they can be very scary.

Unfortunately, too many people stop using an alternative cancer treatment when the treatment is actually working for them, because they don't have a doctor telling them it is working. When you think about it, if chemotherapy were a self-administered approach, how many people would stay with it after their first bout of vomiting, hair loss, or other symptoms? Patients only stay with treatments such as chemotherapy because their doctors tell them that the symptoms they are experiencing are necessary to go through in order to get well. So, too, must you be informed about possible discomforts you may experience with an alternative cancer treatment. Although these discomforts will generally be *much* less severe than those experienced with toxic conventional treatments and will not cause damage to the body, they still may occur at times due to cancer breakdown.

The good news is that, when you *do* go against the grain and use an alternative approach to treat your cancer, you play a much bigger role in your own recovery. You may need to do more of your own research and thinking than you would with a conventional approach, but taking a bigger role in your own healing is a very empowering process. Even if you have chosen an alternative medical practitioner to work with, you can still be very involved in your own healing. Be sure to ask your alternative practitioner lots of questions. If the approach you choose does *not* offer a doctor's guidance of any type, try to find a support group that can give you experienced advice. There will almost always be ways to find out what you need to know in order to achieve your *best* chance for recovery!

24

Dealing With Fear and the Mind/Body Connection

If you have just been diagnosed with cancer and have not yet chosen a treatment approach, then it may be too soon for you to be dealing with your emotions in any depth. Your priority at this point is to investigate your treatment options so that you can get onto an effective cancer-fighting program as soon as possible. But at some point after you are securely established in your chosen treatment plan, examining your mental and emotional patterns may be an important thing for you to consider as part of your recovery process. And when it comes to healing, fear and negative belief systems are critical to examine because of the detrimental effect they can have on the physical body through the mind/body connection. Actually, since fear comes into play from the very first moment after diagnosis, it is even worth thinking about to some extent right away. This is because you don't want overwhelming fear to influence your decisions about treatment any more than necessary.

Dealing With Fear

Very few things are better at generating fear than a cancer diagnosis. The challenge for the cancer patient is to not let one's fear influence the decisions one makes when it comes to treatment. This can result in disaster. Managing the fear and making a treatment decision need to be two very separate processes.

From my years of working with clients in individual and family therapy settings, as well as in hypnotherapy sessions, I developed what I believe are some very helpful ways to look at and deal with the above-mentioned "F" word. The truth is that fear is something to be *highly respected*. Too often, we are afraid of fear and minimize it or try to push it away. But it is much more helpful to *not* minimize and push away fear. Instead, it is best to *acknowledge* fear and give it the respect it deserves as a very important "signal." In other words, it is just as important as your car's dashboard light which comes on when the oil is low. Those of us who wish to drive safely and support the performance of our car don't minimize this dashboard signal—we don't ignore it or push it away from our awareness by placing tape over the light so we can't see it. So, too, must we *not* minimize or ignore the emotional fear signal our bodies give us.

On the other hand, fear is just a signal. That's all it is. *You* are in control, not your fear—just as the light on the dashboard is not in control of your car, but you are.

The best way to deal with fear is to acknowledge it whenever it appears. Notice when it starts. Notice how strong it is, how it feels physically in your body. Notice the thoughts that go on in your head when you are feeling fear. Take a few moments to notice all these things when you start to feel anxiety or worry. Then say to yourself, "It's okay to feel this fear." You might even acknowledge to yourself all the reasons that you are feeling this fear. Many times people who acknowledge fear in this way will notice it quickly dissipate on its own. It may not always go away completely, but by acknowledging that it is an important signal, you are telling your subconscious mind that you have "noticed" the light on the dashboard. You thereby allow your subconscious mind to reply back, "Oh—all right . . . I guess I don't have to flash that signal so much anymore because I now have your attention." Many times, your subconscious mind will then relax a bit more.

Sometimes, when you acknowledge your fear, it may feel like you are *more* vulnerable and helpless than before. Tears may flow. This is also okay. It takes a lot of energy to suppress strong feelings, and if you allow them to come out, you can actually free up some extra energy for your body to use in healing itself. If you feel comfortable enough to share your fears with those close to you, this may also help. And, of course, whenever possible, asking close friends or family whom you trust and feel safe with to help you make decisions or help you start on treatment can be invaluable in relieving some of the fear that comes with facing an illness.

Here's the next step. Once you have acknowledged and looked at your fear more clearly than before, then you can learn to remind yourself that you are *more* than your fear. Your fear may feel like the biggest and strongest part of you, but it is really just a very small part of you. You can take control of your own body and life with the decisions that you make. If you have already acknowledged your fear rather than suppressing it, you are less likely to have the fear subconsciously driving your decisions. Remember, acknowledging your fear does not mean you are letting it make your decisions for you. Quite the contrary. Acknowledging your fear actually *undermines* its power over you and places you more in control!

But also remember that dealing with your fear and other emotions is a long-term process. It is not something you do just once or twice, and then you're done. Thus, you may notice the fear cropping up again at various times over the weeks or months. (Or maybe it never completely goes away.) When this happens, it will be helpful to just periodically acknowledge the fear and remind yourself that it is just a light on your "mental/emotional dashboard," that you are *more* than your fear, and that you *are* handling the problem and *are* in the process of adding the appropriate oil, so-to-speak.

Another helpful tip is that, whenever making important decisions for your recovery, it can be very constructive to ask yourself, "Is this decision based on fear? Or is it based on rationally weighing the information I have gathered?" Try to avoid going with choices that seem to be based mostly on fear. Or at least try to give yourself extra time to make those decisions.

The Mind/Body Connection

The mind/body connection is an amazing aspect of each of us that is very powerful. It is the psycho-physical force behind the "placebo effect." When the mind speaks, the body listens and obeys on some level. In fact, the Latin word "placebo" simply means "I shall please." Because there can be a very real effect even on the cellular level from this force, it is widely accepted as an important force in any healing process.

What many people do not realize, however, is that the mind/body connection only remotely involves the rational, conscious mind. The biggest part of one's consciousness involved in this force is the deeper, subconscious and emotional mind. Only this deeper level of mind has the power to command the body on a cellular level. Yes, we can command our bodies on a "surface level" quite easily with our rational mind. For instance, I can command my arm to lift my hand and reach over and pick up a coffee cup. Or I can think, "I want to slow my breathing and then hold my breath," and I can do that if I wish. But I cannot consciously, in a normal state of mind, command my blood flow to slow down or my white cell activity to speed up, or my cancer cells to die off. This, however, *can* be done by the subconscious mind.

It is well known that a person working with a hypnotherapist or in a self-induced trance state can effectively command changes in his or her body down to the cellular level. This is because these situations involve getting into a state where the conscious mind takes a back seat and the subconscious mind can be accessed and directed. In this sort of situation, the conscious mind plays only a small role in communicating to the subconscious mind. Many emergency medical workers, such as 911 personnel or firemen, have been trained in certain emergency hypnosis techniques to help accident victims survive critical situations. This can work very effectively since a traumatized person in shock is already in a sort of trance state. For instance, when faced with an accident victim who is in a lot of pain the medic might give the victim a hypnotic suggestion to make his or her perception of pain go down. One true story involved a medic who came across a car accident victim with a very bad head injury. The man was at risk of bleeding to death before reaching the hospital. The medic directed the man to greatly slow his own blood flow to reduce the loss of blood. It worked and the man's head stopped bleeding. When the medic got this man to the hospital he then gave him another suggestion to now allow his blood to flow normally since the doctors were there to work on him and the wound started bleeding again.

Meditation can also promote a deep connection to the subconscious mind and this is why yogis and other spiritual masters can often perform amazing physical feats, such as slowing their heart rates down to where they appear almost dead. Another well-known example comes from Tibetan initiates into priesthood who learn to control their body heat so effectively that they can crouch outside in winter snow with no more than a wet sheet wrapped around them. They have learned to make their own body heat rise so high that the sheets quickly dry and they can then spend the night in the snow in just a sheet without freezing to death.

Similarly, many people with cancer have experienced remarkably positive results in their recovery through meditation, hypnotherapy, or guided imagery. All of these examples simply show the power of the mind/body connection.

Working with your *own* mind/body connection can support and enhance your healing process. To do this, some people may want to seek out a therapist or guided imagery specialist who has experience working with cancer recovery. Part of working with your mind/body connection may involve dealing with your emotions, such as fear; part of it may involve active visualization of the cancer cells going away; and part of it may involve examining your own personality dynamics.

Examining Your Personality Dynamics

On a daily basis, our thoughts and behavior patterns can affect our physical bodies. As an example, just think about how you would feel if you entered a dinner party and suddenly realized you didn't have your clothes on! Your muscles would probably immediately tense up, you would feel adrenaline running rampant, and you might even break out in a sweat. The body can very quickly respond to certain thoughts or feelings with strong physical responses.

Although you are not likely to find yourself in the above situation, you may be in many more similar situations on a regular basis than you realize. When you are attempting to pick up your child from after school practice and you are stuck on the freeway starting to experience the physical effects of anxiety, you are in a similar situation. When you are panicking about getting something done at work before a deadline and you feel your blood pressure rise, you are in a similar situation. When you are angry at someone but cannot resolve the conflict in some way, you are in a similar situation. Anxiety in stressful situations *always* produces some type of physical response in the body. This is due to the mind/body connection.

Our bodies are designed to handle anxiety and physical stress reactions as long as they don't occur too often. It is when these reactions occur chronically, or habitually, that our physical bodies run into trouble. Some types of personality characteristics can produce habitual physical stress responses on a daily basis that overstress the body.

One way that chronic stress is physically hard on us is by causing the body to secrete stress hormones on a daily basis that deplete our bodies' stores of vitamin C. Another way that chronic stress is hard on us is by promoting the dehydration of healthy cells. This can happen as a result of the increased metabolic activity involved with hyper-vigilance, or worry. Constantly worrying about what others think of you, how well you are performing at something, what you are going to do next week, and so forth, can produce constant triggering of the physical "fight or flight" mechanisms of the body, such as adrenaline and other responses. Holding emotions in for fear of expressing oneself can also deplete much-needed energy from the body. These are just a few of the examples of how personality dynamics can be a factor that plays a role in how well your body's immune system functions, or how well your body recovers from illness.

Although there is no one-to-one correlation, a number of studies appear to have validated the reality that personality dynamics can play a role in both the development of and recovery from illness. The most common finding in all the studies done on this subject was that people who tend to "suppress" their feelings are more likely to develop cancer than those who tend to "express" their feelings. In other words, your physical body will more often fare better if you do *not* hold your feelings in.

One of the longest studies to focus on the relationship between personality characteristics and cancer was begun in 1946. A group of 972 students at Johns Hopkins School of Medicine was divided into five subgroups based on various psychological measures, then followed for three decades. Results showed that those students who were initially characterized as the type that suppressed their emotions behind a bland exterior of facial expression were actually 16 times more likely to develop cancer than those who generally expressed their feelings.[1]

Dr. Douglas Brodie of Nevada spent over three decades working with cancer patients and specializing in alternative and integrative medicine. He supported the idea of a "cancer-prone personality." In fact, he compiled seven common characteristics of people who develop cancer. Dr. Brodie wrote the following.[2]

> In dealing with many thousands of cancer patients over the past 32 years, it has been my observation that there are certain personality traits which are rather consistently present in the cancer-susceptible individual. These characteristics are as follows:
>
> 1. Being highly conscientious, dutiful, responsible, caring, hardworking, and usually of above average intelligence.
>
> 2. Exhibiting a strong tendency toward carrying other people's burdens and toward taking on extra obligations, often 'worrying for others.'

3. Having a deep-seated need to make others happy, tending to be 'people pleasers.' Having a great need for approval.

4. Often having a history of lack of closeness with one or both parents, sometimes, later in life, resulting in lack of closeness with spouse or others who would normally be close.

5. Harboring long-suppressed toxic emotions, such as anger, resentment and/or hostility. Typically the cancer-susceptible individual internalizes such emotions and has great difficulty expressing them.

6. Reacting adversely to stress, often becoming unable to cope adequately with such stress. Usually experiencing an especially damaging event about two years before the onset of detectable cancer. The patient is unable to cope with this traumatic event or series of events, which comes as a 'last straw' on top of years of suppressed reactions to stress.

7. Showing an inability to resolve deep-seated emotional problems and conflicts, usually arising in childhood, often even being unaware of their presence.

What can be very helpful in reducing the body's stress responses is learning to "let go" of worrying about unimportant things. In other words, "Don't sweat the small stuff!" One woman, while fighting breast cancer, made up a list of all the things she needed to do each day as part of her alternative treatment program for healing. Then, whenever she felt a stress reaction triggered inside her due to outside time crunches, issues with her children, and so forth, she would simply say to herself, "Stress is not part of my program!" This simple technique always reminded her to let go of the little worries and greatly helped her to keep her physical stress reactions down.

Another woman realized, while fighting spinal cord cancer, that she was suffering from too much anxiety and worry about the future. She had a type of cancer that her doctors claimed would take her life in just a few months, but she also had four small children who needed raising. The "what ifs" plagued her mercilessly. She finally developed an effective way to let her worry go while she was recovering from her cancer. Every morning when she woke up, she would say to herself, "I got through yesterday . . . I can get through today." Then, every night before bed, she would say to herself, "I got through today, I can get through tomorrow."

(This woman *did* fully recover using an effective alternative approach and has been cancer-free for the past 18 years.)

When it comes to fears and worries, it is unrealistic to expect anyone with cancer to *not* worry or be afraid at all. But trying to suppress, or ignore the fears and worries is probably the most damaging thing an ill person can do. This is because the body feels and *responds to* the suppressed fears and worries anyway! In other words, you can suppress a thought or feeling so that it is no longer in your conscious awareness. But you cannot suppress a fear or worry so that it is no longer in your *subconscious* awareness and therefore in your physical body's awareness. So, acknowledging your fears or worries whenever they come up, and then learning ways to let them go or to deal with them more constructively is most often the best way to support your healing.

Along with resolving chronic stress, a person who has a history of always taking care of others to the exclusion of themselves, must learn to take care of himself or herself. This is sometimes one of the biggest challenges a person with cancer must face. One must learn to take care of one's physical needs of adequate sleep, nutrition, water, and emotional support. And through dealing with and changing some of one's personality characteristics or patterns, a person can often learn to take care of these needs much better than they did before.

Other than simple stress reactions, our thought patterns and emotional baggage can also create other types of damaging messages that get sent to our bodies' cells and physiological systems. Many alternative and conventional practitioners who work with cancer agree that a patient's attitude, level of hope, and active participation in their own healing are all very *real* factors in recovery. In fact, Dr. Nicholas Gonzalez of New York has been quoted as saying, "I've had patients whose cancer didn't get better no matter how perfectly they did my program . . . until they resolved serious emotional issues in their lives."[3]

The physical body is accustomed to fulfilling instructions that emanate from the mind. Often, we are very aware of these mental thought instructions, such as when we decide to walk across a room, pick up a book, and sit down on a couch. However, we also have mental thoughts that we are not normally aware of. These are usually on a deeper, more subconscious level. (But they are not totally out of conscious access.) For instance, a person may be avoiding dealing with an important issue in his or her life—sweeping the problem under the rug, so-to-speak. The resultant suppression of feelings about the issue then leaves the person with the deep subconscious mental thought that the issue is "eating" him or her up on the inside. The mental concept of being eaten up inside can then possibly translate as a message to the *physical* body, which might result in the physical body fulfilling that message as if it were an instruction and thereby creating a cancer that eats them up. Or, if a person feels on a mental/emotional level that they are "weak and falling apart," there is reason to believe that the cells and systems of the body may at times comply with these instructions as well.

There are many ways to deal with one's emotions, personality dynamics, and subconscious thought messages. Seeking professional counseling is one way. Simply sharing one's fears and thoughts with other caring people is another. Cancer treatment specialist, Dr. W. John Diamond, also believes it is often important for his patients to address some very difficult psycho-spiritual questions. He even talks about the importance of cancer patients addressing whether they have a deep-seated will to live or not. This may seem an odd question to ask a person with a life-threatening illness, because the first reaction is usually, "Well, of course I want to live!" But the question is actually very pertinent when you consider that some cancer patients may have been struggling with extremely difficult issues or situations in their lives previous to their cancer diagnosis. They may have been suffering through problematic marriages, constant financial stress, working at jobs they hate, or possibly trying desperately to emotionally survive the death of a child or spouse.

In his book, *An Alternative Medicine Definitive Guide to Cancer*, Dr. Diamond states,

> A rather hard question must be posed: Is it the patient's personal priority to eliminate the cancer? This may sound absurd at first glance, but it isn't. In some instances, people may not want treatment at all despite the fact that they are sitting in the physician's office. They may desire to pass on to another reality; they may wish to weather the storm using their own resources; they may be seeking encouragement and ways to reduce their pain and suffering.[4]

In other words, it is not uncommon for a person to put on a good face and just tough it out through hard times, while deep inside, they subconsciously wish their struggles were over. Unfortunately, cancer is capable of fulfilling that subconscious wish and may be your body's way of listening to your subconscious mind and obeying.

Thus, Dr. Diamond's emphasis on cancer patients looking at whether they truly want to live or not is very important. But I would add one point to that. From a mind/body perspective, the desire to live is most effective in helping a person to recover from cancer if that person wants to live *for himself or for herself*. In other words, if you have cancer and you do get in touch with a deep desire to live, then you might ask yourself, "Do I want to live for *myself*, or do I want to live for my children, my spouse, or my parents?" Are you hoping to recover because someone else needs you and you want to be there for *them*? Is your reason to live based on the thought, "What would they do without me?" If so, your physical body may be getting "mixed" messages. Your conscious mind may be saying "I want to live" (for Joan or John), but your subconscious mind may be saying "I don't really want to live for myself; I just want to be there for someone else."

There is nothing wrong with wanting to be there for others. But when it comes to overcoming a difficult disease such as cancer, your body's power to heal and fully recover will be best supported if you can get in touch with a desire to live *for yourself*. This is because, in terms of the mind/body connection, the body only responds to messages for "self." It does *not* respond to altruistic messages on a higher philosophical plane.

Thus, if you find out that you are only trying to recover from your illness because you want to be there for your daughter and see her graduate college and get married, or because you want to help your son mature into a fine young man and give him the support and help you never had, or because your fragile parent would die if anything ever happened to you, and so forth, then you may have more introspection and psychological work to do. You will need to go deep inside and find reasons to live *for yourself*. Sometimes this may simply involve a little "re-framing." For example, you can realize that your interest in seeing your daughter get married is *for your own pleasure*, or that *you will be satisfied* if you can give your son the support and guidance you never got, or that *you want* to be there for your parents because you care about them and you also care about yourself. Re-framing is basically just a process of re-stating and re-feeling something from a different reference point—this time from the reference of self.

In order for this process of re-framing to be effective on the mind/body level, however, it must be honest. You can't "fool" the mind/body connection any more than you can fool Mother Nature. The body only responds to what you *truly* feel or think.

Once you have gotten used to your daily cancer treatment program, making an effort to include fun in your day whenever possible is also a good idea. If fun is too much to ask for, then just do something that gets your mind *off* your cancer every day. This, in itself, can be a helpful way to let go of the fears that having cancer has triggered. To a certain extent, just being active in your own healing process can also help to lessen those fears. This is one of the great aspects of all the alternative treatments—every one of them involves active participation on the patient's part, and thereby sends the message to the mind/body connection that the person is in control, not the illness

Last, but not least, participating in some form of meditative activity while you are following your alternative cancer treatment can greatly help you to relax on the emotional and mind/body level. Thus, if you do not already practice one of these, you might consider learning some form of meditation, gentle yoga, tai chi, or qi gong. The healing benefits of these mind-quieting activities cannot be overstated.

The Negative Placebo Effect

One aspect of the mind/body connection, which is too rarely addressed, is the "negative placebo effect." (Also sometimes referred to as the "nocebo" effect.) It is the flip side of the "positive placebo effect" that we have all heard about. The positive placebo effect occurs when someone heals because they *think* they are being given an effective treatment, and therefore they *think* themselves well. Countless studies have proven the positive placebo effect to be a powerful healing force. Yet, the positive placebo effect is simply the wondrous power of the mind/body connection. It is simply the physical body saying, "I shall please" as it responds to a person's genuine thoughts and feelings.

But the negative placebo effect is the exact same wondrous force! It occurs when a person thinks they are *not* going to recover, so they don't. This can happen when a doctor communicates in various ways to a patient that there is nothing more that medical science can do for them and that they, the patient, will soon die. Too often, doctors tell their patients they only have "X" number of months to live and often that is exactly how many months those patients *do* live.

When it comes to dealing with cancer, however, it is not only the doctors who can cause a negative placebo effect to take place. It is also friends, relatives, society, and even ourselves. On a societal level, cancer carries a high fear factor (or expectation of death). This is because, with modern conventional medicine in the U.S. the way it is, most of the people we ever know or hear about with cancer *do* die from their disease. Many of us have witnessed cancer deaths among close friends or family members. This can cause us to be surrounded by negative expectations for recovery, and promotes in the cancer patient's mind a subconscious belief system full of negative expectations. In terms of the mind/body connection, it can be very helpful to the healing process if the cancer patient can *counteract* these negative thought patterns.

I am not saying that you cannot get well unless you have a positive attitude—that would simply be incorrect. But by maintaining a genuinely positive and *proactive* attitude about your own healing process, you can greatly counteract the negative messages that are all around you, that are bombarding you all the time. It is one way you can support your own healing process on the mind/body level.

The gist of this chapter is this. To enhance your own healing, you may want to practice dealing with your fear in constructive ways so that you make informed decisions for yourself and don't get caught in the trap of making decisions based on fear. You may want to look at any personality characteristics you have that could be causing chronic physical stress reactions in your body. You may want to stop holding in your feelings so much, which is exhausting to your body, and learn to take care of yourself if you have had a pattern of not doing so. You may want to practice letting go of worry, or not sweating the small stuff, if this is an issue for you. And you may want to ask yourself the hard question of whether you really want to live *for yourself.* All of this may require some extra courage and honesty, but it is usually well worth it.

German New Medicine

All of the above information in this chapter is important for anyone dealing with cancer to understand, and can help many people to create changes in their thinking and behavior that will enhance their healing. However, any write-up about dealing with the mind/body connection in relation to cancer would not be complete without a reference to German New Medicine. (For more information on this approach, please refer to the section on German New Medicine in Chapter 17.)

Unfortunately, German New Medicine is quite new in the U.S. and there are few American practitioners who are trained experts. But those cancer patients who can find a German New Medicine practitioner to work with may be able to access the *Rolls Royce* of methods for dealing with the mind/body connection. Some remarkable results in making cancer and metastases go away have been achieved through this impressive approach that focuses on the brain's responses to mental/emotional traumas in life. And easy techniques have been developed to help patients stop those responses of the brain that appear to be perpetuating their disease. Thus, for anyone wishing to add a mind/body therapy to their treatment protocol, German New Medicine is a powerful approach to pursue.

Louise Hay and Affirmations

Another powerful approach to enlisting the aid of the mind/body connection for healing comes from the teachings of a woman named Louise Hay. Hay has been a foremost leader in the self-healing movement for decades. A best-selling author many times, Hay popularized the idea of doing "Affirmations" and has helped countless people heal their bodies and lives through effective techniques including examining one's thinking patterns, releasing emotional blocks, and doing mirror work. At first, these techniques may seem superficial or weak to someone facing a life-threatening disease. However, it is quite remarkable that many people have actually healed themselves of cancer in large part by using Hay's techniques. Louise Hay, herself, recovered from cancer without the use of any conventional treatment but, instead, employed her own methods along with diet changes, nutritional therapy, emotional clearing, and detoxification.

For more information about Louise Hay and her self-healing techniques, I highly recommend the informative DVD called "You Can Heal Your Life – The Movie: Expanded Version," a two DVD set which can be ordered from her website www.LouiseHay.com or from Amazon.com for about $24. Other inspirational books and CDs are also available. Hay does not suggest that people should rely on the mind/body connection only when dealing with a life-threatening disease, but her techniques are a powerful adjunct to other therapies a person may be using, and are easy to learn from her DVD, books, and CDs.

Having to fight cancer is never, in itself, a welcome battle. But many people who have done so and won have felt they received positive side benefits, or gifts, as a result. Sometimes these gifts include being more in touch with one's *true* self than before and having a deeper appreciation of everything in one's life.

25

Concluding Comments

The primary point of this book is to make it abundantly clear that you do have a wide variety of treatment options, even though all of these options may not be sanctioned by mainstream medicine or paid for by your health insurance company. You are not limited to the big three conventional cancer treatments of chemotherapy, surgery, and radiation (often referred to as poison, slash, and burn.) You are also not limited to the alternative, non-toxic treatments listed in this publication since there are more alternative treatments out there than this book has space for.

How you decide to treat your cancer should be *your* choice, and you have a right to make that choice an informed one. If you are one of the many people who have heard their doctor say, "There is no cure for your type of cancer," you now know that what that *really* means is, "There is nothing that *conventional* medicine currently has that can cure you." And you also now know there is very real hope in the world of alternative cancer approaches. Although there is never a 100 percent guarantee for recovery, countless people have "outsmarted" their cancer with alternative, non-toxic treatments and gone on to live normal cancer-free lives!

Changes Need To Happen

It is time that cancer treatments be prescribed by mainstream medicine based on what truly works. It is time that our FDA function as the

447

protector of the American people (as it was designed to function), instead of as a protector of big corporations. If the many effective, non-toxic approaches to cancer known today were finally approved by the FDA and supported by the ACS and NCI, there would be many more people starting to use these approaches in earlier stages of their illness. This factor alone could make recovery rates for non-toxic approaches soar to record highs, and cause cancer deaths to decrease dramatically.

Some people believe that if effective alternative treatments were to become mainstream, millions of people would then suddenly be out of work who are currently employed by the conventional cancer industry. I do not think this would have to happen. Oncologists, nurses, technicians, and medical researchers would still be needed to help patients use the alternative approaches. Even with alternative, non-toxic approaches, patients still need medical care. They need frequent diagnostic tests to monitor their progress. They need qualified practitioners helping them to understand their treatment approach. And they often need side complications of their cancer to be dealt with by medical professionals and/or hospitalization. Plus, many of the conventional surgical techniques will still play an important role, as well as some of the conventional fast-acting toxic treatments (when fast-acting damage control is necessary).

The personnel in medical research laboratories could also remain employed. But instead of researching toxic approaches that don't bring long-term recoveries, they could do further research on the best non-toxic approaches and learn about how to improve them or combine them for optimal results. (There is no doubt that these treatment approaches work, so proving they work need no longer be the focus.) Moreover, with public opinion about cancer therapy changing, the first health insurance company to fully cover alternative cancer treatments would probably make a fortune!

Killing Cockroaches With Cannons

Why must there be a paradigm shift from toxic to non-toxic cancer treatments? Because the indiscriminately toxic approaches such as chemotherapy and radiation *rarely work for long-term recovery!*

A crude but helpful way of explaining why toxic treatments fail so often is the following analogy. Let's say you live in a house infested with cockroaches. The bugs are hiding in the walls and beneath the floors. Using an indiscriminately toxic treatment is like trying to kill off all the cockroaches in your house with a cannon. Sure, you could blast away at one or two of the most infested walls and kill a *lot* of cockroaches all at once. (Like getting rid of tumors through surgery, radiation or chemo.) You could even rebuild those walls and it would appear for a while that all the bugs were gone.

But there would still be small nests and colonies of roaches in other walls, or eggs under the floor that you can't see. And these would eventually breed new bugs that would spread throughout the house again. Soon, you're seeing the bugs scurry across the kitchen floor once more and you're discovering new nests (tumors) in new places. Sure, you could try a *different* cannon. Maybe you'd be eligible for the latest, shiniest, most new and improved cannon available that "they" are just doing a new trial on. Still, you'd have to blast the entire house to smithereens in order to get rid of every last cockroach with your cannon. The problem with that scenario is, of course, that you would then no longer have a house! (*Or a body!*)

Sadly, this is what happens when cancer patients are put through the roller coaster of treatment-remission-treatment-remission using toxic approaches, until their bodies eventually just give up. What is *really* happening is that the cancer was never completely gone when the person was pronounced in remission. The clinical signs of cancer may have been absent, but scans and other diagnostic tests cannot see every last cancer cell. So, some cancer cells are virtually always left standing and ready to grow back again—just like those eggs under the floor that you can't see and that were never completely gone.

Non-toxic treatments, on the other hand, can *avoid* this vicious cycle because they can be administered continuously for as long as it is necessary to get rid of every last cancer cell.

In other words, people using alternative methods for cancer can put themselves into remission (the point where diagnostics tests can't see any more cancer and all clinical signs of cancer are gone), but they don't have to stop treatment at that point. Because what they are doing is non-toxic, they can continue the treatment that is getting rid of their cancer for six months or a year or more AFTER the remission point to be sure they get every last cancer cell. Nobody would want to do this with chemo or radiation because prolonged use of chemo or radiation would kill the patient! The countless cases of people who have cured themselves of cancer with non-toxic approaches, when toxic treatments could not cure them, proves that the conventional paradigm has to change.

Misconceptions About Alternatives

Unfortunately, when a cancer treatment is denied mainstream acceptance and labeled "alternative," then the biggest obstacle to people being open to that approach is the *disbelief factor*. As discussed in Chapter 1, this disbelief factor occurs in the minds of physicians as well as patients. Most medical experts know very little, if anything, about alternative non-toxic cancer treatments because these approaches are *not* discussed in medical schools or written about in medical journals. It is understandably difficult for physicians to believe that an alternative approach to cancer could be more successful at achieving long-term recoveries than conventional methods and yet *not* be taught to them.

But just because most conventional doctors don't know about them, that does not mean alternative approaches don't work. Aside from the many documented cases of politically suppressive events that have blocked alternative methods from mainstream medicine, there is also the fact that it is prohibitively expensive for most of these methods to become "accepted" approaches without pharmaceutical financial backing. (As things are set up now, it costs at least $800 million for a new cancer treatment to fully go through the institutionalized processes required for official approval.) Thus, the fact that alternative approaches are not FDA-approved says little about their effectiveness, and more about how much money the developers of that approach had.

One direct outcome of the disbelief factor is the common mistake of assuming that whenever anything unconventional *does* work, it must be the result of "spontaneous remission." It is medically inaccurate to assume that most or all of the recoveries using alternative approaches are attributable to spontaneous remission when the point in time that cancer patients start to recover virtually always coincides closely to the point in time they start the alternative treatment. As you probably noticed in the testimonials presented in this book, many recoveries happened to people whose cancer was getting *worse* while they were on conventional treatments. It was not until after these people started using an alternative approach, that they began to show signs of recovery, and then finally recovered.

Another common mistake is the assumption that alternative approaches must have been developed by "non-scientific people" in "non-scientific ways." However, just the opposite is true. For example:

- The Hoxsey Therapy was clinically evaluated by an independent group of 10 physicians from various parts of the United States. These physicians formally concluded that the Hoxsey treatment was superior to any cancer treatment being used by the medical establishment at the time.

- Essiac tea not only resulted from Native Americans testing and using herbs for hundreds of years, but was also clinically proven by Canadian and American physicians. This included Dr. Charles A. Brusch who had been the personal physician to John F. Kennedy. After 10 years of studying Essiac, Dr. Brusch concluded that Essiac was "a cure for cancer, period."

- Dr. Gerson was a highly esteemed physician in his home country of Germany, whom the famous humanitarian doctor, Albert Schweitzer, called "one of the most eminent medical geniuses in the history of medicine." Known in New York as someone who could cure "incurables", Dr. Gerson's clinic showed astounding results, which he even presented to a sub-committee in Congress known as "the Pepper Commission."

- Dr. Krebs and his son, Dr. Ernst T. Krebs, Jr., (developers of Laetrile), were both prominent physicians and renowned medical researchers. Besides their own meticulous laboratory research, Laetrile was tested clinically on humans and shown to be successful by many physicians around the world as well as by Memorial Sloan-Kettering's research group.

- Dr. Kelley's metabolic therapy involving the powerful use of enzymes was independently evaluated and proven effective for many types of cancer. And for pancreatic cancer, it was proven to be "off-the-charts" better than any current conventional method.

- Dr. Stanislaw Burzynski gained recognition as one of the youngest people in the history of Poland to receive both an M.D. and Ph.D. diploma, and later scientifically researched his antineoplastons at the Baylor College of Medicine in Texas. Independent clinical evaluation has proven antineoplaston therapy to be more effective than current conventional medical approaches, especially for brain cancers and lymphomas.

- Jim Sheridan was a chemist who obtained a private grant to work at the Detroit Cancer Institute where he tested his early versions of Protocel® in a formal, scientific laboratory environment. Later, Sheridan worked on his formula in the Biosciences Division of the Battelle Institute in Columbus, Ohio. There, he tested his formula using the same rigorous standards that were being used to test new chemotherapeutic agents for the National Cancer Institute. Finally, in 1990, the NCI tested Sheridan's formula in vitro on many different cancer cell lines and all the results were excellent.

- The mechanism of anaerobic functioning in cancer cells was scientifically proven by the famous biochemist, Otto Warburg, who received a Nobel Prize for his contributions to science.

- Dr. Johanna Budwig was a brilliant biochemist who was nominated for a Nobel Prize seven different times. Her impeccable laboratory research on essential fatty acids was a monumental contribution to science and her own clinical work reportedly demonstrated over 1,000 documented cases of cancer recoveries using her dietary approach.

- Aubrey Keith Brewer, Ph.D., was the pioneering physicist for cesium high pH therapy. He was highly qualified for his research that focused on the study of cell membranes and, for a time, was chief of the National Bureau of Standards Mass Spectrometer and Isotope section. Clinical trials later proved his approach using cesium to be effective at bringing about late-stage cancer recoveries in humans.

- Royal Rife and Gaston Naessens were considered by many to be two of the greatest geniuses of the 20th century. Their contributions to microbiology and the understanding of micro-organisms were immeasurable. Brilliant inventors, they each independently developed new types of microscopes to aid them in their work. Rife's "Universal Microscope" and Naessens's "Somatoscope" were far more powerful than any microscope being used at the time and both allowed observation of virus-size organisms in their alive state, something that still cannot be done today with current technology.

Thus, the belief that alternative cancer treatments are "non-scientific" is simply as wrong as it could be!

Medical Freedom

Some physicians *are* open to alternative approaches and to their patients using them. More and more oncologists and other doctors are overseeing patients using a non-toxic approach for their cancer. Many of these physicians are seeing the alternative approach work and are saying to their patients, "Keep doing what you're doing!" But a very real obstacle to any physician *prescribing* an alternative approach for cancer is that most states in the United States do not legally allow physicians to do this. Many doctors are in the unenviable position of having to say, "Keep doing what you are doing because it is working, but don't tell me the details of what you are doing because I can't prescribe it anyway."

As a result of state laws restricting doctors to only prescribing certain types of treatments, medical freedom is not yet secure for us in the United States. Moreover, medical freedom is not yet protected as a "right" in the Constitution. However, at least one signer of our Declaration of Independence had the foresight back in 1776 to proclaim that medical freedom should be a protected right, and should be in our Constitution. Benjamin Rush, M.D., was the Pennsylvania delegate to the Continental Congress as well as a prominent medical doctor of his day. Dr. Rush wisely stated:

> Unless we put medical freedom into the Constitution, the time will come when medicine will organize into an undercover dictatorship to restrict the art of healing to one class of men and deny equal privileges to others; the Constitution of this republic should make a special privilege for medical freedom as well as religious.

Hopefully, the day will come when *all* effective medical approaches are available to us. But until that time, how you choose to treat your cancer is still *your* decision, not someone else's. Don't let others push you into doing something you don't want to do, whether they happen to be doctors, friends, or family. And don't let your own fear push you either. Instead, take a deep breath and do your research as quickly as you can. Get someone you trust to help you, if possible. Listen to your heart. Once you have started treatment (whether conventional or alternative), *keep* doing research at a slower pace. There may be even more you can do for yourself as you start to recover.

Cancer is never easy, but many others have "outsmarted" their cancer with alternative non-toxic treatments that work, and you can pursue the same methods, too!

Recommended Resources

Multiple Alternative Cancer Treatments

Options: The Alternative Cancer Therapy Book, by Richard Walters (Avery/Penguin Putnam, New York, 1993).

An Alternative Medicine Definitive Guide to Cancer, by W. John Diamond, M.D. and W. Lee Cowden, M.D., with Burton Goldberg (Future Medicine Publishing, Inc., Tiburon, California, 1997).

Cancer Therapy: The Independent Consumer's Guide to Non-Toxic Treatment and Prevention, by Ralph W. Moss, Ph.D. (Equinox Press, New York, 1996).

Cancer-Free: Your Guide to Gentle, Non-toxic Healing, 3rd Edition, by Bill Henderson (Booklocker.com, Inc., 2008).

Cancer: Step Outside the Box, 2nd Edition, by Ty M. Bollinger (Infinity 510 Squared Partners, 2006).

Painless Cancer Cures and Preventions Your Doctor May Not Be Aware Of, by Deanna K. Loftis, R.N., B.B.A. (JADA Press, 2005).

I Beat Cancer: 50 People Tell You How They Did It, by Zack Vaughan (Awareness Publishing, Oxnard, California 2003).

Alternatives in Cancer Therapy, by Ross Pelton, R.Ph., Ph.D., with Lee Overholser, Ph.D. (Simon and Schuster, New York, 1994).

Natural Strategies for Cancer Patients, by Russell Blaylock, M.D. (Kensington, 2003).

Specific Alternative Cancer Treatments

Antineoplastons

The Burzynski Breakthrough, by Thomas D. Elias (Lexikos, Nevada City, California, 2001).

Cesium High pH Therapy

Cancer Cover-Up, by Kathleen Deoul (Cassandra Books, Baltimore, 2001). www.cassandrabooks.com.

Essiac Tea

The Essiac Report, by Richard Thomas (The Alternative Treatment Information Network, Los Angeles, 1993).

Essiac Essentials, by Sheila Snow and Mali Klein (Kensington Books, New York, 1999).

Flaxseed Oil and Cottage Cheese

How to Fight Cancer and Win, by William L. Fischer (Agora Health Books, Baltimore, Maryland, 2000).

Fats That Heal, Fats That Kill: The Complete Guide to Fats, Oils, Cholesterol and Human Health, by Udo Erasmus (Alive Books, British Columbia, Canada, 1993).

Flax Oil as a True Aid Against Arthritis, Heart Infarction, Cancer, and Other Diseases, by Dr. Johanna Budwig (Apple Publishing, Vancouver, Canada, 1994).

Gerson Therapy

A Cancer Therapy: Results of Fifty Cases, by Max Gerson, M.D. (The Gerson Institute, Bonita, CA, 1999).

Censured For Curing Cancer: The American Experience of Dr. Max Gerson, by S. J. Haught (The Gerson Institute [under the P.U.L.S.E. imprint], Bonita, California, 1991).

The Gerson Therapy, by Charlotte Gerson and Morton Walker, D.P.M. (Kensington Publishing, New York, 2001).

Hoxsey Therapy

When Healing Becomes a Crime: The Amazing Story of the Hoxsey Cancer Clinics and the Return of Alternative Therapies, by Kenny Ausubel (Healing Arts Press, Rochester, Vermont, 2000).

Issels's Approach

Cancer—A Second Opinion, by Josef Issels, M.D. (Avery Publishing Group, New York, 1999).

Kelley's Enzyme Approach

Cancer: Curing The Incurable Without Surgery, Chemotherapy, or Radiation, by Dr. William Donald Kelley, D.D.S., M.S., with Fred Rohe (New Century Promotions, Bonita, California, 2000).

Laetrile

World Without Cancer: The Story of Vitamin B_{17}, revised edition, by G. Edward Griffin (American Media, Westlake Village, California, 1997).

Alive and Well: One Doctor's Experience with Nutrition in the Treatment of Cancer Patients, by Philip E. Binzel, Jr., M.D. (American Media, Westlake Village, California, 1994).

Poly-MVA

First Pulse: A Personal Journey in Cancer Research, 2nd Ed., by Dr. Merrill Garnett (First Pulse Projects, Inc., 1998).

Robert D. Milne, M.D., & Melissa L. Block, M.Ed. *Poly-MVA: A New Supplement in the Fight Against Cancer,* by Robert D. Milne, M.D. (Basic Health Publications, Inc., 2004).

Fire in the Genes: Poly-MVA—the Cancer Answer? By Michael L. Culbert, ScD. (Foundation for the Advancement of Medicine, 2000).

Protocel®

The Breast Stays Put: No Chemo—No Radiation—No Lumpectomy—No Thank You, by Pamela Hoeppner (Xulon Press, 2008).

Rife Machine

The Cancer Cure That Worked! Fifty Years of Suppression, by Barry Lynes (Marcus Books, Ontario, Canada, 1987).

Video: "The Royal Rife Story: Historical Documentary." 1-888-486-4420.

Cancer Politics and/or Conventional Treatments

The Cancer Industry, by Ralph W. Moss (Equinox Press, Brooklyn, New York, 1999).

Questioning Chemotherapy, by Ralph W. Moss, Ph.D., (Equinox Press, Brooklyn, New York, 2000).

Racketeering in Medicine: The Suppression of Alternatives, by James P. Carter, M.D. (Hampton Roads Publishing Company, Inc., Charlottesville, PA, 1992).

Politics in Healing: Suppression and Manipulation in American Medicine, by Daniel Haley (Potomac Valley Press, Wash., D.C., 2000).

The Healing of Cancer: The Cures, the Cover-Ups, and the Solution Now!, by Barry Lynes (Marcus Books, Queensville, Ontario, Canada, 1989).

The War on Cancer: Anatomy of Failure, A Blueprint for the Future, by Guy B. Faguet (Springer, 2008).

Video: "Cancer Doesn't Scare Me Anymore!" by Lorraine Day, M.D. 1-800-574-2437, or www.drday.com. (Dr. Day also speaks about her own battle and approach.)

Other Medical Issues Relating to Cancer Recovery

Women's Hormones

What Your Doctor May Not Tell You About Breast Cancer, by John R. Lee, M.D., David Zava, Ph.D., and Virginia Hopkins (Warner Books, New York, 2002).

What Your Doctor May Not Tell You About Menopause, by John R. Lee, M.D., with Virginia Hopkins (Warner Books, New York, 1996).

Video: "Managing Your Hormones at Menopause and Beyond." Can be ordered from www.johnleemd.com.

Alkalizing the Body

The Calcium Factor: The Scientific Secret of Health and Youth, by Robert R. Barefoot and Carl J. Reich, M.D. (Deonna Enterprises Publishing, Wickenburg, AZ, 2001).

The pH Miracle: Balance Your Diet, Reclaim Your Health, by Robert O. Young and Shelley Redford Young (Wellness Central, 2008).

Toxic Teeth

Root Canal Cover-Up, by George E. Meinig, D.D.S., F.A.C.D. (Bion Publishing, Ojai, California, 1998).

It's All in Your Head: The Link Between Mercury Amalgams and Illness, by Dr. Hal A. Huggins (Avery Publishing Group, Inc., Garden City Park, New York, 1993).

Fluoride

The Fluoride Deception, by Christopher Bryson, (Seven Stories Press, 2006).

APPENDIX

Five Big Environmental Cancer Triggers

In Chapter 2, we looked at many cancer-causing factors of modern living. Some of these factors involve insufficient dietary nutrition, others involve environmental pollutants, and still others occur as a result of life-style choices. This Appendix goes into extra detail about five big *environmental* cancer-causing factors that are extremely important today. They are:

1. Chlorine byproducts

2. Fluoride

3. Asbestos

4. Fiberglass

5. Nuclear radiation

Chlorine Byproducts

Right up there with pesticides and herbicides is another *huge* threat to public health in our modern world. However, unlike the issue of pesticides and herbicides, it happens to be an issue that most people are not the least bit aware of. It is the issue of chlorine byproducts. Since about 1908, chlorine has been used in the United States to treat public water supplies. For a long time, this was seen as a great advance in public welfare because chlorinating water greatly reduced the risk of disease from waterborne microbes that could cause cholera, typhoid fever, and other devastating illnesses. Dow Chemical Company was the leading producer of chlorine for water disinfecting, and Dow's business soared even more when the paper and plastics industries skyrocketed. Paper mills use chlorine for bleaching purposes and the plastics industry uses chlorine in their production of polyvinyl chloride (PVC plastics).

For many years, chlorine was thought to be quite safe because under controlled laboratory conditions it harmlessly breaks down into salt and water. In truth, chlorine in its pure form does *not* cause cancer in laboratory animals. However, what was not originally looked at, was a host of *unintentional byproducts* that resulted from the chlorine used in industry. It wasn't until about 1974 that scientists discovered that the chlorine used to disinfect public water supplies was combining in the water with organic material from plant and animal sources to produce byproduct compounds in our drinking water. These byproduct compounds are called "organochlorines," or "chlorine byproducts."

The problem is that when chlorine combines with organic material in water, the majority of the resulting organochlorine compounds are extremely toxic. These toxic compounds are a bigger problem in water supplies that come from surface water sources (such as reservoirs, lakes, and rivers) than they are from well-water sources. This is because the surface water sources tend to have more natural organic material (algae, leaves, and other plant materials) to which the chlorine can bind. The well water, or groundwater sources have much less organic material and therefore, when chlorinated, result in far fewer organochlorines than the surface water sources.

Organochlorine compounds are not found naturally anywhere in the world, but once formed as a byproduct of water chlorination, they are not only toxic, they are also extremely stable. Most organochlorines don't break down in nature for hundreds of years. Yet, organochlorines are easily absorbed into the bodies of virtually all animals and tend to *accumulate* over time in fat cells. With enough exposure, they can produce birth defects, reproductive disorders, immune system breakdown, and cancer.

These toxic chlorine byproducts are a more and more alarming problem to authorities. One type of organochlorine that has been heavily studied in recent years is a group of compounds called "trihalomethanes." Epidemiological studies have shown that the number of years a person drinks water with certain levels of trihalomethanes directly correlates with an increased risk of bladder and rectal cancer. Yet, the first trihalomethane limits in public water were not set by the U.S. Environmental Protection

Agency (EPA) until 1979. Since then, specific types of filters have been set up in many water supplies to finely filter out organic material before chlorine is added to the water. But not all water companies currently meet the standards and the EPA still has not regulated *other* chlorine byproducts in public water supplies that may also cause cancer.

If you think you have not been exposed to dangerous organochlorines because you only drink pristine well water, think again. We are exposed to organochlorines in other ways than through the water we drink. For instance, there are often high levels of organochlorines in swimming pools. Once again, the chlorine in the swimming pool water combines with organic material in the water. These organochlorines can enter the body through the skin. We can also inhale them from fumes near the surface levels of swimming pools and hot tubs. And it is not uncommon to breathe in organochlorines every time we open our dishwasher at home. In this case, the chlorine compounds that originate from both the dishwashing soap and the water are *volatized* and released with the steamy mist when the dishwasher door is opened. In the same way, organochlorines are also released into the air after chlorine from laundry detergents mixes with organic material from clothes in our washing machines.

Unfortunately, organochlorines are so persistent in our environment now that probably all humans on Earth, as well as almost all animal and marine life, have been contaminated with them. In fact, people considered to be average Americans have been shown to have 177 different organochlorines in their bodies when tested. These dangerous compounds are found in the fat cells, mother's milk, semen, blood, and breath of probably every person alive today. Because organochlorine molecules are shaped like some of our own hormone molecules, they can easily slip into our cells in place of hormones, and this is partly why there is an alarming increase of infertility in people these days. Some scientists are now relating the dramatic decrease in men's sperm counts to organochlorines. It is no small matter that the average man's sperm count has dropped by about 50 percent over the last 50 years. One has to wonder whether or not humans will be able to reproduce naturally at all within a few decades.

But the most toxic type of chlorine byproduct does not come from our public water systems. This most toxic type of compound is a family of organochlorines called "dioxins." The chemical category called "dioxin" *is the single most carcinogenic type of manmade chemical known to science.* The EPA considers dioxin to be 300,000 times more potent as a carcinogen than DDT. No level of dioxin is considered safe.

Most of the dioxin we are exposed to is released into our environment from the following three sources:

1. Industrial incinerators that burn chlorinated wastes

2. Industrial production of plastics

3. The paper production industry

Modern living involves lots of paper. Chlorine is used in the paper industry in two ways. Firstly, it is used to dissolve the lignan in the wood pulp before the pulp can be turned into paper. Secondly, after the paper is made, chlorine is used again to bleach the paper white. Dioxin results as a byproduct. Strangely, the most common way we are exposed to this sort of dioxin is through the food we eat. This is because the dioxin waste from paper mills and other industries is dumped into streams and waterways where it is easily absorbed into fish and food crops. It then bioaccummulates up the food chain into the beef, dairy products, chicken, pork, fish, and eggs that we buy at our supermarkets. The most concentrated amounts of dietary dioxin are found in beef and dairy products!

Some of the dioxin we are exposed to, however, comes from paper itself. Studies have shown that dioxin from paper milk cartons leaches into the milk we drink and that dioxin from white (bleached) coffee filters leaches into the coffee we drink. This is why many people choose to only use unbleached paper coffee filters. The deadly carcinogen, dioxin, even crosses the placental barrier into growing fetuses and is fed to infants through their mother's milk. This may be another reason so many children these days are developing cancer.

Of course we can't go back to drinking totally untreated water, but there *are* alternatives to the chlorination of public water supplies. For example, most of Europe is now using ozonation to purify their water, and some cities in the United States, such as Seattle, are already starting to use that procedure. Hydrogen peroxide is also a possible alternative to using chlorine in the paper industry. Although Europe is leading the way in this type of progress, millions of dollars are spent every year in the United States on federal lobbying by the chemical industry to keep chlorine in use.

Fluoride

Another common health hazard in our environment, and primarily in our water, is fluoride. This is still a controversial issue, but it is well documented that fluoride is an extremely toxic and carcinogenic substance. It is added to many of our public water supplies which means that many people are drinking it in on a daily basis. It can also be found in countless common foods and dental products.

Just how water fluoridation in the United States got started is an interesting story. Our more than 50-year history of water fluoridation started with the atomic bomb industry during World War II. Developing atomic bombs required the processing of uranium. And the processing of uranium produced toxic fluoride waste. Initial problems of fluoride waste were evident early on when New Jersey chemical industries producing bomb-grade uranium allowed fluoride waste to escape into the air. This event resulted in severe damage to fruit trees and animal life downwind of the factories. The early chemical factories also allowed fluoride waste to run off into local waterways, which resulted in "dead" lakes (after the fluoride killed everything in the lakes).[1] Mistakes like these and their damages were covered up at the time, but it quickly became apparent to uranium manufacturers that toxic fluoride waste was going to be a serious problem for them.

Other industries that created fluoride waste were also developing in the mid-1900s. For example, steel-producing was becoming big business. The steel industry has historically produced fluoride waste and emitted fluoride air pollution. Zinc mills also produce fluoride waste. One well-known disaster occurred in Donora, Pennsylvania, in 1948 when a zinc mill emitted a fluoride-rich smog so deadly that about 6,000 people became ill, 20 people died, and numerous pets and livestock were adversely affected or killed over a five-day period.

In the mid-20th century, aluminum manufacturing was also developing. Aluminum manufacturing is a big producer of fluoride and, with the use of aluminum cans rapidly rising, the aluminum industry soon became a huge source of industrial fluoride waste. At the same time, aluminum manufacturers and other fluoride-producing industries (steel, zinc, aluminum, phosphate fertilizers, glass, and others) were facing extremely high costs involved with safe disposal of their fluoride waste.

Physician John R. Lee was chairman of a 1972 environmental health committee that was tasked with evaluating water fluoridation for an area in California. In the "John R. Lee, M.D. Medical Letter" of February 1999, Dr. Lee reports that it was one man, the chief legal counsel for the Aluminum Company of America, who got the concept of water fluoridation started. His name was Oscar Ewing. It was in 1947 that Ewing hatched an insidious plan to allow the aluminum industry to avoid high costs of safely disposing their deadly fluoride, and to actually make money on their fluoride waste instead. Apparently, it was such a good idea, the other fluoride-producing industries followed in the aluminum industry's footsteps. According to Dr. Lee, here is how it happened.

Oscar Ewing was named head of an organization that oversaw the governmental Public Health Safety (PHS) Department. This department is now called Health and Human Services. Ewing then made it an official policy of the PHS to promote the concept of water fluoridation under the guise of reducing dental cavities. This was based on the understanding that a certain amount of dietary fluoride is important for the development of healthy teeth. Ewing influenced changes in federal regulation, which resulted in the establishment of all drinking water fluoride levels to be under the control of the PHS Department.

Ewing's idea was an ingenious profit-maker because, instead of paying high costs to dispose of their toxic waste, the aluminum manufacturers and other industries could now sell it to public water companies for a huge profit. With more and more industries developing that produced toxic fluoride waste, a big public campaign touting the benefits of fluoridated water was widely supported by big money interests, and scientific researchers soon found that it was career suicide to oppose water fluoridation. Soon, countless toothpaste companies jumped onto the bandwagon and became new markets to which industries could sell their toxic fluoride waste.

But there was a deadly "bait and switch" involving the *type* of fluoride studied for dental health versus the type of fluoride put into our water and toothpaste. The original tooth decay prevention tests were done using *calcium fluoride* (CaF_2), or dietary fluoride. Calcium fluoride is the type of fluoride found naturally in water and plants. Yet, the type of fluoride from industrial waste that got added to our public water supplies and dental products was *sodium fluoride* (NaF). Sodium fluoride is highly toxic. To give an idea of just how toxic it is, back in the 1930s, before the big water fluoridation campaign was launched, the only way the aluminum industry could sell off its toxic fluoride waste (sodium fluoride) for a profit was by selling it to companies that made *rat poisons* and *cockroach poisons*! Sodium fluoride, in other words, does a great job of killing off rats and cockroaches.

So the public campaigners were putting one type of toxic fluoride into our country's water supplies while referring to research done on a totally *different* type of fluoride that has some benefit for teeth. And all of this to save the toxic fluoride-producing industries the expense of disposing their toxic fluoride waste!

The public campaigners working for the fluoride waste-producing industries knew very well how toxic sodium fluoride was and still is, so they were not referring to calcium fluoride by mistake. Moreover, the toxic type of fluoride waste from industrial sources which is used in public water fluoridation and toothpaste (primarily sodium silicofluoride and fluosilicic acid) has *not* been tested in any widespread way as to general safety or benefit for teeth.

This deadly fluoridation scam was so successful it still thrives in the United States today, and prodigious amounts of toxic sodium fluoride continue to be put in our water supplies and dental products. You will be hard-pressed to find a brand of toothpaste at your local drug store that does *not* contain fluoride in it. And many children are still given fluoride washes in the dental chair and/or fluoride supplements to protect their teeth. Yet, large studies have shown there is *no* significant reduction in dental cavities through the use of this type of fluoride. In fact, it often causes damage to the teeth in the form of "dental fluorosis," which results in mottled, yellowish teeth for life.

Clinical toxicology organizations list sodium fluoride as more toxic than lead poisoning. Even Proctor and Gamble, the makers of Crest toothpaste, have admitted that the fluoride in a family-sized tube of Crest toothpaste could, if ingested all at once, be enough *to kill a small child*! Of course, it is not likely that a small child is going to ingest a whole tube of toothpaste at once, but they do ingest much more than that amount of fluoride from fluoridated toothpaste *over time*.

It is truly amazing that fluoride supplements for children are still being marketed under the guise of helping their teeth when the companies selling these supplements have *never* been required to demonstrate that their supplements are safe. This is because fluoride supplements were developed and sold before 1962, which is the year that the FDA started requiring new drug applications to demonstrate safety and effectiveness. The FDA chose to *exempt* products marketed before 1962 from this safety requirement and continues to allow them to be sold.

We should at least learn from the many cases where children have actually *died* as a direct result from fluoride treatments done on their teeth. In 1979, a large settlement was awarded the parents of a three-year-old child who was unnecessarily killed this way. In this case, the court found the dentist and dental hygienist to be at fault but did *not* find the American Dental Association to be at fault. Apparently, the ADA took the following defensive stance:

> The ADA owes no legal duty of care to protect the public from allegedly dangerous products used by dentists . . . The information it disseminates is intended for the benefits of its membership only. Dissemination of information relating to the practice of dentistry does not create a duty of care to protect the public from potential injury.[2]

From the above statement, one must conclude that the ADA only feels obligated to protect its members (the dentists), and that any dental advertisements or products claiming the support of the American Dental Association are simply giving the public a false sense of security.

Not only does public water fluoridation *not* protect teeth, it has now been officially linked to dental fluorosis, skeletal fluorosis, increased hip fractures, increased infant mortalities, lowered IQ, increased hyperactivity in children, and cancer. Numerous studies have proven that fluoride can cause damage to chromosomes in concentrations as low as one part per million, and *one part per million is the average target level used in fluoridating public water supplies.*

One of the insidiously dangerous effects of fluoride on the body is its ability to interrupt, or interfere with the functioning of many different enzymes, thereby disrupting a variety of important processes in the body. The U.S. National Academy of Sciences and the World Health Organization have published lists of *over 100 enzymes* in the body that are inhibited at the fluoride levels common in drinking water. Studies have also shown that fluoride adversely affects the migration rate of white blood cells in the human body and causes a breakdown in collagen, which is a protein that helps to hold every cell in our bodies together.

Various studies have linked sodium fluoride to bone cancer, bladder cancer, liver cancer, oral cancer, lung cancer, and other types of cancer. And there have been many epidemiological studies linking water fluoridation with increased cancer incidences in various geographical areas. In 1977, one top fluoride researcher told a congressional committee that unless something were done to stop the fluoridation of water in the United

States, more than 500,000 people alive at the time of his speech could be expected to die from fluoridation-linked cancer!

It is also suspected that fluoride may be a contributing factor to the development of Alzheimer's disease. This is because aluminum in the brain has been suspected to be a factor in this debilitating disease. The connection here is that elemental aluminum cannot pass the blood-brain barrier by itself. But elemental aluminum *can* interact with sodium fluoride in our bodies to form "aluminum fluoride." And aluminum fluoride *can* pass the blood-brain barrier.

The really scary part is that even in a country like the United States, where not all communities have fluoridated water, the effects of water fluoridation are nevertheless *everywhere*. In other words, you may not live in an area that has fluoridated water for drinking purposes, but many of the fruits and vegetables you buy at the grocery store have been grown using fluoridated water. These fruits and vegetables absorb the fluoride from the water through their roots. The amount of toxic fluoride in fruits and vegetables may then be compounded by the fact that artificial fertilizers and pesticides used in agriculture often contain sodium fluoride to keep the level of insect activity down. This fluoride then gets washed into the soil and absorbed by the roots of our food plants as well.

Moreover, even though you may not live in a fluoridated drinking water area, you may drink common commercial beverages such as sodas, juices, beer, and wine. These beverages may have been made with fluoridated water. Keeping in mind that chromosome damage to cells can occur at fluoride amounts as low as one part per million, or 1.0 ppm, here are a few examples of the levels of fluoride in some common food and beverage products:[3]

Beverage	Fluoride in Parts Per Million
Diet Coke	2.6 ppm
Beer, Wine	15 ppm
Gerber's First Year's Juices	3 ppm
Kellogg's Fruit Loops Cereal	2.1 ppm

The public health danger of fluoridated water is astronomical, and will only get worse as it builds up in our environment. Americans should consider following the lead of most European countries when it comes to water fluoridation. Here is what some countries in Europe have already done:[4]

— **Sweden** banned and discontinued fluoridation in 1971.

— **Norway** and **Germany** rejected fluoridation in 1975 as *'foreign to nature, unnecessary, inefficient, irresponsible and harmful to the environment.'*

— **Holland** banned fluoridation in 1976 and changed their country's constitution so that fluoridation could never be re-introduced.

— **Denmark** rejected fluoridation in 1977. The Minister for the Environment stated that *no 'adequate studies had been carried out on the long-term effect on human organ systems.'*

— **France** rejected fluoridation in 1980. The Chief of Public Health in France declared it was too dangerous.

— **Finland** rejected fluoridation in 1992.

— All Councils in **Northern Ireland** have rejected fluoridation.

— **Italy, Austria, Belgium** and **Luxembourg** have all rejected water fluoridation.

Currently, less than 2 percent of the people in Europe drink fluoridated water, and studies have shown that people with the best teeth in Europe are from those countries that do not fluoridate their water.[5] Getting toxic fluoride out of our water, common foods, beverages and dental products is one of the *best* things we can do for ourselves and our environment.

Asbestos

Another highly carcinogenic substance in our environment, that the average person has very little control over, is asbestos. Asbestos is a curious substance. It is actually a family of minerals that can be spun into fibers and woven into cloth. Thus, asbestos is basically a rock that has been spun into fabric. Once discovered, it became a highly sought after substance, because *asbestos will not burn.*

Around the beginning of the 1900s, the asbestos industry had become big business. Asbestos was looked at as a magical substance that gave people a sense of safety from fire. Before long, asbestos was being manufactured into thousands of different commercial products as a fire retardant. Some of these common products were potholders, floor tiles, stove linings, table paddings, coffee pots, toasters, irons, electric blankets, and hair dryers. But about 75 percent of all the asbestos produced was used in the construction of buildings. After all, what could be better than a fire-retardant building insulator?

The only problem was, and still is, that asbestos is extremely hazardous to everyone's health. The reason is that microscopic asbestos fibers are easily released into the air from the many asbestos-containing products or building insulation materials. These fibers are so microscopic, they cannot be seen by the human eye. And each of the unseen fibers can break down even further into a multitude of smaller particles, called "fibrils." These fibrils are so small, they can only be detected by an electron microscope.[6]

Once released into the air, asbestos fibers and fibrils take a very long time to settle and are virtually indestructible. Anyone can breathe them into their bodies without knowing it. Once in the body, these microscopic, indestructible fibers and fibrils get caught in the sensitive membranes and linings of the lungs and other parts of the body. They irritate the tissues, causing microscopic lesions and eventually scar tissue. Finally, cancer may form in and around this scar tissue.[7]

The danger of asbestos fibers to lungs has been well known for many decades. As early as the 1920s, studies revealed that many asbestos factory workers were dying at very young ages from lung ailments. Originally, many of these ailments were classified as "asbestosis." For decades, however, the dangers of asbestos were not made public. Then, in the 1960s, studies began to reveal alarmingly high rates of lung cancer and other lung diseases among building insulation workers. These lung diseases were also surfacing among asbestos-mining workers and shipyard workers.

The reason that early studies did not show a significant lung cancer connection to asbestos was that researchers did not realize at the time that it could take *twenty years or more* for lung cancer to develop after exposure to asbestos. In the words of Dr. Irving Selikoff, a physician who studied the asbestos to lung cancer relationship among shipyard workers,

> For lung cancer the percentage of all deaths that occurred at 10 years or less was trivial; it was not until 25 years after onset of employment that deaths [from lung cancer] became common [among shipyard workers].[8]

In 1977, after completing another study, this time involving men belonging to the New York pipefitters union, Dr. Selikoff presented his conclusions to a medical meeting. After discussing the details, he summed up the cancer risk by saying, "One out of every three asbestos workers dies of lung cancer. This is simply a disaster!"[9] Selikoff also noted a small rise in deaths from esophageal, stomach, colon, and rectal cancers among the men of the pipefitters union. He attributed these intestinal tract cancer deaths to asbestos as well, pointing out that when people breathe in asbestos fibers and fibrils from the air, they also *ingest* a certain amount of them, thus contaminating the intestinal tract.[10]

In the 1970s, U.S. government agencies had finally begun to regulate permissible exposure limits to asbestos fibers in factories, construction, and shipyards, and to enact safety regulations in building demolition policies for all buildings containing asbestos. However, the danger has not gone away. Although modern appliances in the United States, such as toasters and irons, no longer contain asbestos, many buildings still do.

The use of asbestos to insulate new buildings has been banned since the mid-1970s, but millions of office workers in this country still work in asbestos-laden older buildings. It is difficult to know just how many buildings this is, but it has been estimated, for instance, that about *half* of the country's skyscrapers still contain asbestos insulation. And about two-thirds of all the buildings in New York City have been found to contain asbestos.[11] Air-conditioning systems in many of these buildings still circulate air right over sprayed-on asbestos insulation, which causes fibers and fibrils to be picked up and circulated directly into myriads of offices and employees' breathing spaces.[12]

Even more disturbing is the issue of asbestos in schools. In 1972 a Wyoming elementary school was ordered to be closed after the school librarian brought attention to a layer of asbestos dust that covered most of the furniture in the school. The dust turned out to be from a deteriorating ceiling that had been sprayed with asbestos 11 years before. This spraying technique was a fairly common practice from the 1950s to the 1970s. In 1977, six New Jersey elementary schools were also closed due to asbestos exposure to the children. In 1978, Harlem parents forced two New York City schools to be shut down for the same reason. Moreover, the Harlem investigation revealed that hundreds more schools in New York City were still contaminated with asbestos.[13]

In 1986, the "Asbestos Hazard Emergency Response Act" was passed, which provided for standards and timetables to clean up asbestos in 30,000 schools in this country. But this type of task cannot be done overnight. Meanwhile, many of these schools may be exposing about 50 million children today to the hazards of asbestos.[14] How many of these children or employees in skyscrapers will be developing cancer 20 to 25 years after exposure?

At this point in time, virtually every man, woman, and child has already been exposed to asbestos-contaminated air, even if they have not spent time in asbestos-laden office buildings or schools. The fibers and fibrils are already just about everywhere in our environment. The best we can do at this point is to give our support to clean-up projects and public awareness, thereby minimizing future health risks as much as possible. It is also important to know that other countries may be less aware of the dangers of asbestos. In fact some countries, such as Chile, Argentina, and parts of Brazil, do *not* have bans on asbestos and still allow the sale of many asbestos-containing household products.

Fiberglass

Similar to asbestos, but a much less studied substance at present, is fiberglass. Fiberglass shares many of the characteristics of asbestos, but instead of being rock that can be spun into fibers, it is *glass* that can be spun into fibers and then woven into material. Just like asbestos, microscopic pieces of fiberglass (which are really just needle-shaped pieces of glass) get into the air. As early as the 1970s, Dr. Mearl F. Stanton of the National Cancer Institute concluded from his experiments that glass fibers less than 3 microns across and more than 20 microns long were "potent carcinogens" in rats.[15]

The problem is that the health risks of fiberglass have not been as well studied as asbestos, and with the banning of asbestos, the production of fiberglass in the United States has been quickly increasing as an alternative. Now, fiberglass is being used for thermal and acoustic insulation in buildings and homes, in automotive parts, and in air filters. Tens of thousands of commercial products currently contain fiberglass, and it is estimated that *most of the homes in America now use fiberglass insulation*!

Fiberglass products can directly pollute the air around them with tiny glass fibers the way asbestos can. Putting either of these substances into air filters or insulating homes and buildings with them will only accelerate the release of the dangerous microscopic particles as air rushes past the material. Fiberglass and asbestos can also pollute the air around landfills after these materials have been discarded. Like asbestos, microscopic fiberglass fibers can now be measured in the air just about anywhere on the planet—whether it be in cities, rural areas, or remote mountains. As fiberglass products are being produced in ever-increasing quantities, this pollution is quickly getting worse. Yet, there is every reason to believe that the cancer-causing mechanism of fiberglass is similar to that of asbestos and just as deadly.

Already, some researchers believe that a ban on fiberglass is long overdue. But despite this, and even though numerous studies have shown elevations in lung cancer rates among fiberglass factory workers, public health officials have claimed that there is *no evidence* that fiberglass is a health risk to humans. As to the truth of this unbelievable claim, only time will tell.

Nuclear Radiation

The fifth big cancer-causing environmental factor of modern living is environmental radiation left over from nuclear testing and other bomb-related activities. There are many people who have filed lawsuits against the U.S. government for their exposure to nuclear radiation, and they call themselves "downwinders." These people lived in areas of the country that were downwind of nuclear testing done primarily in the 1950s and 1960s. Many of these downwinders have already died of cancer or are currently fighting cancer as a result. Epidemiological studies on high-exposure areas of the country also indicate a strong correlation between nuclear exposure and higher incidences of cancer. Yet it still remains a problem that it is virtually impossible to *prove* any particular person's cancer was caused by nuclear fallout. Because of this difficulty, the government has been able to remain vague on the subject of how much cancer nuclear radiation from bomb testing has really caused.

According to one downwinders website (www.downwinders.org), the National Cancer Institute *did* finally admit in 1997 that the fallout from atomic bomb tests carried out in the 1950s blanketed this country with much higher levels of radioactive material than was previously admitted by the government.[16] But the government report only went so far as to include the statement that ". . . there *could* be between 10,000 and 75,000 cases of thyroid cancer among those exposed."[17]

Research done by many concerned downwinders indicates that the problem is much, much worse than the NCI is willing to admit. For one thing, many more bomb tests were conducted on land *after* the 1950s, and also offshore in the Pacific. Tiny particles of radioactive material were blown high into the atmosphere from these tests, then carried on the wind for thousands of miles to where they could be deposited in other places. Another issue upsetting downwinders is that the government study referred to by the NCI only looked at the effects of iodine-131, which is only one of *dozens* of radioactive isotopes emitted during nuclear testing!

Iodine-131 tends to cause thyroid cancer. This is because the chemical structure of this particular radioactive isotope causes it to be readily absorbed into and stored by the thyroid gland. Breast tissue in women also uses a lot of natural iodine, so radioactive iodine would be sent there by the body as well, potentially causing breast cancer. But scores of *other* radioactive isotopes in the same fallout are also absorbed into the body and are equally or even more deadly. For instance, strontium and plutonium are usually absorbed into and stored in the bones of anyone exposed to them. (Because strontium-90 mimics calcium, it generally ends up in the bones and teeth.) On the other hand, radioactive plutonium may end up in the bones, liver, lungs, or other body organs and may remain there over the lifetime of the person.[18] Once in the bone, these isotopes can damage the bone marrow and blood cells. Unlike radioactive iodine-131, which tends to cause thyroid and breast cancer, radioactive strontium and plutonium can result in cancers of the bone marrow and blood, namely the multiple myelomas and leukemias.

Because of their different chemical structures, different radionucleides from nuclear fallout tend to concentrate in different organs of the body. Once there, they continue to irradiate that organ until the radiation either fully decays, or they are eliminated from the body. Unfortunately, the decay period for many of these substances is extremely long. Iodine-131 has one of the shortest time periods for decay, with a half-life of only eight days. But strontium-90 has a half-life of 30 years, and plutonium has a half-life of 24,000 years!

One downwinders organization is now making the point that, ". . . if the iodine-131 resulted in 10,000 to 75,000 cases of thyroid cancer alone, how many cases did the other isotopes produce, and of those hundreds of thousands of cases (of cancer) that they would induce, how many innocent, unwitting, and unsuspecting Americans died?"[19] Cesium-137, zirconium, and other radioactive isotopes are *also* extremely dangerous substances emitted by nuclear detonations, and they have yet to be studied!

Radioactive fallout became a known contaminant issue as early as 1945. On July 16, 1945, the first atomic bomb test was successfully carried out at Alamogordo, New Mexico. Back then, scientists knew very little about the dangers of radiation. They had the technology to create the bomb, but did not have all the technology needed to study the dangers of radioactive isotopes. Only gamma ray and X-ray radiation were understood. The more dangerous radioactive contamination issues from nuclear testing, such as beta radiation and neutrons, were a mystery. There was no technology or device that could measure some of these new radioactive particles. In fact, scientists and government officials were so naive about the dangers of fallout back then that, right after the test at Alamogordo in 1945, two physicists were sent out in a car to follow a cloud of radioactive material blowing east across the country. These physicists discovered for the first time that radioactive fallout did not fall evenly when blown by wind. Instead, it tended to fall more heavily in certain "hot spots" due to various weather and geographical conditions.

Even more far-reaching effects from the first detonation in Alamogordo were discovered three years later, in 1948. This occurred when customers of the Eastman Kodak Company complained about "fogged" film. The investigation that followed this complaint revealed that ". . . the film had been packed in paper made from straw that had been washed in water from the Wabash River, which had been contaminated by the explosion at Alamogordo, more than 1,000 miles away."[20]

On August 6, 1945, the nuclear bomb detonation occurred over Hiroshima, Japan. Three days later, on August 9, another bomb was detonated over Nagasaki. No studies on the widespread fallout of these wartime detonations were *ever* done, partly because scientists at that time did not have the technology to detect or measure many of the radioactive particles. We still do not know how much of the fallout from those two war-time bombs actually circulated via wind over the United States and other parts of the world and was deposited on land and in waterways.

Later, more was learned about the wind-blown distribution of nuclear fallout from tests done in Nevada in the 1950s and 1960s. For instance, in April 1953, *just two days* after an atomic bomb test had been conducted in the Nevada desert, a professor and his students in Troy, New York, discovered that the gamma radiation measurements on their campus suddenly shot up to 500 times the normal amount. And they found that the beta ray radiation was even higher than that in some hot spots, such as in rainspouts and puddles. This professor later discovered that the mushroom cloud created at the Nevada test site had reached 40,000 feet in the atmosphere and had then drifted 2,300 miles across the country to the northeast in just two days. The cloud of radioactive material had passed over (and mostly likely contaminated) parts of Utah, Colorado, Kansas, Missouri, Illinois, Indiana, Ohio, and Pennsylvania before it got caught up in a rain system that dropped radioactive precipitation onto upstate New York, southern Vermont and parts of Massachusetts.[21]

Over the years, about 1,000 nuclear devices were tested in Nevada, three were tested in Alaska, three in New Mexico, two in Mississippi, and two in Colorado. As early as 1953, scientists knew that a lot of the radioactive elements from these explosions were settling down to earth and contaminating not only the air and soil, but also the waterways from which we drink. From these waterways, the radioactive isotopes were then getting into our food crops and livestock. Thus, we began "eating" and "drinking" radioactive compounds. In fact, a 1960 study done at the University of Michigan revealed that, due to drinking milk from contaminated cows, children were getting radiation doses to their thyroid glands that were 10 to 100 times greater than doses to adult thyroid glands. This was due, in part, to the children's higher consumption of milk and also due to the higher concentration of radioactivity in the children's smaller thyroid glands.

There are two basic ways that exposure to radiation from nuclear fallout occurs: (1) externally, and (2) internally. External exposure occurs when radiation enters through the skin from the surrounding air. Internal exposure occurs when radioactive by-products are directly inhaled or ingested from food or water. It is now known that radioactive isotopes from nuclear fallout concentrate more and more as they move up the food chain. Algae concentrates it out of the water, plants concentrate it out of the soil, and birds, fish, and other animals concentrate it even more when they drink the water and eat the plants. The radioactive isotopes that are concentrated in dairy animals then concentrate even *more* in their milk. Even human mothers concentrate these isotopes in the milk their own bodies produce to feed their babies.

In other words, because each step up the food chain helps to accumulate and concentrate dangerous radioactive isotopes, the actual internal exposure to humans from what they eat can be *many times greater* than the external atmospheric exposure around them. And there is no amount of nuclear radiation that is safe. Any amount can cause cell damage!

The areas most highly contaminated by U.S. domestic nuclear testing were to the east and northeast of the Nevada test sites. This is because detonations were generally scheduled when wind directions were moving toward the east or northeast. The schedulers of these tests apparently knew enough about the dangers of nuclear fallout to want to avoid exposing the more densely populated areas to the south and west (such as around Las Vegas and southern California). Residents in the less populated areas subjected to the direct path of wind-blown fallout in the east and northeast (such as eastern and northern Nevada and southwestern Utah), suffered *epidemics* of cancer, infertility, miscarriages, and birth defects.

Iron County, Utah, was one of the populated areas particularly hard hit by radioactive fallout. According to the website, www.historyto go.utah.gov/:

> Scott M. Matheson, governor of Utah from 1977 to 1984 and a former Parowan and Cedar City resident, recalled life in Iron County during the early 1950s: 'People in southern Utah were mainly concerned with making a living, and I don't recall anyone being too upset about the brilliant flashes and thunder-like blasts that were part of the 1953 atomic testing. The Upshot-Knothole series, conducted from March to June 1953, included the 'Dirty Harry' exposure that carried an enormous amount of debris downwind, over southern Utah. People were concerned about the sheep deaths that occurred in May 1953, but when the AEC said there was nothing to worry about, we all just shrugged our shoulders. No one really accepted the malnutrition rationale, but we were used to accepting whatever the government said, especially during that very nationalistic period.'
>
> As part of a test site public-relations program in March 1953, some 600 observers were invited to view a test shot and its effect on manikins, typical homes, and automobiles in an effort to get Americans more interested in civil defense. Klien Rollo represented the *Iron County Record* at the media event. Observers watched the detonation seven miles from ground zero and later were taken into the test area, after debris and dust had settled. Rollo at first thought it was 'his good fortune' to be invited to the test site, but not many weeks later the newspaper began questioning the safety of nuclear fallout. It printed a long article by University of Utah student Ralph J. Hafen of St. George, in which he wrote that he felt 'morally obligated to warn people of the irreparable damage that may have occurred or may in the future occur' from exposure to radiation. He also called upon the AEC to explain why cars entering St. George were washed after the shot. Predicting later problems, he cautioned that 'damage done to an individual by radiation often does not make itself known for five to ten years or a generation or more . . .'

Finally, in 1982, Congress passed legislation calling for a government study on human exposure to iodine-131 caused by Nevada nuclear testing done in the 1950s and 1960s. The results of the study did not come out until 15 years later. Finally, in 1997, the National Cancer Institute released the results of their county-by-county report. Their conclusion was that *every person and animal living in the 48 contiguous states* was exposed during those two decades to iodine-131. The NCI report also concluded that the highest areas of exposure from the Nevada tests were in Iowa, Nebraska, South Dakota, Kansas, Montana, Wyoming, Colorado, Utah, Missouri, Idaho, Nevada, and Arkansas.[22]

And that study was done on just one radioactive isotope that was emitted by domestic nuclear testing. No big studies have ever been undertaken to assess the radioactive exposure caused by: (1) "Cold War" nuclear testing in the former Soviet Union that might have blown over the United States, (2) exposure from our own nuclear testing in the Pacific that might have blown back over our country, or (3) radioactive fallout from the detonation of the bombs over Hiroshima and Nagasaki which might have blown back to our country. Some researchers believe that parts of California and the Pacific Northwest may have suffered significant fallout from these three additional sources, which may have put these locations at the top of the list of most exposed U.S. areas if these sources of nuclear radiation had been studied.

But we also need to be aware of the fact that *nuclear contamination does not only result from detonating bombs.* This is because bombs don't just create themselves. They have to be made and the nuclear explosive material used to make them has to be produced. For example, the plutonium for the bomb dropped over Nagasaki was produced at the Hanford Plutonium Nuclear Reservation in central Washington State. It is now known that the Hanford facility regularly released radioactive iodine-131 into the atmosphere between the years of 1944 to 1972 as part of their process of developing nuclear bomb material. And it is a little known fact that, in 1945, the Hanford facility "accidentally" released an amount of radioactive iodine into the American skies that was equivalent to the amount released in the 1986 Chernobyl disaster![23]

The Hanford site downwinders group is a very large group of people. The areas exposed include eastern Washington, northeastern Oregon, most of Idaho, and parts of Montana and Canada. It is estimated that more than 2 million people were exposed to radioactive iodine-131, plutonium, cesium, strontium, and ruthenium.[24] One Department of Energy study, which looked at 30,000 workers at Hanford, showed cases of multiple myeloma and pancreatic cancers to be clearly correlated with exposure to radiation.[25]

Moreover, the Hanford operation used water from the Columbia River to cool its reactors. This water became contaminated with radiation and then was discharged back into the Columbia River. One researcher wrote:

> According to a formerly classified 1954 technical report by Herb Parker, former Director of the Health division at Hanford, the operators at Hanford knowingly discharged at least 8,000 curies of radioactive material per day into the Columbia River. The discharges from Hanford exposed people who ate fish and waterfowl, swam or boated on the river, irrigated their fields with water from the river, or simply drank the water from the Columbia River (such as residents of Pasco). The exposures to radioactive materials through the water pathway increase a person's total exposure to radiation when coupled with exposure through the air emissions.[26]

We also need to be aware that radioactive contamination starts even *before* the plutonium-producing facilities are involved. Environmental contamination actually starts at the uranium mining sites. Uranium ore must be mined to fuel not only nuclear weapons, but also to fuel nuclear reactors in power plants. What happens is that when uranium ore is first extracted from the ground, it is dug up then crushed at the mining site. The problem is that the process of crushing the uranium ore, or rock, leaves behind a certain amount of pulverized material, which is approximately the consistency of flour. This is part of the uranium "tailings." These tailings are left on the ground after the mining is done, where they are free to be blown by the wind or washed into surface and ground water supplies by rain. This material is very light and can be blown a thousand miles in just a few days. It is estimated that 85 percent of the radioactivity of the uranium ore remains in these powdery tailings. And the half-life of this material is about 80,000 years!

Uranium mine sites are located in many states in the United States, including Arizona, Colorado, Idaho, New Mexico, Oregon, Pennsylvania, Texas, Utah, Wyoming, and North Dakota. Currently, investigations are going on as to how much radioactive contamination, including groundwater contamination, has occurred in these areas.

In 1990, Congress passed the "Radiation Exposure Compensation Act." This act was passed to provide millions of dollars of compensation to citizens who lived downwind of above ground atomic tests, as well as to test site workers and uranium miners. Quoting from this legislation, Congress finally declared that:

> The United States should recognize and assume responsibility for the harm done to these individuals. And Congress recognizes that the lives and health of uranium miners and of innocent individuals who lived downwind from the Nevada tests were involuntarily subjected to increased risk of injury and disease to serve the national security interests of the United States . . . The Congress apologizes on behalf of the Nation to the individuals . . . and their families for the hardship they have endured.[27]

Thus, the risk factors for cancer and other illnesses due to radioactive fallout are not gone just because we are no longer testing nuclear weapons or detonating war-time bombs. Much of this radioactive material is *still* in our environment, still contaminating all of us, and a lot of it will not go away for thousands of years. There is also a great deal of "clean up" of uranium mine sites that still needs to be done. All of the issues of radioactive fallout are important for the public to know about. Probably hundreds of thousands of people, maybe even millions of people, have already become cancer victims as a result of nuclear radioactive isotopes. Unfortunately, even though it is *known* that radiation exposure can cause virtually any type of cancer (blood, breast, lung, bone, thyroid, digestive system, and others), the National Cancer Institute continues to play down the health risks of this exposure.

References

Chapter 1—The Cancer Reality Today

1. Moss, Ralph W., Ph.D. *The Cancer Industry*. New York: Equinox Press, 1999, p. 21.
2. *Ibid.*, p. 22.
3. *Ibid.*, p. 39.
4. *Ibid.*
5. *Ibid.*
6. Brodie, Douglas, M.D. (with Michael L. Culbert, D.Sc.). *Cancer and Common Sense: Combining Science and Nature to Control Cancer*. White Bear Lake, Minnesota: Winning Publications, 1997, p. 47.
7. Day, Lorraine, M.D. Video: "Cancer Doesn't Scare Me Anymore." (www.drday.com, or 800/574-2437).
8. Moss, *op cit.*, p. 38.
9. www.alkalizeforhealth.net/

Chapter 2—Why So Much Cancer and What Causes It?

1. Stoff, Jesse A., M.D. and Dallas Clouatre, Ph.D. *The Prostate Miracle*. New York: Kensington Books, 2000, p. 18.
2. Diamond, John W., M.D. and W. Lee Cowden, M.D. (with Burton Goldberg). *An Alternative Medicine Definitive Guide to Cancer*. California: Future Medicine Publishing, Inc., 1997, p. 570.
3. *Ibid.*, p. 571.
4. Pickrell, J. "Cancer Causer?", *Science News*. Vol. 162, no. 12, Sept. 21, 2002, pp. 179–180.
5. Diamond et al., *op cit.*, p. 579.

6. www.lightparty.com/Health/Pestacides.html.
7. Diamond et al., *op cit.*, p. 568.
8. Diamond et al., *op cit.*, p. 582.
9. *Ibid.*
10. *Ibid*, p. 585.
11. *Vitamin Research News*, Aug. 2002, vol. 16, No. 8, p. 5.
12. Martini, F., et al., "Human Brain Tumors and Simian Virus 40," *Journal of the National Cancer Institute*, vol. 87, Sept. 6, 1995.

Chapter 3—The Hoxsey Therapy

1. Ausubel, Kenny. *When Healing Becomes a Crime: The Amazing Story of The Hoxsey Cancer Clinics and the Return of Alternative Therapies.* Rochester, Vermont: Healing Arts Press, 2000, p. 57.
2. *Ibid.*, p. 93.
3. *Ibid.*, p. 96.
4. *Ibid.*, p. 106.
5. *Ibid.*, p. 41.
6. Walters, Richard. *Options: The Alternative Cancer Therapy Book.* Avery Penguin Putnam, 1993, pp. 98–99.
7. *Ibid.*, p. 96.
8. *Ibid.*, p. 100.
9. Ausubel, *op cit.*, p. 169.

Chapter 4—Essiac Tea

1. www.vegan.swinternet.co.uk/articles/health/Essiac_info.html
2. *Ibid.*
3. *Ibid.*
4. Olsen, Cynthia. *Essiac: A Native Herbal Cancer Remedy.* Pagosa Springs, Colorado: Kali Press, 1996, pp. 19–20.

Chapter 5—The Gerson Therapy

1. Walters, Richard. *Options: The Alternative Cancer Therapy Book.* Avery Penguin Putnam, 1993, p. 190.
2. www.gerson.org/clientservices/whatisthegersontherapy.htm
3. Haught, S.J. *Censored for Curing Cancer: The American Experience of Dr. Max Gerson.* The Gerson Institute, 1991, p. 6.

4. Carter, James P., M.D. *Racketeering in Medicine: The Suppression of Alternatives*. Virginia: Hampton Roads, 1993, p. 31.
5. www.sawilsons.com/gerson.htm
6. Carter, *op cit.*, p. 31.
7. *Ibid.*
8. www.sawilsons.com/gerson.htm

Chapter 6—Laetrile

1. Griffin, G. Edward. *World Without Cancer*. California: American Media, 1997, p. 112.
2. *Ibid.*, p. 105.
3. Binzel, Philip E., M.D. *Alive and Well: One Doctor's Experience With Nutrition in the Treatment of Cancer Patients*. California: American Media, 1994, p. 114.
4. *Ibid.*, pp. 117–118.
5. *Ibid.*, p. 123.
6. *Ibid.*, p. 111.
7. *Ibid.*
8. *Ibid.*, p. 113.
9. Griffin, *op cit.*, p. 105.
10. *Ibid.*, p. 102.
11. *Ibid.*, p. 130.
12. Moss, Ralph W. *The Cancer Industry*. New York: Equinox Press, 1999, p. vii.
13. Griffin, *op cit.*, p. 110.
14. *Ibid.*, p. 108.
15. *Ibid.*, p. 106.
16. *Ibid.*, p. xvii.
17. Griffin, *op cit.*, p. 26.
18. Moss, *op cit.*, p. 132.

Chapter 7—Dr. Kelley's Enzyme Therapy

1. Moss, Ralph, Ph.D., WeeklyCancerDecisions.com Newsletter, #82, 5/14/03.
2. Griffin, G. Edward. *World Without Cancer*. California: American Media, 1997, p. 83.
3. *Ibid.*, p. 84.
4. *Ibid.*, p. 78.

5. Mitchell, Terri, "War on Cancer: One Physician is Winning—Dr. Nicholas Gonzalez," *Life Extension Magazine*, October 1996.
6. *Ibid.*
7. *Ibid.*
8. *Ibid.*
9. *Ibid.*
10. *Total Health Magazine*, vol. 22, no. 5, October 2000.

Chapter 8—Burzynski's Antineoplastons

1. Moss, Ralph W., Ph.D. *The Cancer Industry*. New York: Equinox Press, 1999, p. 290.
2. Elias, Thomas D. *The Burzynski Breakthrough*. Nevada City, California: Lexikos, 2001, p. 100.
3. *Ibid.*, p. 123.
4. *Ibid.*, p. 129.
5. Moss, *op cit.*, p. 313.
6. Whitaker, Julian, M.D., *Dr. Julian Whitaker's Health and Healing Newsletter*, Mid-February 1996 Supplement, p. 3.
7. Elias, *op cit.*, p. 87.
8. *Ibid.*, p. 91.
9. Whitaker, *op cit.*, p. 3.
10. *Ibid.*, p. 4.
11. *Ibid.*
12. *Ibid.*, p. 6.
13. www.burzynskipatientgroup.org
14. Whitaker, Julian, M.D., *Medical Alerts*, vol. 11, no. 4, 2002, p. 12.
15. www.burzynskipatientgroup.org/burdickreport.htm
16. Elias, *op cit.*, p. 76.
17. *Ibid.*
18. *Ibid.*, p. 220.
19. *Ibid.*
20. www.burzynskipatientgroup.org
21. Burzynski, Stanislaw, personal communication, April 2003.
22. Elias, *op cit.*, p. 181.
23. *Ibid.*, p. 60.
24. *Ibid.*, p. 74.
25. *Ibid.*, p. 75.
26. Whitaker, Julian, M.D., *Dr. Julian Whitaker's Health and Healing Newsletter*, April 1997 Supplement.

Chapter 9—Protocel®: History and Theory

1. Sheridan, James Vincent. Personal Writings.
2. *Ibid.*
3. Sheridan, James Vincent and Sheridan, James Edward. "How Does Entelev/Cancell Work: A Layman's Explanation." *Journal of the Bio-Electro-Magnetics Institute*, vol. 3, no. 3. April 1992, p. 37.
4. *Ibid*, p. 40.

Chapter 11—Protocel®: Suppression of the Formula

1. Galluppi, Marcello. "Entelev/Cancell: In Search of the Holy Grail." *Journal of the Bio-Electro-Magnetics Institute* (BEMI), vol. 3, no. 3. April 1992, p. 24.
2. *Ibid.*
3. Sheridan, James Edward. "Entelev: The Latest Controversy. What Is the Significance of the NCI Graphs?" *Journal of the Bio-Electro-Magnetics Institute*, vol. 3, no. 4. March 1993, p. 9.
4. Galluppi, Marcello. "Entelev/Cancell: In Search of the Holy Grail." *Journal of the Bio-Electro-Magnetics Institute* (BEMI), vol. 3, no. 3. April 1992, p. 27.
5. Sheridan, James Edward, Personal Communication. May 2002.

Chapter 12—Protocel®: How To Use It For Best Results

1. Sheridan, James Vincent and Sheridan, James Edward. "How Does Entelev/Cancell Work: A Layman's Explanation." *Journal of the Bio-Electro-Magnetics Institute*, vol. 3, no. 3. April 1992, p. 41.

Chapter 13—Flaxseed Oil and Cottage Cheese

1. Fischer, William L. *How To Fight Cancer and Win*. Baltimore, MD: Agora Health Books, 2000, p. 140.
2. Budwig, Dr. Johanna. *Flax Oil As a True Aid Against Arthritis, Heart Infarction, Cancer and Other Diseases*. Vancouver, Canada: Apple Publishing Co., 1994, p. 17.
3. Fischer, *op cit.*, p. 143.
4. www.mnwelldir.org/docs/cancer1/budwig.htm
5. www.houseofsteed.com/sons/budwig.htm

6. www.enviro_healthtech.com/flax.htm
7. Erasmus, Udo. *Fats That Heal, Fats That Kill.* Canada: Alive Books, 1993, p. 301.

Chapter 14—The Rife Machine

1. Video—"The Royal Rife Story: Historical/Documentary." (Produced by AAA Production, Utah. 888/486-4420.)
2. *Ibid.*
3. *Ibid.*
4. *Ibid.*
5. Lynes, Barry. *The Cancer Cure That Worked: Fifty Years of Suppression.* Ontario, Canada: Marcus Books, 1987, pp. 17–18.
6. *Ibid.*, p. 17.
7. *Ibid.*, p. 18.
8. *Ibid.*, p. 50.
9. Video, *op cit.*
10. Lynes, *op cit.*, p. 45.
11. Video, *op cit.*
12. Lynes, *op cit.*, p. 60.
13. *Ibid.*, p. 88.
14. *Ibid.*, p. 30.
15. *Ibid.*, p. 51.
16. *Ibid.*, p. 25.

Chapter 15—714X

1. www.sonic.net/sentine/gvcon4.html
2. www.bccancer.bc.ca/pg_g_05.asp?PageID=1708&ParentID=2
3. www.sonic.net/sentinel/gvcon4.html
4. www.sph.uth.tmc.edu/utcam/therapies/714x.htm
5. www.bccancer.bc.ca/pg_g_05.asp?PageID=1708&ParentID=2
6. www.sonic.net/sentinel/gvcon4.html
7. www.essiac-resperin.com/en/report01.html
8. *Ibid.*
9. www.cerbe.com/en/web_review.html
10. *Ibid.*
11. www.cancerinform.freewebsites.com/naessens.html
12. *Ibid.*
13. *Ibid.*
14. www.prevention.com/cda/feature/0,1204,3847,00.html

Chapter 16—Cesium High pH Therapy

1. Brewer, A. Keith, Ph.D., "The High pH Therapy for Cancer, Tests on Mice and Humans," *Pharmacology Biochemistry and Behavior*, vol. 21, suppl. 1, 1984, pp. 1–5.
2. www.cancer-coverup.com/fighters/cesium_a.html
3. *Cancer: The Mechanism Involved and a High pH Therapy, 1978 Papers of A. Keith Brewer, Ph.D., and coauthors.* A. Keith Brewer Foundation, 325 N. Central Avenue, Richland Center, WI 53581.
4. Deoul, Kathleen, *Cancer Cover-Up*. Cassandra Books: Baltimore, MD, 2001, p. 37.
5. www.advancedhealthplan.com/2cesiumchlorideforcancer2.html ("Cesium Therapy in Cancer Patients," by H. E. Sartori.)
6. Deoul, *op cit.*, p. 37.
7. *Ibid.*, p. 38.
8. *Ibid.*
9. Brewer, A. Keith, Ph.D., *op cit.*
10. *Ibid.*
11. *Ibid.*
12. *Ibid.*

Chapter 17—Ten More Treatment Options

1. Garnett, Merrill. *First Pulse: A Personal Journey in Cancer Research, 2nd. Ed.* New York: First Pulse Projects, Inc., 2001, pp. 43–45.
2. *Ibid.*, p. 81.
3. Diamond, W. John, M.D., W. Lee Cowden, M.D., and Burton Goldberg. *An Alternative Medicine Definitive Guide to Cancer*. California: Future Medicine Publishing, Inc., 1997, P. 506.
4. Milne, Robert D., M.D. and Melissa L. Block, M.Ed. *Poly-MVA: A New Supplement in the Fight Against Cancer*. New Jersey: Basic Health Publications, 2004, p. 11.
5. www.cancure.org/CAAT/htm
6. Howenstine, James A., M.D. *A Physician's Guide To Natural Health Products That Work*. Florida: Penhurst Books, 2002, p. 352.
7. *Ibid.*
8. www.germannewmedicine.com/documents/verifications.html
9. Dr. David Holt, DVD entitled "Introduction to German New Medicine," Reno Integrative Medical Center, April, 2007.
10. www.ldninfo.org/ldn_and_hiv.htm
11. *Ibid.*
12. www.geocities.com/HotSprings/Villa/5443/alts/naltrexone.html

13. www.lowdosenaltrexone.org/ldn_and_cancer.htm
14. *Ibid.*
15. Diamond, *op. cit.*, p. 834.
16. www.pau-d-arco.com/Dr. Mowry.html
17. *Ibid.*
18. *Ibid.*
19. www.oralchelation.com/taheebo/lapacho3.htm

Chapter 18—To Alkalize or Not to Alkalize

1. Aihara, Herman. *Acid and Alkaline.* California: George Ohsawa Macrobiotic Foundation, 1986, p. 1.
2. www.cocoonnutrition.org/consult.html
3. Barefoot, Robert R. and Carl J. Reich, M.D. *The Calcium Factor: The Scientific Secret of Health and Youth.* Arizona: Deonna Enterprises Publishing, 2001, p. 137.
4. Aihara, *op cit.*, p. 17.
5. Barefoot, *op cit.*, pp. 135–136.
6. www.cocoonnutrition.org
7. www.gethealthyagain.com
8. Barefoot, *op cit.*, p. 13.
9. *Ibid.*, p. 97.
10. *Ibid.*, p. 133.
11. *Ibid.*
12. *Ibid.*, p. 111.
13. *Ibid.*, p. 67.
14. *Ibid.*, p. 122.

Chapter 19—What Women Must Know About Hormones

1. Lee, John R., M.D., David Zava, Ph.D. and Virginia Hopkins. *What Your Doctor May Not Tell You About Breast Cancer: How Hormone Balance Can Help Save Your Life.* New York: Warner Books, 2002, p. 7.
2. Lee, John R., M.D., Jesse Hanley, M.D. and Virginia Hopkins. *What Your Doctor May Not Tell You About Premenopause.* New York: Warner Books, 1999, p. 212.
3. *Ibid.*, p. 215.
4. www.johnleemd.com/
5. Lee, John R., M.D., David Zava, Ph.D. and Virginia Hopkins, *op cit.*, p. 27.
6. *Ibid.*, p. 50.
7. *Ibid.*, p. 73.

8. *Ibid.*, p. 299.

9. *Ibid.*

10. *Ibid.*, p. 99.

11. *Ibid.*, p. 35.

12. *Ibid.*, p. 78.

13. www.lightparty.com/Health/Pestacides.htm

14. Lee, John R., M.D., David Zava, Ph.D. and Virginia Hopkins, *op cit.*, p. 29.

15. www.lightparty.com/Health/Pestacides.htm

16. Lee, John R., M.D., David Zava, Ph.D. and Virginia Hopkins, *op cit.*, p. 53.

17. *Ibid.*, p. 53.

18. *Ibid.*

19. Moss, Ralph W., Ph.D. *Questioning Chemotherapy: A Critique of the Use of Toxic Drugs in the Treatment of Cancer.* New York: Equinox Press, 1995, p. 91.

20. Moss, Ralph W., Ph.D. *The Cancer Industry.* New York: Equinox Press, 1999, p. 51.

21. Lee, John R., M.D., David Zava, Ph.D. and Virginia Hopkins, *op cit.*, p. 5.

22. Moss, Ralph W., Ph.D. *(Questioning Chemotherapy), op cit.*, p. 95.

23. *Ibid.*, p. 91.

24. Brownlee, Shannon, "Bad Science + Breast Cancer," *Discover Magazine,* vol. 23, no. 8, Aug., 2002, p. 78.

25. Lee, John R., M.D., David Zava, Ph.D. and Virginia Hopkins, *op cit.*, p. 182.

26. *Ibid.*

27. *Ibid.*

28. *Ibid.*, p. 182–183.

29. *Ibid.*, p. 8.

30. *Ibid.*, p. 185.

31. *Ibid.*, p. 184.

32. *Ibid.*, p. 190.

33. Lee, John R., M.D., Jesse Hanley, M.D. and Virginia Hopkins, *op cit.*, p. 212.

34. Lee, John R., M.D. Video: "Managing Menopause."

35. Lee, John R., M.D., David Zava, Ph.D. and Virginia Hopkins, *op cit.*, p. 227.

36. Lee, John R., M.D., Jesse Hanley, M.D. and Virginia Hopkins, *op cit.*, pp. 59–60.

37. Lee, John R., M.D., David Zava, Ph.D. and Virginia Hopkins, *op cit.*, p. 198.

Chapter 20—What Men Must Know About Prostate Cancer, the PSA, and Hormone-Blocking Drugs

1. www.rcog.com/questions_and_answers.cfm?SubCat_ID=28
2. www.cancer.org/docroot/NWS/content/NWS_1_1x_Does_PSA_ Fight_Prostate_Cancer_.asp
3. *Ibid.*
4. Lee, John R., M.D. *Hormone Balance For Men.* 28-page Booklet from www.johnleemd.com, 2003, pp. 15–16.
5. *Ibid.*, pp. 17–18.
6. Navar, Paul D., M.D. "Optimizing Testosterone Levels in Aging Men." *Life Extension Magazine,* July, 2008, p. 38.
7. www.msnbc.msn.com/id/6818019
8. *Ibid.*

Chapter 21—Toxic Teeth

1. www.curezone.com/diseases/cancer/cancer_dental_risk.html
2. *Ibid.*
3. Levy, M.D., Thomas, "Teeth—The Root of Most Disease?," *Extraordinary Science,* Apr./May/June, 1994.
4. *Ibid.*
5. www.curezone.com/diseases/cancer/cancer_dental_risk.html
6. *Ibid.*
7. *Ibid.*
8. Issels, M.D., Josef. *Cancer—A Second Opinion.* New York: Avery Publishing Group, 1999, p. 121.
9. Diamond, W. John., M.D. and W. Lee Cowden, M.D. (with Burton Goldberg). *An Alternative Medicine Definitive Guide to Cancer.* California: Future Medicine Publishing, Inc., 1997, p. 153.
10. Shallenberger, Frank, M.D. Personal Communication.

Chapter 22—Evaluating Conventional Methods

1. Moss, Ralph W., Ph.D. *The Cancer Industry.* New York: Equinox Press, 1999, p. 43.
2. Moss, Ralph W., Ph.D. *Questioning Chemotherapy: A Critique of the Use of Toxic Drugs in the Treatment of Cancer.* New York: Equinox Press, 1995, p. 163.
3. *Ibid.*, p. 56.
4. Diamond, W. John., M.D., W. Lee Cowden, M.D. and Burton

Goldberg. *An Alternative Medicine Definitive Guide to Cancer.* Tiburon, California: Future Medicine Publishing, Inc., 1997, p. 840.

5. *Ibid.,* p. 848.
6. *Ibid.,* p. 846.
7. Moss, *op cit.* (The Cancer Industry), p. 64.
8. Moss, *op cit.* (Questioning Chemotherapy), p. 16.
9. *Ibid.,* p. 18.
10. Ausubel, Kenny. *When Healing Becomes a Crime: The Amazing Story of the Hoxsey Cancer Clinics and the Return of Alternative Therapies.* Rochester, Vermont: Healing Arts Press, 2000, p. 234.
11. *Ibid.,* p. 239.
12. Griffin, G. Edward. *World Without Cancer: The Story of Vitamin B_{17}.* California: American Media, 1997, pp. 154–155.
13. Moss, *op cit.* (Questioning Chemotherapy), p. 70.
14. www.whale.to/cancer/quotes1.html
15. *Ibid.*
16. Moss, Ralph, W., Ph.D., *Weekly CancerDecisions.com Newsletter #86,* June 7, 2003.
17. Moss, Ralph, W., Ph.D., *Weekly CancerDecisions.com Newsletter #87,* June 13, 2003.
18. Moss, Ralph, W., Ph.D., *Weekly CancerDecisions.com Newsletter #88,* June 21, 2003.

Chapter 24—Dealing With Fear and the Mind/Body Connection

1. Diamond, W. John., M.D., W. Lee Cowden, M.D. and Burton Goldberg. *An Alternative Medicine Definitive Guide to Cancer.* Tiburon, California: Future Medicine Publishing, Inc., 1997, p. 617.
2. www.drbrodie.com
3. Mitchell, Terri, "War On Cancer: One Physician Is Winning— Dr. Nicholas Gonzalez," *Life Extension Magazine,* October, 1996.
4. Diamond, *op cit.,* p. 136.

Appendix—Five Big Environmental Cancer Triggers

1. The John R. Lee, M.D. Medical Letter, February 1999, p. 4.
2. www.alaskawellness.com/archives/flouride-pt3.htm
3. *Ibid.*
4. http://greenparty.ennis.ie/press/column/fluoride-poison-1_june00.html
5. *Ibid.*

6. Moss, Ralph W., Ph.D. *The Cancer Industry*. New York: Equinox Press, 1999, p. 382.
7. *Ibid.*, p. 372.
8. *Ibid.*, p. 377.
9. *Ibid.*, p. 378.
10. *Ibid.*
11. *Ibid.*, p. 386.
12. *Ibid.*, p. 385.
13. *Ibid.*, p. 384.
14. *Ibid.*, p. 386.
15. http://consumerlawpage.com/article/fiber.shtml
16. www.downwinders.org/nci/html
17. *Ibid.*
18. www.akitarescue.com/hiroshim.htm
19. www.downwinders.org/nci.html
20. www.akitarescue.com/hiroshim.htm
21. *Ibid.*
22. *Ibid.*
23. Diamond, W. John., M.D., W. Lee Cowden, M.D. and Burton Goldberg. *An Alternative Medicine Definitive Guide to Cancer*. Tiburon, California: Future Medicine Publishing, Inc., 1997, pp. 567–568.
24. www.akitarescue.com/hiroshim.htm
25. *Ibid.*
26. www.downwinders.com/pathways.htm
27. http://historytogo.utah.gov/nuctest.html

Index

Y

Z

Give the Gift of
Outsmart Your Cancer
To Family, Friends and Colleagues

TO ORDER

PHONE: **(800) 266-5564**

— Order line available Monday–Friday, 7 a.m. to 11 p.m. Eastern Time —

<u>Paperback Discounts Through Above Phone Number Only:</u>

1–2 books	no discount	($26.95 each + S/H)
3–5 books	15% off	($22.90 each + S/H)
6–9 books	25% off	($20.21 each + S/H)
10 or more books	40% off	($16.17 each + S/H)

ONLINE: Go to **www.OutsmartYourCancer.com**
or **www.Amazon.com**

BOOKSTORE: If your local bookstore does not yet carry this book, simply ask them to order it and mention ISBN #978-0-9728867-8-9.

For **WHOLESALE ORDERS**, call (800) 266-5564 and receive up to 50% off ($13.48 per book).

Media/Publicity: Call Thoughtworks Publishing at (888) 679-2669.

INVITATION TO SHARE YOUR STORY OR COMMENTS

If you have a cancer recovery testimonial using an alternative approach discussed in this book that you would like to share with the author, or to simply share how this book impacted your life, you can email your story or comments to:

info@outsmartyourcancer.com

Some stories or comments may be chosen to be posted online or printed in published material. If you would like yours to be considered for this, please include the following release statement in your letter:

"My comments and/or story may be posted online or used in print as I have written them, using my first name only to protect my privacy."

Please be sure to sign and date the letter and include your phone number if possible.

NOTE: Please do NOT email inquiries for advice about a particular case. The author is not a doctor and cannot answer these types of questions.

EVERYDAY MIRACLES

How 12 Ordinary People Outsmarted Their Cancer

AUDIO CD (1 hr. 16 min.)

Track 1:   Stream of Excerpts from Testimonials

Track 2:   Author Discussion

Track 3:   Merille's Story — Ovarian Cancer (Mets to Lymph and Abdomen)

Track 4:   Author Discussion

Track 5:   LaVaughn's Story — Advanced Stomach Cancer

Track 6:   Author Discussion

Track 7:   Gerry's Story — Localized Prostate Cancer

Track 8:   Author Discussion

Track 9:   Betty's Story — Localized Breast Cancer

Track 10: Author Discussion

Track 11: Dylan's Story — Infant Brain Tumor (Diffuse Pontine Glioma)

Track 12: Sydney's Story — Childhood Leukemia

Track 13: Author Discussion

Track 14: Mary's Story — Bladder Cancer (Mets to Urethra)

Track 15: John's Story — Melanoma (Mets to Lymph and Possibly Lung)

Track 16: Pam's Story — Aggressive Breast Cancer

Track 17: Author Discussion

Track 18: Arch's Story — Lung Cancer (Mets to Neck and Possibly Throat)

Track 19: Tricia's Story — Breast Cancer (Mets to Hips, Legs, Ribs, Shoulder, Spine and Skull)

Track 20: Herb's Story — Prostate Cancer (Mets to Pelvis, Femur, Ribs and Spine)

Track 21: Author Discussion